The Nurse As Executive

Fourth Edition

Barbara Stevens Barnum, PhD, RN, FAAN
Consultant/Editor
The Presbyterian Hospital of New York City
and
Editor
Nursing Leadership Forum
New York, New York

Karlene M. Kerfoot, PhD, RN, CNAA, FAAN
Executive Vice President of Patient Care
Chief Nursing Officer
St. Luke's Episcopal Hospital
Houston, Texas

AN ASPEN PUBLICATION®
Aspen Publishers, Inc.
Gaithersburg, Maryland
1995

Library of Congress Cataloging-in-Publication Data

Barnum, Barbara Stevens.
The nurse as executive / Barbara Stevens Barnum, Karlene M.
Kerfoot. — 4th ed.
p.   cm.
Includes bibliographical references and index.
ISBN 0-8342-0571-8
1. Nursing services—Administration.   I. Kerfoot, Karlene M.
II. Title
[DNLM: 1. Nursing, Supervisory.   WY 105 S844n   1995]
RT89.B287   1995
362.1'73'068—dc20
DNLM/DLC
for Library of Congress
94-40830
CIP

Aspen Publishers, Inc., grants permission for photocopying for limited personal or internal use.
This consent does not extend to other kinds of copying, such as copying for general
distribution, for advertising or promotional purposes, for creating new collective
works, or for resale. For information, address Aspen Publishers, Inc., Permissions
Department, 200 Orchard Ridge Drive, Suite 200, Gaithersburg, Maryland 20878.

Editorial Resources: Jill A. Berry
Library of Congress Catalog Card Number: 94-40830
ISBN: 0-8342-0571-8

Printed in the United States of America

1   2   3   4   5

Contents _____

Preface to the Fourth Edition

One of the profound and career-shaping experiences is that of having the opportunity to learn from a mentor who truly shapes and molds your practice. As a fledgling manager, I followed closely the writings of a person I had never met, Dr. Barbara Stevens Barnum. I read everything she wrote. I was struck by the reality-based focus of what she wrote and by the way she always visualized nursing at least 5 years into the future. I found everything she wrote to have a profound effect on me and my practice.

Finally, I had the opportunity to study with Dr. Barnum when I was in the Doctoral Program at the University of Illinois School of Nursing in Chicago where she was directing the Department of Nursing Administration. The experience of being her student was challenging. She not only bombarded my brain with volumes of new information but also challenged my models of thinking and decision making, which in many instances had become very hard-wired. Because of Barbara's very broad conceptual skills, I saw nursing and health care through the eyes of someone who was not steeped in the rigidity of nursing dogma. I experienced Barbara as a renaissance woman who had an incredible breadth and depth of knowledge of nursing, as well as many other disciplines and life in general.

I have tried to describe to many people the experience of working with Barbara as her student, but it is an experience that cannot be adequately put into words. She helped me solidify a personal vision for nursing that has become the broad conceptual framework that has guided my practice throughout the years. Barbara taught through theory, research, and specific details. But she also taught through real-life examples. Because she had lived in the trenches of life as a nurse executive and because she had studied, taught, and researched the field as an academic, she provided for me a unique conceptual overlay and way of thinking. She provided me with the tools to face any situation. She taught the style and grace, positioning and presentation that, coupled with the hard-core academic knowledge and conceptual framework she demanded, has served me very well in my executive practice.

The opportunity to look thoughtfully at the third edition and to update it for the new world of health care has been a wonderful experience. It has provided me the opportunity to review again the knowledge base of my practice and to face today's challenges. There is little of Barbara's book that needs to be changed. Her work, like the Constitution of the United States, will endure in principle through many editions and many generations of nurse executives.

The fourth edition is intended to continue the tradition of a practical theory-based text to provide an overlay for nursing administration students and for the practicing nurse executive.

The additions to the text are from our practice and teaching and, it is hoped, follow from Barbara's tradition of a reality-based text that is grounded in theory and research. Her influence can be felt throughout what I have done in the text and in my practice. She is truly one of the greatest influences in the field of nursing administration. It is hoped that this text will provide as much energy and guidance to you as Barbara's works have provided for me.

Karlene M. Kerfoot

Note:

There is an old saying that if you meet the Buddha on your path, you should kill him. Obviously, I failed to instill that message in Karlene. She gives me more credit for her career development than I deserve. Anyone who has followed Karlene's career will recognize that she has charted it in her own unique style and set her own directions. Her instinct for effective administration surpassed mine early in her career.

In truth, the recognition must go the opposite direction. I was hesitant to revise this book because many years have passed since I held an executive nursing post in a health care delivery institution. I was relatively certain that I had kept up to date by providing consultation for various nurse executives, but one never feels the same pressures in coaching from the sidelines.

I am grateful to Karlene for agreeing to join me in this fourth edition to make sure the text stayed on course—on today's course, a very different course than the one that pertained when earlier editions of this book were written.

Barbara Stevens Barnum

A FINAL WORD ABOUT GENDER

Much of what is written here addresses the nurse executive, singular. Instead of playing word games, trying to fit or misfit ideas into neutral plural phrases, we have elected to use consistency within each chapter. In some chapters the nurse executive will be *she*, in others *he*. It's the best we could do with the eternal gender predicament.

Part I

Introduction to the Model

Underlying this fourth edition of *The Nurse As Executive* is an assumption that nursing administration has truly become a corporate function in today's health care management. Indeed, the corporate perspective must extend downward through nursing management even to the head nurse level.

The change requiring this widely dispersed corporate perspective is the press for fiscal economy in every aspect of care delivery. The health care corporation must do everything with an eye to monetary efficiency. For nursing, this has required a new approach, a strategy that makes compatible its enduring focus on quality of care and the superimposed need for austerity. In this era, the nurse executive must balance quality and quantity in his managerial designs. Such a balancing act called for a new practice model.

Nor are the results of this model as bleak as it might sound. Along with the demand for fiscal restraint is the possibility of competition, creativity, and even the big win that comes from bold new moves, creative strokes. Even these high points, however, arise from considering the financial status of an organization and developing a quick eye and clever response to environmental opportunities.

This book is based on the resource-driven model, a model for patient care management in which the quantity and quality factors of man-agement and patient care are carefully meshed in continuous sensitivity to environmental conditions. The model starts with a scan of one's environment. For that reason, Chapter 1 reviews the social and legislative context of today's health care, including a brief examination of historical developments and trends that led to today's situation.

Many of these same factors come into play in other nations, but this book focuses on conditions in the United States. The reader from elsewhere will need to make his own translations.

Nor are the national social and legislative milieus the only environments the nurse executive will need to consider. Each institution has many environments: its city or town, local politics, the needs and expectations of the multiple communities it serves, and the various groups that play a part in the life of the organization. The national situation was selected for review here simply because it is one milieu we share.

Chapter 2 explains the resource-driven model and applies it to the nurse–patient interface. This is where the ultimate nursing goals are reached and where most resources devoted to nursing are spent.

Much of the nurse executive's work today takes place on a corporate level that seems removed from nursing care. We must be grateful that nursing has earned its seat at the corporate table, debating institutional issues and goals. Yet the nurse executive cannot forget that his chief contribution to the corporation is the effective organization of nurse–patient interactions. Chapter 2 begins, then, with nursing's endpoint: patient care.

The chapter concludes by showing how the same resource-driven model may be applied to the business end of the enterprise. Indeed, it explains how many newer managerial trends exemplify a resource-driven stance. The nurse executive's job is a lot more complex today than it was even a decade ago. He needs more complex tools for successful management; the resource-driven model is one such tool.

1

Environment: The Health Care System and Its Institutions

The structure of a nursing division is shaped by the structure of its parent institution and by the formalized patterns through which that institution relates to the rest of the world. Nationwide, structures of health care institutions are undergoing a period of radical change. The relationship of a health care institution to the society also is in a state of major reorganization. Looking at some of these changes helps us to gain perspective on the work of the nurse executive in today's world.

SOCIETAL REORGANIZATIONS OF HEALTH CARE

To understand today's health care environment, it is helpful to review events shaping health regulation during the past two decades. In any era, society, through its governmental systems, makes decisions concerning what aspects of life will be valued and how those values (and their related products and activities) will be distributed among its populations. Health is one value among many to be considered in this system.

With rare exception, every nation—certainly ours—works in an environment of scarcity. That is, the society does not have the capability to implement all the worthy goals to which it as-

pires. Hence, resources put into health are not available for the advancement of other values such as education, leisure, and arts. In this nation, when health care costs continued to increase exponentially in the past two decades, legislators and citizens expressed concern. When health care costs reached close to (and later exceeded) 10 percent of the gross national product, that concern was translated into action.

Early actions included voluntary and not-so-voluntary cost-containment measures imposed on the health care industry. Originally, these controls were encouraged at the federal level but enacted on state levels. Although some gains were made in controlling costs of health care, overall results did not stabilize or contain increasing health care costs.

The causes of increasing costs were easy to identify and understand—increasing technology, for example. No one is against advances in medical technology (especially if the technology is helpful to one's own family member). Yet, the resultant technology, as well as the related research, constitute major cost factors.

Other increases in health care cost had to do with the internal organization of health care. Until recently, many work groups within health care were undercompensated. Most of us would argue that nurses were among those groups. An era of unionization did much to raise worker remuneration in the industry but not without a major impact on total health care costs.

Advancing medical technology had another indirect effect on health care costs: It enabled large numbers of persons to live longer. A new statistical group was created: the older old. But many required constant medical monitoring as well as long periods of intensive medical care. When people live longer, their declining days tend to be fraught with more medical problems, incurring more cost to the society.

Also, this increase in life span occurred in an era when the numbers of active workers to retired or older persons was declining. Today, those who carry the costs of society are decreasing in relation to the numbers of heavy users of societal resources.

More recently, costs of health care were exacerbated by growing numbers of acquired immune deficiency syndrome (AIDS) patients and increasing life-style problems brought on by addictions and substance abuses. Only the addiction to smoking showed a temporary decline, with some studies now showing new increases among the younger population.

It was inevitable that such a situation would reach crisis proportion. The crisis was brought to the forefront even before the AIDS crisis: It was projected that the social security health fund, the national funding of Medicare and Medicaid, would become insolvent.

This projected failure brought, in rapid fashion, a change in the federal reimbursement process. Providers of care for Medicare patients would be reimbursed through a prospective payment system that tightly controlled costs. Organizations would have to manage in extremely frugal ways to recover costs. Of course, there was a carrot: Institutions that were clever could keep unused reimbursement funds if they managed to give care at less than the reimbursed cost. The diagnosis-related group (DRG) system entered the scene.

The imposition of the DRG system at the federal level caused all institutions to reanalyze their health care delivery systems and structures. The system effectively enforced cost reduction, even at the expense of other values near and dear to those in health care. The system imposed a business mentality on the health care provider, with bottom-line solvency as a driving force in all health care decisions.

The DRG system was not the only force driving health care into an industrial, bottom-line model. Indeed, the DRG system itself was a partial response to a trend already underway. Whether it was cause, effect, or more accurately, both, the DRG system accentuated the trend toward industrializing health care.

At present, there are indications that the DRG system itself may be replaced, but the notion of prospective payment has solidly taken hold in most reimbursement plans. Nor should we expect a return to the old payment-for-costs-incurred system in which costs were accepted at face value.

With the Clinton administration, there has been a return emphasis placed on health as a social value. A plan for national health care may yet emerge. Yet, the intensive demand for controls on health care costs has not declined as the pendulum swung back toward health as a major societal value. The goal of improving the health care of the nation remains solidly tied to the notion of bottom-line management.

THE MANAGED CARE ENVIRONMENT

Whether by decision or default, managed care has become the environment in which we all practice. As early as the passage of the Medicare legislation in 1965, it became apparent that continuing attempts would be made to manage the cost and quality of patient care. As we said, initial methods of management by various controls gave way to the DRGs in which the prospective payment system gave a lump sum to pay for the care based on the discharge diagnosis.

With the passage of the Health Maintenance Organization Act in 1973, many other opportunities became available for prepaid plans. This signaled the shift of medical care delivery to corporate arrangements and introduced many new concepts of organization into the health care environment.

Today, the list of variations in managed health care organizations is extensive. The abbreviations read like a confusing collection of unrelated letters: HMO, IPA, PPO, EPO, and others. Although the distinctions between the various types of managed care organizations have blurred over time, there are several basic organizational structures from which they have all evolved. They vary in their organizational structures and in the loose or tight affiliation with physicians and other people in the practice.

Overview of Managed Care Organizations

Managed care is the generic term for a system that attempts to control and influence the way in which health care is provided and paid for. One can argue that the country is moving toward a comprehensive managed care package during the Clinton administration. As this book goes to press, we have yet to see a final version of such a plan. Hence we will look at the extant forms of managed care already in effect throughout the United States.

The most common form of managed health care is that of the health maintenance organization (HMO). Not only do these organizations deliver comprehensive health services, but they also provide the financing and enroll a population for a fixed prepaid fee. HMOs take several forms. The most common are listed below:

- *Independent/individual practice association (IPA):* In this model, a group of physicians who are in practice for themselves join to form an association offering the full spectrum of services to managed health organizations. Within these associations, the necessary peer review and utilization review can be performed as is required by the HMOs. Also, some IPAs will take capitated payments from HMOs and distribute a fee-for-service arrangement within the association. IPAs provide an opportunity for physicians who want to remain in individual practices to form an association that can interact and negotiate with HMOs.

- *Preferred provider organization (PPO):* In this model, employers and insurance companies set up certain standards and criteria for practice. The physician, when joining the organization, agrees to abide by these standards and the reimbursement structure. In essence, the PPO corporation guarantees service at an established reduced cost (for some payers). What is given is the reduced cost; what is gained is a guaranteed patient population.

- *Independent practitioner organization (IPO):* In this model, the physicians also form an organization through which they can interact with an HMO. However, the organization also takes the responsibility for providing information to their member physicians about HMOs.

- *Exclusive provider organization (EPO):* In this model, the physician organization becomes the exclusive provider of care. Participants are not allowed to receive coverage from any other providers. By developing an exclusive provider situation, an exclusive employer provider can often negotiate better rates because the system can guarantee a certain volume of business.

Hospitals are reimbursed in essentially four methods under managed care. Historically, a discount-off-charges was common in the early phases of managed care. A per diem rate is common today. In this arrangement, HMOs and PPOs pay a fixed rate per day per patient, regardless of the amount of equipment, the number of supplies, the number of procedures, or the use of ancillary services required. In a per case or per stay reimbursement system, reimbursement is provided as a fixed sum regardless of the length of stay. This is similar to the DRG system of payment.

Capitation arrangements pay the hospital a fixed amount each month per member enrolled per month whether the member uses hospital services or not. In this arrangement, hospitals reap financial rewards if no one uses the hospital or its services.

Different financial rewards are realized by the hospital when fees depend on the cases handled. Different payment schemes exist side by side at present. For example, discount-off-charges and per diem contracting encourage longer lengths of stays if the hospital is able to make a positive margin on the dollars available to care for the patient. In contrast, in payment on a per case basis, shorter length of stays and reduced resource consumption would lead to greater profit margins. And in a capitated system, low hospital usage means greater financial gain for the hospital.

In addition to understanding payment schemes, it is important to know how physicians relate to managed care. There are many ways for an HMO to affiliate with physicians. In a staff model, the physicians are employees of the HMO. Physicians who are not employed by the HMO are not allowed to participate in this organization.

Group model HMOs do not employ physicians. Instead, they negotiate with physicians' practices. In the network model, the HMO contracts with many different physician practices. In the IPA, their physicians become members of the organization but also remain in their individual practices.

Finally, in the direct contracting mode, the HMO contracts directly with physicians on a fee-for-service basis or through capitation with a managed care organization.

The growth of managed care is in what Boland (1993) called the third generation. In the first generation, freedom of choice for the patient was common with discounts. Because of the lack of effective cost accounting systems, it was difficult to determine the accuracy of costs and pricing. In Boland's second generation, this stage has been driven by employers demanding lower costs and the application of utilization management techniques and technology to control costs.

The third generation, according to Boland, is the one we are just now entering. He predicted that this era will see the necessity for documenting cost-effective care and developing a delivery system that goes beyond just managing the cost to managing the care as well. Individual treatment patterns and approaches will be examined and revised. With the increase in availability of information technology, the ability to document and describe will be much greater in this third era.

The future will provide many variations on the emerging forms of managed care. With the trend toward managing the care, clinicians are in great demand to work both in and with HMOs to determine the most cost-effective opportunities for giving care. Managing the care for high-quality and cost-effective outcomes becomes the goal with the advent of the third generation of managed care.

ORGANIZATIONAL RESPONSE TO BOTTOM-LINE HEALTH CARE

Some organizations have been better prepared to cope with health as a bottom-line industry than others. For example, proprietary for-profit institutions already had a business orientation. Also, some organizational forms were better prepared to be cost-effective than others. Notably, the multi-institution corporation had advantages over the freestanding single institution. Those advantages had to do with (1) the ability to borrow capital for future expansion, (2) economies of scale, and (3) ability to expand easily by acquiring additional institutions. The health care chain had great advantages in terms of growth potential and profit making.

It is not surprising that not-for-profit institutions soon followed this pattern, and most health care institutions will probably be part of multi-institution corporations soon, a move for survival and for profit.

All sorts of multi-institution conglomerates are being created and assessed. Two major organization designs are described as *vertical* and *horizontal integration* of health care services. Horizontal growth occurs in a corporation that builds around like institutions, typically acute care hospitals. Vertical integration occurs when a corporation is comprised of different types of health institutions. Often these institutions serve as feeders for each other. For example, a corporation might own an acute care hospital, several nursing homes, and several surgicenters. All sorts of combinations can be devised in a vertical integration plan.

Nor are these two designs the only corporate structures to be found. As in industry at large, health care corporations are diversifying beyond a central theme or purpose. One corporation may include health care institutions as well as institutions with goals that have nothing to do with health care. Others may have institutional linkages within health care but not limited to provider services. Hence a corporation might own patient facilities as well as a business that supplies surgical equipment, hospital equipment, or some other product line that interfaces with provider facilities.

Interestingly, many single institutions or small chains find themselves diversifying as a way to support the costly health care provision component of their operation. Nor have we seen the end of all the possible corporate forms to arise. Horizontal and vertical integration and diversification are recurrent themes, however.

Another important variable is size. Corporations range from the combination of two facilities to the corporate ownership of hundreds. Similarly, geography may be a factor: Some chains are geographically limited, others are nationwide or even international. Profit versus nonprofit is another dimension, although this factor may or may not be reflected in corporate decisions.

In addition to the move toward multi-institutional corporations for health care, there is growth in new types of care provider organizations. Most of the growth here is outside of the acute care setting. Growth patterns include the development of ambulatory care centers, outpatient surgicenters, emergency care centers, hospices, rehabilitation institutes, home care organizations, diagnostic volunteers, and substance abuse centers. Such providers may be freestanding or related to a hospital or chain. The growth of these providers reflects the fact that profits flow from keeping patients out of hospitals. HMOs also show growth. PPOs may span both acute care and outpatient care.

Not only has the move toward bottom-line management in health care changed the structure of health care organizations, but it has changed the tactics and strategies of management as well. The DRG system clearly rewards a reduced length of stay for a given patient. However, each institution must strive to keep its beds filled for profit. Thus, institutions are all striving for an increased volume of business. This means competition for the customer.

Competition means assessing one's own strengths as opposed to those of one's potential competitors. Competition also involves marketing oneself in ways that attract customers. Competition and marketing are new notions to much of the health care industry. They also involve learning new managerial skills.

Competition for customers in the acute care health institution is further complicated by an already extant situation of overbedding (usually traceable to Hill-Burton funding in the recent past). Sometimes, this situation can be ameliorated by using some excess beds for new purposes (e.g., for conversion to a nursing home facility or to a rehabilitation center). Correction of the overbedding situation obviously is compatible with a strategy of diversification or at least of vertical integration.

Not only are more customers needed, but in an environment of declining resources (lowered reimbursement rates), one must learn to use resources more effectively and economically. Hence a focus on productivity becomes important in health care. Productivity in a labor-intensive field such as health care usually means learning to do with fewer workers. Decreases in staff force institutions to consider new ways of doing things. All old traditions and patterns of behavior must be reviewed for inefficiencies. Further, there is a need for new kinds of measurement. How will the health care institution determine whether its changes actually are more efficient?

Such questions bring into play the management information systems. What data are needed? To make what decisions? How are those data to be acquired? How distributed? Often the computerized information system is the source of much revision and updating. Many institutions have had to do major computer system revision simply to be able to accumulate the sort of data required by the DRG system. Increased use of computer capability also may help in gathering other productivity information.

Changes in the health care system have brought about other dislocations and opportunities. Obviously, the ultimate aim of the prospective payment system is to decrease, nationally, total patient days in acute care. If this does not happen, then health costs ultimately will not be contained.

IMPACT ON THE NURSING DIVISION

The nurse executive in each institution may see the challenge of combining qualitative and quantitative measures of nursing achievement. The challenge, of course, is for nursing management to derive these systems on its own, creating measurements and systems that meet its own needs. Clearly, the first problem is that of coming to grips with the nursing ethos of comprehensive patient care as *the* standard. The resource-driven model for nursing practice is the model on which this text is based. Briefly, this model has a philosophy like that practiced in battlefield nursing or in emergency department triage. It seeks to get the best possible nursing care from the resources at hand. Professionalism is based on achieving this goal rather than the idealistic goal of comprehensive nursing care.

Here then are two intermixed goals for nursing: (1) goals for cost accountability and cost reduction, and (2) acceptance of various levels of nursing care as professional, with context and resources as mediating factors in determining reasonable levels.

Organization of Nursing Divisions

Not only are goals of nursing changing, but those goals are achieved in changing structures. The institutional organizational changes have already been discussed, but what changes are unique to the nursing division? The most obvious change is the new matrix design in which

many nurse executives find themselves reporting to two bosses: the institution administrator and the corporate-level nurse executive. The term *nurse executive* applies accurately to two layers of nurse managers in the multi-institution corporation.

Also, the nurse executive in the multi-institution corporation has a new group of peers: his fellow nurse executives within the corporation. The nurse executive of a care institution now relates to many more persons. Furthermore, he is not able to act as independently as before. A decision on his part may affect other nursing divisions within the corporation. A consultative mode of management becomes a necessity.

Not only must the nurse executive in the multi-institution corporation relate to new numbers of nurse executives, but also he must relate more closely with institutional management as a whole. The nursing division cannot afford to act in isolation. And if nursing does not have a major part in the corporate planning, it will be seriously disadvantaged as a division.

Suffice it to say, horizontal and vertical integration of services create new interfaces among nurse executives. The new patterns also create powerful nursing managerial roles that span various services and are offered in various geographic locations and even in various different sorts of linked institutions. What most of these new nurse executive roles share is that they are high-powered positions in large corporations. They will not be filled by nurses unable to hold their own in business management.

Processes of Nursing Management

The nurse executive, like other health care executives, must learn new tactics and strategies of management. Like the chief executive officer, he must learn to market his own division as well as participate in the marketing of the institution as a whole. Similarly, he must deal with nursing competition for the client. In the past, institutions were seldom selected by a patient because of the quality of the nursing care offered. Today's competitive marketplace offers interesting challenges to the nursing division. One can readily imagine the increased power of a nursing division that has managed to establish itself as a major drawing card in attracting consumers.

Other new skills are required of today's nurse executive. He must learn to be effective in public relations as well as interpersonal relations. He is more highly visible, and he often is a spokesman for his institution or corporation. His communications also must be effective downward. In a rapidly changing environment, the nurse executive has a responsibility to keep staff informed about the organization and nursing's participation in it. If there are too many changes, with staff alienated through isolation, the nurse executive may find himself set up as scapegoat for the dissatisfactions of many groups.

Not only will the nurse executive find himself in a competitive mode with other institutions, but he may find himself the object of internal competition. Many other groups and individuals would like to control the nursing operations of an institution. Because of its size, the nursing division is seen as a powerful acquisition by the upwardly motivated health care manager. Also, other professional groups, especially medicine, often have sought to control nursing practice. In a time of new economic constraints and problems, the nursing operation may be vulnerable to takeover attempts if nursing is not prepared to regulate itself according to the new rules.

SUMMARY

It is an era of change for health care organizations and for the nursing divisions within them, an era of opportunity for nursing, and an era of challenge. It is critical that nurse managers be able to interpret correctly what is happening locally and nationally. Their responses must not be reactionary but appropriate to the times and the context in which they operate. It is essential that the nursing management decisions also keep a clear eye on the goals of the profession. The context in which care is given must be rec-

onciled with professional goals. Advancement of the profession should not be the price paid, and it need not be.

REFERENCE

Boland, P. 1993. *Making managed care work*. Gaithersburg, Md.: Aspen Publishers, Inc.

SUGGESTED READINGS

Clinton, H.R. June 1993. Nurses in the front lines. *Nursing and Health Care* 14, no.6: 286–288.

Davis, C.K. 1992. Who will pay? The economic realities of health care reform. *Scholarly Inquiry for Nursing Practice* 6, no.3:217–219.

Drew, J.C. 1990. Health maintenance organizations: History, evolution, and survival. *Nursing and Health Care* 11, no.3:144–149.

Gale, B.J., and B.J. Steffl. 1992. The long-term care dilemma: What nurses need to know about Medicare. *Nursing and Health Care* 13, no.1:34–41.

Goldsmith, J.C. 1981. *Can hospitals survive?* Homewood, Ill.: Dow Jones-Irwin.

Grace, H. 1990. Can health care costs be contained? *Nursing and Health Care* 11, no.3:124–130.

Haddon, R. 1990. An economic agenda for health care. *Nursing and Health Care* 11, no.1:20–26.

Perkins, C.B., and K.C. Perkins. 1992. Uncompensated care: The millstone around the neck of U.S. health care. *Nursing and Health Care* 13, no.1:20–23.

Phillips, E.K., et al. 1989. DRG ripple and the shifting burden of care to home health. *Nursing and Health Care* 10 no.6:324–327.

Rantz, M. 1990. Inadequate reimbursement for long-term care: The impact since hospital DRGs. *Nursing and Health Care* 11, no.9:470–472.

Rosenberg, C.E. 1987. *The care of strangers: The rise of America's hospital system*. New York: Basic Books.

Schroeder, P. 1993. We've come a long way, maybe. *Nursing and Health Care* 14, no.6:292–293.

Shalala, D.E. 1993. Nursing and society—The unfinished agenda for the 21st century. *Nursing and Health Care* 14, no.6:289–291.

Sharp, N., et al. 1991. Public policy: New opportunities for nurses. *Nursing and Health Care* 12, no.1:16–22.

Starr, P. 1982. *The social transformation of American medicine*. New York: Basic Books.

Stevens, P.E. 1992. Who gets care? Access to health care as an arena for nursing action. *Scholarly Inquiry for Nursing Practice* 6, no.3:185–200.

2

The Resource-Driven Model

This chapter examines the basic patient care delivery system, the crux of nursing's work. The organization for the nurse–patient interaction (i.e., the assignment system) must be understood as the most important work design the nurse executive oversees.

Nursing has a long history of teaching its students to provide total patient care—comprehensive patient care in some coinage. Every student begins by learning this ideal. We call total patient care idealistic because it is based on goals set in the abstract. The nurse is responsible for providing everything deemed good for the patient. Hence we label total patient care a *goal-driven model* (Stevens 1985; Barnum and Mallard 1989). Success implies identifying all the potential patient needs, setting all the relevant goals, and achieving them.

In most cases, this ideal level of care is not possible in today's delivery environments. Yet, the notion dies hard. One version of total care that still prevails today is nursing care applying the nursing process and using nursing diagnoses. In this common formulation, the nurse assesses the total patient, coming up with a comprehensive list of nursing diagnoses. These diagnoses cumulatively dictate the substance of her nursing care. Treatment plans are set for every diagnosis. Unless this concept is modified

by a notion of prioritizing, it may be seen as today's version of total patient care.

Whatever their source, we label such models of care as *goal-driven models* because they originate in patient needs translated without mediation into desired goals and therapeutic interventions. With equal justification, one could call them needs-driven or intervention-driven models. The key defining principle is that the work flow originates in the patient or more accurately in the nurse's assessment of him. There is no notion of compromise or limitation in these models, no sense that the patient is only paying for a given amount of care, and certainly no sense that the institution has the ability to deliver on only part of the package.

Yet, the truth is that few institutions have the available resources, especially nursing staff-hours, by which to provide all the care that might be envisioned for every patient in the system. That is the problem that arises under goal-driven models: They are only effective in ideal conditions. Goal-driven models assume that the resources to deliver on the comprehensive package of patient needs will be forthcoming. Whether nurses ever actually practiced under ideal circumstances is not the point. Nurses educated and working under a goal-driven ideology are supposed to "do everything."

Models advocating delivery of comprehensive care are vulnerable to failure when the control of the nurse's environment and its resources is partial. And nurses who have learned to place their self-worth in the inclusiveness of their work for each patient find that they must change that investment or judge themselves to be failures.

Today, goal-driven care has been replaced in many places with *resource-driven* care. In this model, the nurse first takes into account her environment and the resources it holds. Then, she determines what goals she reasonably can take on for a patient or group of patients. The resources drive the goals, not the other way around.

Any nurse who has served in a combat zone will recognize the model; emergency triage makes similar assumptions. There have always been resource-driven models in nursing. In any form of resource-driven care, environmental resources have a major impact on what one does. Decisions, sometimes hard ones, are required in making the best selection of goals and using scarce resources appropriately.

Further, a resource-driven model is more complex: It demands more choices, an accurate fit between available resources and work to be performed. If goal-driven care took its origin in quality factors, then resource-driven care demands a mesh of quality and quantity factors. The chief quantity factor, because it is the chief cost in the system, is the nurse's time. The question becomes how much and what sort of care can be given with a limited number of man-hours.

Many nurses recall school assignments in which they spent hours in the library completing a nursing care plan for a single patient. The student took as much time as required. She poured everything into the care plan, being careful not to skip a single patient need or goal. Resource-driven care does not have that luxury. Today's nurse must make more complex professional decisions, determining what things she will do for which patients, knowing that her priorities are critical, and accepting that she must often make hard choices between the essential and the merely beneficial.

COMPARISON OF NURSING CARE MODELS

Goal-driven and resource-driven models may be compared on many dimensions. First, their *underlying assumptions* are different. The goal-driven model assumes that all worthy goals should be tackled and that with the proper initiative the nurse will find the necessary resources to achieve the goals.

In contrast, the resource-driven model takes the system's resources as a given, expecting work to conform to the available assets. Certainly, creativity and cleverness may help the nurse make the best of a situation when resources are limited. But she accepts and works within the assets rather than seeking to alter them. By being flexible in the methods she selects to achieve goals, she may stretch resources in many cases.

The *processes* by which the two models work are significantly different also. The goal-driven model begins by setting goals derived from patient assessment and diagnosis. The nurse then determines the methods to achieve the goals and implements her plan. Finally, she evaluates to what extent the goals have been achieved.

In contrast, the process of applying resource-driven care begins with an assessment of the resources at hand. Only then is the nurse in a position to determine what goals (from a plethora of potential ones) can be achieved given her assets.

In resource-driven care, the choice of methods may affect the number of goals that can be tackled. When there are few nurses, for example, a charge nurse might select a less favored method if it is known to be a time-saver. For example, a functional care assignment method might be substituted for a primary care design in a staffing crisis. Similar shifts might take place in how individual treatments were designed.

Evaluation also differs in the two models. In a goal-driven model, the nurse simply checks to see if she has achieved the patient-related goals. In the resource-driven model, there are many more aspects for evaluation. The nurse must ask if resources were accurately defined, whether an appropriate number of goals were tackled, whether the goals were achieved, and whether the best choice of methods was made.

Similarly, there are *limitations* to both methods. If the necessary resources cannot be found, the goal-driven system breaks down. If all worthy goals cannot be achieved, the nurse is a failure. Worse, in attempting to "do everything" when it is not possible, critical aspects of care may be skipped haphazardly.

One limitation of the resource-driven model is that some or many worthy objectives may not be attempted. A miscalculation may lead a nurse to undertake less than was possible. The nurse must learn to take into account quantitative factors (e.g., one's time constraints).

Another danger in the resource-driven model occurs when there simply are not enough resources for basic safe care. Because of this vulnerability, a nurse using a resource-driven model needs a safety net (i.e., clear criteria for recognizing unsafe levels of care). Without such indices, dangerous deficiencies may be tolerated.

Each system, goal-driven and resource-driven, has some *advantages* over the other. A goal-driven model gives the nurse the satisfaction of practicing exemplary care. And because the nursing process and its evaluation are relatively simple, it is a good model for an inexperienced nurse.

In the resource-driven model, however, a nurse has the advantage of recognizing when she gives good care even in a bad situation. When care prescriptions are reality-based, it also makes for a less frenetic environment, one in which fewer mistakes may be made.

Further, the resource-driven model is more adaptable. It may be applied in a resource-scarce environment or in a resource-rich environment as well. In the case of a resource-rich environment, the nurse simply takes on more goals.

THE REALITY FACTOR

Advocates of the resource-driven model would assert that excellence in nursing practice has never really been separate from its environ-mental resources. Excellent nursing can take place in the most difficult of circumstances. Florence Nightingale in Crimea did not find the best of all possible worlds. Excellence consists of optimizing on the possible; simply put, it is what one does with what one has. A model that demands nurses find the necessary resources to deliver on perfect care may be unrealistic in our era.

However, working with a resource-driven model does not preclude simultaneously seeking to enhance one's resources. Indeed, as one learns to make intelligent decisions in the resource-driven model, one gains experience in weighing the issues of quality and quantity.

Such experience enables the nurse to better estimate the changes that may be expected in relation to any given quantum change in available resources. In essence, a resource-driven model teaches the nurse to estimate with accuracy what sort of nursing may be achieved for a given number of resources.

Although the nurse executive seldom gives direct hands-on care, she does set the stage for the nursing care model that will be accepted and valued in her institution. Because the nursing assignment system has a direct effect on use of institutional resources, the executive should be involved in deciding the model to be used.

To implement a resource-driven model requires that everyone in the system, from supervisors to head nurses to staff nurses, be taught the model and learn to conform to its expectations. If, for example, a staff nurse tries to use a resource-driven model, only to have her head nurse complain that she did not do everything for her patients, then the model cannot succeed.

RESOURCE-DRIVEN MANAGEMENT MODELS

Although it is not essential, it simplifies operations if the nursing care delivery model and the nursing management model correspond. The nurse executive will be wise to consider the fit of these elements in her nursing system.

The preferred managerial approach in the era when goal-driven nursing prevailed was the traditional management by objectives (MBO). Ten years ago, it was difficult to find a nursing service that had not devoted extensive time to setting its yearly to 5-year objectives, laying careful plans for their achievement.

The MBO model functioned much like the goal-driven model of care, beginning by setting goals—ideal ones, determined in the abstract. The managerial question was, What do we want to do? and not, What are we able to do? True, the goals were managerial rather than patient-related, but the process was identical.

After setting objectives, the nurse executive or her management team drew up logical plans for achieving the goals, identifying what resources must be found to make it possible. The plans were drawn up in fine detail, usually subject to a formalized schedule with achievement target dates assigned at each step. The plans were implemented and then evaluated periodically and terminally.

The MBO model assumed a stable world where things did not change very much or very fast—a world where the variables were known and where one could predict the result of implementing action Q instead of action R. The world of MBO was a known world not taken to throwing unexpected curves once a plan was set into motion. MBO worked best when the executive had the ability to predict the future for at least the period of time under review.

Now, we live in an era of shrinking resources and rapidly shifting opportunities, so we should not be surprised to find management models changing to fit the new reality. MBO is rapidly being replaced by strategic management as the predominant model (Barnum and Mallard 1989). Like resource-driven patient care, strategic management starts by assessing the environment. The manager assesses her organization's strengths and weaknesses in comparison with those of the competition. The model starts with the resources and the immediate situation.

Only after the environment is carefully scanned and assessed are goals selected. They will be goals that can reasonably be taken on given environmental constraints, goals that opti-

mize on the opportunities possible in the milieu. The effective organization is the one that makes the most accurate assessment of and most rapid response to the immediate and short-term future situation.

Hence, strategic planning can be seen to be a resource-driven model of management. Not only is the management scheme designed with the environment in mind, but it is made flexible to change as the external environment changes. Quick response is more important than 5-year plans. Of necessity, assessment is ongoing rather than periodic.

In strategic management, the image is always changing—not at all like MBO, in which one assumed that most elements of the situation were in one's control. In strategic planning, the outside world impinges and affects one's plans. The race is to the swift, to the one who most quickly and accurately interprets the changing situation.

Often strategic planning uses alternate scenarios, different plans designed for meeting different environmental contingencies. The strategic plan recognizes that instability and unpredictability are part of today's world.

Strategic management is discussed in greater detail in Chapter 3, but the characteristics given here should be adequate to make the point. We live in an era when economic factors are dominant, resources constrained, and the societal changes that have an effect on health care are not always predictable. In such an era, models of care delivery and models of management tend to be those best qualified to mesh with this milieu.

To a great degree, resource-driven care models and strategic management have replaced goal-driven care models and MBO. This is not to say that one cannot still draw on the best to be offered in both systems. The discussion here can be taken to refer to the dominance of the newer models over the older ones.

For example, strategic management may be superimposed on a traditional MBO system. When this is done, there is an understanding that the more traditional objectives can be set aside or changed when strategic considerations demand it.

SUMMARY

Newer models for care delivery and management have arisen in response to a different sort of health care environment than prevailed in the past. The context in which care takes place has assumed a new central importance in all our efforts. The care provider and the health care organization have less control of the context than was once the case.

No matter where they work, for most nurse executives, the new environment will be burdened by scarcity of resources and simultaneous demands for improvement or maintenance of quality of care. Newer models or care and management enable the nurse executive to make the most of her environment, realistically weighing factors of quality and quantity together.

Chief among those new models is the resource-driven model applied to care assignments and the strategic management approach applied to all aspects of management.

REFERENCES

Barnum, B.J.S., and C.O. Mallard. 1989. *Essentials of nursing management; Concepts and context of practice.* Gaithersburg, Md.: Aspen Publishers, Inc.

Stevens, B.J. 1985. *The nurse as executive,* 3rd ed. Gaithersburg, Md.: Aspen Publishers, Inc.

SUGGESTED READINGS

Armstrong, D.M., and C.B. Stetler.1991. Strategic considerations in developing a delivery model. *Nursing Economics* 9, no.2:112–115.

Barnum, B.J.S. 1994. *Nursing theory: Analysis, application, evaluation,* 4th ed. Philadelphia: J.B. Lippincott Co.

Curtin, L. 1991. Strategic planning: Asking the right questions. *Nursing Management* 22, no.1:7–8.

Hillebrand, P.L. 1994. Strategic planning: A road map to the future. *Nursing Management* 25, no.1:30–32.

Ives, J.R. 1991. Articulating values and assumptions for strategic planning. *Nursing Management* 22, no.1:38–39.

Liedtka, J.M. 1992. Formulating hospital strategy: Moving beyond a market mentality. *Health Care Management Review* 17, no.1:21–26.

Servais, S.H. 1991. Nursing resource applications through outcome based nursing practice. *Nursing Economics* 9, no.3:171–179.

Shamian, J., et al., 1992. Nursing resource requirements and support services. *Nursing Economics* 10, no.2:110–115.

Smith, H.L., et al. 1990. *Strategic nursing management: Power and responsibility.* Gaithersburg, Md.: Aspen Publishers, Inc.

Part II
Building a Nursing Program for the Future

The nurse executive is always building toward the future. This is true for every element in her organization and management. But Part II focuses on those aspects that explicitly require an eye to the future. In this part of the book, we discuss the nurse executive as a strategist (Chapter 3), her use of nursing theories (Chapter 4), the model or models she selects for nursing practice (Chapter 5), and her underlying philosophy of nursing and nursing management (Chapter 6).

Part II also explores the mission and objectives (Chapter 7) and nursing goals and management goals of the nursing division (Chapter 8) as well as the operating documents that capture these ideas. In essence, Part II looks at the intellectual underpinnings of a nursing division, the driving beliefs, direction, and purposes.

Although such ideas are driven by a view of the future, they might better be described as a look at the present through future-colored lenses. The ideas and guiding documents cannot merely represent pie-in-the-sky wish fulfillment. They must chart a realistic path, beginning from where the institution is now.

3

Nurse Executive As Strategist

At one time, it was expected that the nurse executive was only accountable for the division of nursing. The position of nurse executive was conceptualized as an internal position, one that was strictly operational. Those times have changed. The nurse executive is no longer merely an operational manager of the division of nursing. He now is involved in institutional strategic planning in many of the hospitals in the United States. If he is not now involved in strategic planning, he soon will be, because the life of the health care facility depends on people with expert knowledge of patient care being at the forefront of strategic planning. The chief nurse executive position has become much more than the operational position of a few years ago. Consequently, the nurse executive requires new knowledge, meets new challenges, and applies high levels of thinking, in addition to exercising know-how about operations.

Strategists are people who can survey the environment, understand the trends, assimilate vast amounts of information into a plan for direction, and manage the change that direction implies. Strategists design organizational structures to support the strategic plan and keep the organization focused on the important issues. Nurse executives do all this from the perspective of their own division and from the perspective of their facility as well as from a commitment to

professional values. Skills of forecasting, negotiating, and influencing are a few of the many requirements for this kind of role.

Not only does the nurse executive strategize with people at the corporate level about what the organization should be, but he also thinks strategically for the areas for which he has responsibility. Day-to-day operational responsibility has been replaced by long-range thinking and planning that drives the daily operations. The nurse executive is expected to understand strategic planning and to operate in this way.

This textbook prepares the nurse executive for strategic thinking and planning. Each of the chapters guides the reader through the necessary process. As the reader thinks through each chapter, the programmatic outcomes become clear as well as the strategic planning capacity he must develop. The analysis and synthesis of material in each of these chapters guides the nurse executive in becoming the strategist mandatory in today's positions.

RETHINKING MARKET ORIENTATION/COMPETITIVE ADVANTAGE

For the nurse executive, becoming a strategist involves switching away from traditional thinking in which the outcome of nursing care was the primary drive in the system. That outcome is still important, but so is a view of the big picture external to the division, a view based in the market and the competitive advantage that is necessary for success.

No longer can the nurse executive merely provide excellence in the quality of care. He must be now aware of what the market wants, how the market defines quality, what the market is willing to pay for, and what the market considers essential. A nursing organization that looks like all the other organizations in the same area will not work. Instead, the nurse executive must clearly delineate and differentiate how his program differs from other competitive nursing programs based on what the market is seeking and what it is expecting in health care.

In today's market, successful facilities fulfill specific niches; the nurse executive must consider this in planning a program. Nor can personal agendas be sustained if they do not fit the environment. Suppose, for example, the nurse executive wants his staff to contribute regularly to nursing research, but the environment is not supportive of this kind of productivity. The executive will falter in his ability to achieve this objective.

The nurse executive as strategist thinks first in terms of developing a competitive advantage. He is strategically driven by the market to carve out a competitive position and advantage. This is a major switch in tactics for many executives who have been educated to think in terms of day-to-day operations.

As health care changes from a cottage industry with many small players to the corporatization of health care with the market dominated by a few large players, characteristics of the market take on critical importance. The nurse executive's job is to provide greater value for the customer than the competition can provide.

Not only must the nurse executive provide a greater value for the customers (patients, payers, physicians, etc.), but he must also provide a greater value than the person who might be his replacement. In the resource-driven model, a cost-effective approach means that the nurse executive achieves better outcomes for a given

cost than can someone else. Or that he achieves a given outcome (achievable by others) but at a lower cost. The successful nurse executive in this era of health care must provide evidence of value.

The way the nurse executive gets the job done is to work strategically through others. He is no longer in a position to do all the work himself. Instead, strategic leadership involves bringing diverse groups of people together to work for the articulated mission and goals.

The nurse executive who operates as strategist is able to develop a mission and vision for the division of nursing that articulates with the facilities' mission and vision. He is able to manage the programs and changes necessitated by the strategic vision and plan.

In a market-driven environment in which competitive advantage is one key success factor, the typical nurse executive must manage within an environment that is progressively more resource-driven. This is the challenge for the nurse executive: to assimilate and synthesize a program of excellence within the confines of the environment, the resources, and the market.

Getting the Job Done

Market research is essential to the success of the nurse executive. He must know the strengths and weaknesses of his areas of accountability, but he must also know the same information about competitors. Further, he needs similar information about other departments in the hospital and about key groups and individuals such as physicians.

Beyond the internal workings of the facility, the nurse executive must be knowledgeable of the external market in terms of payer expectations and 3- to 5-year trends in the marketplace. He will also need to acquire any other information vital for building a base on which the vision for the nursing division can be achieved.

Developing the Program

Developing a strategic program for success is only where the work begins. Not only must the nurse executive be a strategic planner, but he must be an implementer as well. To be successful, he must create the need for change by unfreezing old thought patterns and ways of doing the work.

Many organizations become hard-wired in their approach to change. Traditionally, health care was allowed to remain relatively stable, but now it is in the midst of a dramatic revolution driven by the corporatization of health care. The nurse executive must help everyone see the necessity for change so that his program will be adopted and implemented.

To change, people must feel uncomfortable with the present or at least perceive large rewards on the horizon if they change. Unfortunately, in the resource-driven environment, as costs get ratcheted down, often the only reward is that the facility stays in business and people have their jobs.

Given this pattern of running to stay even, the nurse executive must continually scan the horizon and keep people abreast of the big picture. He cannot minimize the threats or opportunities in the environment. Staff can never be given too much information. Nor should they be protected by lack of disclosure. Staff adjust best when they understand what the nurse executive knows and when the strategic plan addresses the issues on the horizon.

There are many ways to keep staff informed. Experts can be brought into the hospital, and staff can be sent to conferences. Inservice programs and the continual updates through newsletter and facility publications can also serve this purpose. Communication is a service issue for the nurse executive to address.

Creating a Shared Vision

Staff respond best to the challenges of this new era of health care if they believe that they share the vision of the nurse executive. A sense of joint ownership of that vision is a powerful incentive; it enables staff to see a better future. Even when the nurse executive is very visible in the organization, he is dependent on communication channels (direct reports and other people)

to teach, educate, and sell the vision. High-performing, synergized management teams that closely involve the staff help them to feel a part of the vision and to develop a commitment to the organization's future.

Once the strategic vision is articulated and well known throughout the organization, the skills of project management on the part of the nurse executive ensure its implementation. By delegating, continually working through others, and constantly assessing and benchmarking progress, the plan is implemented. The work of the nurse executive then becomes the work of managing the strategic plan and making sure that everyone is accountable for their share of the implementation.

Of course, implementing a strategic plan is not a smooth process. There will be setbacks and many challenges. If the vision of the strategic plan is constantly at the forefront of what everyone does, however, the organization will be able to assess the progress. Even with setbacks, the executive can tell when progress is being made.

There is also a danger of being locked into a strategic plan so that the organization is not free to improvise and to change course when the market and the environment demand. Markets can change suddenly. Without warning, payers can make demands that were not anticipated, and resources such as staff can suddenly be in dramatic over- or undersupply.

If the nurse executive and the executive team work together in a high-performing, synergistic team, they will manage. As new information is made available, the system can adjust quickly and cope with the new input. If the nurse executive and other corporate executives work as an integrated team, the success of the facility is ensured.

NURSING STRATEGIC PLAN

It is common custom for a nursing division to create a document that expresses its most immediate strategic goals, along with the action plans designed to achieve them. Assigned deadlines included in the plan keep things moving. Unlike the divisional goals which tend to be enduring and comprehensive of all the division's responsibilities, the strategic plan represents only a few major thrusts, those bold efforts designed to produce substantial changes or optimize on immediate opportunities.

Preparing a new program, investigating a new computerized nursing information system, or expanding one's markets into a new neighborhood might be examples of items found on such a list. There is no right or wrong for inclusion. The chief reason for committing a strategic divisional plan to paper is to solidify one's thinking about it.

Furthermore, to pin down a strategic plan the nursing management team must come together and ask, Where are we going? Where do we want to be 2 years from now? How will we be different then than we are today? Such meetings not only define a strategic plan, but they place responsibility and accountability among the managerial members.

Like any strategic plan, the document may require revision any time that circumstances change. Meanwhile, it serves as a clear guideline for the more entrepreneurial, innovative plans of the division.

SUMMARY

Strategic leadership involves the ability to survey the environment, to analyze and synthesize information into a viable plan, and to develop a mission and vision that are shared by the entire staff. With unity of purpose, the executive team and the staff will become a learning organization, a well-articulated system that integrates information, plans appropriately, and adjusts to the environment and the market as quickly as needed.

There is much work and thought involved in the process of getting from the strategy of the division of nursing to the implementation of a successful program. Building a program involves a thoughtful design to carry out the plan. Subsequent chapters of this book are building blocks for implementing a successful strategy for the division of nursing.

SUGGESTED READINGS

Anderson, H., and M. Koska. 1992. Hospitals and medical staffs: The concept of planning takes on new meaning. *Hospitals* 66, no.20:22–24, 26–28, 30.

Behrenbeck, J., et al. 1990. Strategic planning for a nursing information system model. *Computers in Nursing* 8, no.6:236–242.

Bryan, L., et al. 1990. Strategic planning: Collaboration and empowerment. *Nursing Connections* 3, no.3:31–36.

Curtin, L. 1991. Strategic planning: Asking the right questions. *Nursing Management* 22, no.1:7–8.

John, J., and A. Miller. 1989. Strategic planning for nursing homes: A market opportunity analysis perspective. *Health Care Management Review* 14, no.4:11–19.

Johnson, L.M. 1992. Structures, strategies, and synthesis: The nurse executive as social architect. *Nursing Administration Quarterly* 17, no.1:10–16.

McLean, R. 1990. A strategic planning framework for endowment management. *Health Care Management Review* 15, no.2:53–60.

Philbin, P. 1993. Strategic planning—from the ground up: Planting the seeds of network development. *Hospital Health Network* 67, no.11:46–52.

Shinn, L. 1993. Action steps to avoid pitfalls in strategic planning. *Aspen's Advisor for Nurse Executives* 8, no.9:1.

Smith, H., et al. 1993. Nursing department strategy, planning, and performance in rural hospitals. *Journal of Nursing Administration* 23, no.4:23–24.

Sovie, M. 1993. Hospital culture—Why create one? *Nursing Economics* 11, no.2:69–75, 90.

Thomas, A. 1993. Strategic planning: A practical approach. *Nursing Management* 24, no.2:34–35, 38.

4

Analyzing Nursing Theories

Because the job of the nurse executive is to make nursing operational by delivering care to patients, it is essential that she understand the theory (or theories) of nursing used in the institution. Indeed, she is likely to exert influence in its selection.

The nursing profession has developed various nursing models, each with its own advantages and limitations. Whatever theory a division or department selects, there are advantages to implementing a theory-based practice. Nursing theory constitutes the intellectual framework for patient care. When carefully chosen and well implemented, a theory-based practice provides a sound basis for patient care.

CHOOSING A THEORY

Because it is selective, any theory is necessarily a partial view, presenting the most salient features of nursing as the theory depicts them. Theories are not so much true or false as useful or impractical. Two or more different theories of nursing can be used to explain the same nursing phenomena. The question is not which theory is right, but which theory best explains and makes clear the nursing phenomena.

The answer to that question may be different in different institutions, with different patients,

and with nurses from different backgrounds. The answers may even vary for discrete patient groups within the same institution.

A theory distills the features of the nursing phenomena according to its own ordering principles. In each case, a theory lays bare an underlying structure that explains or describes the nursing phenomena. In turn, that structure constitutes the categories according to which nursing work is planned and recorded. The categories are used to organize the nurses' plan of care and such diverse documents as quality measurement tools, nurses' notes, and various accreditation reports. The theory, then, sets the mind frame by which nurses using it approach their work.

Many unique theories of nursing have evolved over time. Works of Rogers (unitary, evolving man approach), Roy (stimulus-response orientation), Orem (self-care principle), Johnson (behavioral approach), Newman (evolving consciousness orientation), Neuman (stress/strain vectors design), and Watson (transpersonal caring focus) are cited in the suggested readings section. Capturing their orientations in a word or two does justice to none of these theories, but it makes the point that nursing theories arise from vastly different perspectives on humans, science, and the world. In each case, the orientation colors the ways that nurses working under these premises go about their practice and research. Nor should the theories cited here be taken as all-inclusive. There are close to 20 extant theories of nursing, with varying degrees of popularity.

Some arguments may be given that these generic theories work better in step-down and community facilities (Barnum 1994) than in the high-tech environment of today's acute care facility.

Today's Most Popular Theory

At present, the most popular theory of nursing in acute care is not the work of any individual theorist but instead a theory comprised of the so-called nursing process applied to various patient diagnoses, the most common taxonomy for which comes from the North American Nursing Diagnosis Association (NANDA 1992). Other taxonomies of nursing diagnoses are also available and may differ in format. See, for example, diagnostic taxonomies by Doenges and Moorhouse (1988), Gordon (1982), Kim et al. (1984), and Carpenito (1984).

A concurrent effort by Bulechek and McCloskey (1992) heralds serious work on the next step of this theory: taxonomizing nursing interventions. This endeavor follows the same conceptual plan as the nursing process/nursing diagnosis schema, adding to that design. This highly codified approach to nursing is conceived as part of the effort to create a nationwide nursing minimum data set (Werley and Lang 1988).

What Bulechek and McCloskey are attempting to do for all interventions has already been organized for nurses in home health care by Saba and associates (1991). These nurses developed a computerized classification of nursing interventions for Medicare patients.

The nursing process/nursing diagnosis-based theory mimics the practice of medicine in its attempt to design a complete taxonomy for practice. And because it purports to identify diagnoses that nurses can agree on, the system has potential for nursing research. Its similarity to the design of medical systems may be useful in an environment in which the two professions work closely together, particularly when care/treatment focuses on critical body work.

One of the limitations of the nursing process/nursing diagnosis-based theory is that it requires a grasp of an extensive number of components on the part of the nurse. Another limitation of the system, as noted earlier, is that unless it is combined with a notion of prioritizing goals, it is incompatible with a resource-driven model of care.

As an alternative, some institutions construct theories built around crucial presenting problems. The Weed system (1978) was one early formulation of this problematic approach. The alternative often works well in an institution that admits patients with like diagnoses or problems (e.g., a rehabilitation institution or a cancer care facility).

In problem-oriented nursing, the caregiver views the patient as presenting various overt and covert problems. The nurse's task is to identify the problems accurately and seek solutions. The problem-initiated approach is less systematic and less comprehensive than the nursing process/nursing diagnosis design. In problem-initiated care, only systems identified as disturbed will receive the nurse's attention—a built-in priority system.

ONE THEORY OR MANY?

The nurse executive must decide whether to use one theory throughout an institution (or even in a corporation of various institutions) or whether to allow different departments, units, or even individual nurses to use theories of their own choice. This is a more complicated decision than it first appears.

Adoption of a single theory throughout an institution allows for flexibility in use of staff among the various nursing units and makes inservice education simpler. It also promotes coordination with other professionals (who get to know the basics of the model in time). A single theory approach also helps nonprofessional nursing staff learn the system, even if they are shifted among different units.

The disadvantage of imposing a single theory institutionwide is that any given theory shows differences of fit with different arenas of care. A theory that is excellent for orthopedic care, for example, may be less adequate for maternity care and just plain awkward for emergency department care.

Some nurse executives allow each major department to select a theory appropriate to its patient populations. Because each theory dictates a different set of recording documents (e.g., Kardex forms, nurses' notes, and nursing orders), the cost and managerial complexity involved in creating different forms may be a consideration. Most institutions, however, are used to permitting great variance between and among major departments.

Theories specific to specialty practice are beginning to emerge and may offer an ideal fit in these areas. Some of the older generic theories also may work well in a given specialty.

Few if any nurse executives allow each nurse to choose the theory of her preference. This simply makes care too complex to convey to alternate shifts of varying personnel. Nor is it fair to patients to subject them to radically shifting patterns of nursing care if theories are changed from nurse to nurse or shift to shift.

Furthermore, accrediting agencies will want to know what theory or theories of nursing are used. They will be less than satisfied with an answer that every nurse selects her own theory.

THEORY ELEMENTS IN NURSING PRACTICE

Not all nurse executives believe it is essential to apply a given nursing theory to practice. Some say that they do not theorize. This position fails to recognize that theory elements inevitably underlie the organization of nursing care. Whatever categories the nurse uses to think, chart, and evaluate quality structure her nursing actions whether or not the fact is recognized.

The point is that theorizing is inevitable. A theory viewpoint emerges informally if not formally. Because that is the case, it makes more sense to select a theory or theory elements than

to let them emerge by accident. If a theory is purposefully chosen, then one can check to see that it is systematically applied in all related managerial and care delivery tools.

For consistency, the same conception of nursing can be implemented in nursing care plans, nurses' notes, nursing orders, quality assurance tools, performance appraisal formats, patient acuity systems, and staffing and scheduling plans. Consistency in these structural elements helps improve nursing managerial efficiency and care performance.

SUMMARY

The nurse executive must consider the effect of nursing theory on the practice in her institution. The trend is to be able to identify the theory extant in the practice in a given institution (or the departments therein). Even if the nurse executive elects not to adopt a given theory, her reporting and recording structures of necessity will exhibit certain theory predispositions.

REFERENCES

Barnum, B.J.S. 1994. *Nursing theory: Analysis, application, evaluation*, 4th ed. Philadelphia: J.B. Lippincott Co.

Bulechek, G.M., and J.C. McCloskey. 1992. Defining and validating nursing intervention. *Nursing Clinics of North America* 27, no.2:289–299.

Carpenito, L.J. 1984. *Handbook of nursing diagnosis*. Philadelphia: J.B. Lippincott Co.

Doenges, M.E., and M.F. Moorhouse. 1988. *Nurse's pocket guide: Nursing diagnosis with interventions*, 2nd ed. Philadelphia: F.A. Davis Co.

Gordon, M. 1982. *Manual of nursing diagnosis*. New York: McGraw-Hill Publishing Co.

Kim, M.J., et al., eds. 1984. *Pocket guide to nursing diagnoses*. St. Louis: C.V. Mosby Co.

North American Nursing Diagnosis Association. 1992. *NANDA nursing diagnoses: Definitions and classifications 1992–1993*. St. Louis, Mo.

Saba, V.K., et al. 1991. A nursing intervention taxonomy for home health care. *Nursing and Health Care* 12, no.6:296–299.

Weed, L.1978. *Medical records, medical education, and patient care*. Cleveland: Press of Case Western Reserve University.

Werley, H.H., and N.M. Lang, eds. 1988. *Identification of the nursing minimum data set.* New York: Springer Publishing Co., Inc.

SUGGESTED READINGS

Allison, S., et al. 1991. Nursing theory: A tool to put nursing back into nursing administration. *Nursing Administration Quarterly* 15, no.3:72–78.

Anderson, R., et al. 1992. Theory-based approach to computer skill in nursing administration. *Computers in Nursing* 10, no. 4:152–157, 1992.

Bostrom, I., et al. 1992. Nursing theory based changes of work organization in an ICU: Effects on quality of care. *Intensive and Critical Care Nursing* 8, no.1:10–16.

Brown, B. 1991. The efficacy of nursing models and theories in nursing practice (editorial). *Nursing Administration Quarterly* 15, no.3:v–vii.

Fernandez, R., et al. 1990. Theory-based practice: A model for nurse retention. *Nursing Administration Quarterly* 14, no.4:47–53.

Huckabay, L. 1991. The role of conceptual frameworks in nursing practice, administration, education, and research. *Nursing Administration Quarterly* 15, no.3:17–28.

Jacques, R. 1993. Untheorized dimensions of caring work: Caring as a structural practice and caring as a way of seeing. *Nursing Administration Quarterly* 17, no.2:1–10.

Johnson, D.E. 1980. The behavioral system model for nursing. In *Conceptual models for nursing practice,* 2nd ed., ed. J.P. Riehl and C. Roy, 207–216. New York: Appleton-Century-Crofts.

Lutjens, L. 1992. Derivation and testing of tenets of a theory of social organizations as adaptive systems. *Nursing Science Quarterly* 5, no.2:62–71.

Mayberry, A. 1991. Merging nursing theories, models, and nursing practice: More than an administrative challenge. *Nursing Administration Quarterly* 15, no.3:44–53.

Neuman, B. 1980. The Betty Neuman health-care systems model: A total person approach to patient problems. In *Conceptual models for nursing practice,* 2nd ed., ed. J.P. Riehl and C. Roy, 119–134. New York: Appleton-Century-Crofts.

Newman, M., et al. 1991. Nurse case management: The coming together of theory and practice. *Nursing and Health Care* 12, no.8:404–408.

Newman, M.A. 1986. *Health as expanding consciousness.* St. Louis: C.V. Mosby Co.

Orem, D.E. 1985. *Nursing: Concepts of practice,* 3rd ed. New York: McGraw-Hill Publishing Co.

Rogers, M.E. 1990. Nursing: Science of unitary, irreducible, human beings: Update 1990. In *Visions of Roger's science-based nursing,* ed. E.A.M. Barrett, 1–11. New York: National League for Nursing.

Roy, C. 1980. The Roy adaptation model. In *Conceptual models for nursing practice,* 2nd ed., ed. J.P. Riehl and C. Roy, 179–188. New York: Appleton-Century-Crofts.

Schmieding, N. 1988. Action process of nurse administrators to problematic situations based on Orlando's theory. *Journal of Advanced Nursing* 13, no.1:99–107.

Smith, M. 1991. The contribution of nursing theory to nursing administration practice. *Image* 25, no.1:63–67.

Sorrentino, E. 1991. Making theories work for you. *Nursing Administration Quarterly* 15, no.3:54–59.

Walker, L.O., and K.C. Avant. 1983. *Strategies for theory construction in nursing.* Norwalk, Conn.: Appleton-Century-Crofts.

Watson, J. 1988. *Nursing: Human science and human care: A theory of nursing.* New York: National League for Nursing.

West, P. 1991. Theory implementation: A challenging journey. *Canadian Journal of Nursing Administration* 4, no.1:29–30.

Williams B. 1991. The utility of nursing theory in nursing case management practice. *Nursing Administration Quarterly* 15, no.3:60–65.

5

Model for Nursing Practice

Many different models for nursing practice are available for the nurse executive and her staff. When a model is based on an extant nursing theory, it simply draws on the basic elements of that theory. In other cases, nursing divisions elect to construct their own practice models. This chapter builds a protocol for a practice model, relying generally—and loosely—on formulations of the nursing process model. First, however, we look closely at the most common irregularities in that model.

COMPARING THE NURSING PROCESS MODEL TO THE MEDICAL MODEL

Most nursing process models more or less adopt the basic medical model; that is, they contain some form of the following steps: assessment, diagnosis, prognosis, prescription, therapy, and evaluation. Although nursing has adopted the basic categories of the medical model, it has developed its own terminology (Table 5–1).

The medical model would appear to be well suited to the needs of acute care nursing if one were to judge by its extensive adoption. However, there are differences in the ways the two professions use the model.

Differences in the ways in which medicine and nursing use the model can be detected by looking at nursing's implementing tools. The first difference in adaptation is in the area of nursing diagnosis. Most nursing diagnostic systems derive diagnoses in a way different from that used in medical taxonomies.

After the physician assesses the patient through examination and history taking, he uses the information attained to make a diagnosis. That diagnosis—diabetes, strangulated hernia, or myocardial infarction—is a different entity from those signs and symptoms that were observed in the assessment.

Seldom does the nurse combine all the discrete symptoms she assesses into some further entity called a diagnosis. If, for example, the nurse assesses that the patient has a defect in visual perception and paresis of the left leg, she uses these assessments as diagnoses in her goal setting and care planning. Most diagnostic systems in nursing collapse the two categories of assessment and diagnosis. The nurse treats a patient assessment as if it were itself a diagnosis.

Another difference in nursing's use of the model from medicine is the association between prognosis and prescription. The thinking in the medical model dictates the following sequence of events:

Table 5-1 Common Nursing Terminology and Related Nursing Tools

Category	Nursing Terms	Implementing Tools
Assessment	Patient assessment Identification of patient needs/problems	Nursing interview Nursing history Physical examination
Diagnosis	Nursing diagnosis	Diagnostic taxonomies
Prognosis	Goal setting	Nursing care plan
Prescription	Nursing order Nursing care plans	Nursing order sheet Nursing care plans
Therapy	Nursing intervention	Routine nursing notes Nursing progress notes
Evaluation	Quality assurance	Nursing quality control forms Nursing chart audit

1. Prognosis establishes the realistic outcome to expect for this patient with this impairment.
2. Achieving that realistic outcome or better is the goal of therapy, that is, the prognosis—in its form as the optimal realistic outcome of health—becomes the goal of therapy.
3. Prescriptions are aimed at reaching that optimal goal. Such prescriptions may be partial measures at any particular state in time (e.g., passive exercise with active exercise later), but they all aim toward ultimate attainment of the goal.

In contrast, nursing process models seldom specify the prognosis element. Outcome goals are set, but the concurrent prognosis is seldom defined. Table 5-2 is offered as a guide for the steps of the model as used in most applications.

GENERIC MODEL FOR PRACTICE

Patient Assessment

All nursing practice models tend to use the same tools for assessment of the patient's present and prior health status: physical examination, observation, and interview. Such techniques, singly or combined, appear in tools

termed *nursing interviews, nursing histories,* and *nursing assessments.* Although all nursing models provide for some method of patient assessment, not all use the same approach.

The structure of a system's assessment tools shows how the model categorizes the important aspects of humans (patient) or of nursing. Tools make certain that the assessment process is both systematic and complete. Schemes for categorization are manifold (see Exhibit 5-1); the following are but a few examples.

The reader familiar with nursing theory will recognize the various theories from which these category schemes have been borrowed. The first group of schemes is based on categorizations of patient, whereas the second group uses categories of nursing as its basis.

More complex schemes may use parallel systems, converting an initial patient-based assessment into categories of nursing practice. One's selection of a patient-based or nursing-based category scheme should be consistent with the philosophy and definition of nursing of one's particular institution.

It is important that the organization consider the suitability of the selected topics in each category. Errors of topic selection include deficiencies or excesses in number of topics covered, selection of topics that are unwieldy for practical use, or selection of topics not consistent with the organizational philosophy and definition of nursing.

Table 5-2 Components of the Nursing Process Based on the Medical Model

Steps in the Nursing Process	Objective	Criteria	Prerequisite Knowledge	Activities	Tools
Patient assessment	Develop a knowledge base on which to make nursing decisions	Normal health patterns and normal rehab-adapted patterns	Ability to identify needs and problems, knowledge of norms, and ability to identify deviations	Assessment of physiological, psychological, social, and personal factors	Nursing interview Nursing history Physical exam and observation
Nursing diagnosis	Place a judgment upon assessment data	Implicit or explicit taxonomy of diagnoses (may or may not differ from medical diagnoses)	What signs and symptoms constitute what nursing diagnoses	Place judgments upon assessment data	Nursing taxonomies of diagnoses
Goal setting	Use nursing diagnosis and patient assessment to set realistic health goals	Normal health outcomes for illnesses, patient's motivation, opportunity, capacities	Knowledge of outcome norms, ability to modify outcome norms based on individual factors	Setting long-term and immediate goals	Nursing summaries Nursing care plan
Therapy planning	Identify care measures most likely to meet long-term and immediate goals of nursing and medical regimens	Documented relations between care activities and patient outcomes, logical prediction of care effects on outcome	Nursing theory relating nursing measures to desired outcomes	Identify nursing measures to be taken	Nursing orders Nursing care plan Nursing research studies
Care implementation	Provide care measures needed to meet goals	Implicit or explicit standards of care	Ability to use nursing skills, manipulomotor and psychosocial	Provide needed care activities	Nursing progress notes Routine nurses' charting
Care plan evaluation	Determine if plan is meeting goals	Implicit or explicit patient outcomes	Patient assessment skills	Assess client progress and its relation to care given	Nursing quality control systems Nursing chart audit Case studies

Exhibit 5–1 Schemes for Categorization

Group I

Scheme A
  State of consciousness
  Emotional status
  Intellectual capacity
  Sensory status
  Motor abilities

Scheme B
  Social status
  Mental status
  Emotional status
  Sensory perception
  Motor ability
  Metabolic status
  Respiratory function
  Circulatory status
  Nutritional status
  Elimination status
  Rest and comfort
  Skin and appendages

Scheme C
  Pain and discomfort
  Body positioning
  Mobility
  Fluid and electrolyte balance
  Oxygen supply
  Learning needs
  Psychosocial adjustment
  Skin integrity

Scheme D
  Structural integrity
  Mass and energy conservation
  Social integrity
  Personal integrity

Scheme E
  Physiologic status
  Psychological status
  Sociologic status

Group II

Scheme A
  Disease-related needs
  Therapy-related needs
  Personal needs

Scheme B
  Supportive needs
  Therapeutic needs
  Rehabilitative needs

Scheme C
  Immediate, acute needs
  Chronic maintenance needs
  Rehabilitative needs
  Well-health maintenance needs

Scheme D
  Sustaining needs
  Remedial needs
  Restorative needs
  Preventive needs

Scheme E
  Preserving body defenses
  Preventing complications
  Providing comfort
  Implementing prescribed therapies
  Planning return to the community
  Detecting changes in the body's regulatory system

Several common sense rules can be applied to the evaluation of or construction of assessment tools:

1. The assessment tool should not duplicate investigations already available from other sources. There is no reason nurses cannot use information gained by others for nursing purposes. To submit the patient to unnecessary duplication in examination or interview is wasteful of nursing time and stressful to the patient.

2. Assessment processes should seek only information that will be used in the nursing planning. One often finds such inanities as a careful listing of each patient's food preferences in an organization that allows no variation in menus. There should not be interviewing for interview's sake. No matter how weighty the information, unless it will actually enter nursing care planning, obtaining it is an invasion of privacy.

3. The form should allow for discretion in collection of data instead of compulsive form-filling. One of the most valuable parts of an assessment may be the nurse's decision that certain sections of the assess-

ment tool are not pertinent for this patient and can be omitted without impairing the nursing care planning.

4. The assessment tool should be realistic in terms of the nursing actually practiced or practicable in the institution. Few institutions, for example, allot enough nursing hours per patient for ideal nursing care. If a resource-driven model is used, the assessment tool should reflect the scope of nursing practice that is realistic.

Patient assessment, then, is the first stage of the nursing process no matter what model is used. The raw data collected are selected through a preconceived screen found in the assessment tools and based on the model's description of nursing.

To reduce assessment data to workable size, the method of exception is often used. This means that only health patterns seen as abnormal or deficient are considered. To identify health abnormalities requires that two criteria be built into the assessment process: knowledge of usual health patterns and knowledge of usual rehabilitation-adapted patterns. The second criterion is just as important as the first. For example, the nurse must determine if the patient who has been admitted for another health problem has already adapted to his existing diabetes, blindness, amputation, or other impairment. She must take the patient's state of adaptation to standing deficiencies into account in her assessment.

Nursing Diagnosis

In an attempt to apply the medical model in its entirety, nurses are developing their own taxonomies of diagnosis as discussed in Chapter 4. A nursing diagnosis usually is differentiated from a medical diagnosis as being a label for a condition amenable to treatment by nursing care. What is a diagnosis for one discipline may be a symptom for another. For example, the medical diagnosis, cervical arthritis, might be derived, partly, from an extant limitation in mobility (a nursing diagnosis and a medical symp-

tom). Although there is agreement that a nursing diagnosis is arrived at through assessment data, there is little agreement on just what constitutes a nursing diagnosis. The following entities have been called nursing diagnoses by various authors:

1. states being experienced by the patient (e.g., anxiety, confusion)
2. physiologic deviations from the norm (e.g., irregular bowel function, impaired hearing)
3. patient behavioral deviations from the norm (e.g., obsessive compulsions, continual seeking for attention from nursing staff)
4. combinations of above classes with their underlying causes (e.g., pacing due to anxiety concerning upcoming surgery)

Although many groups and individuals have produced tomes of diagnoses, there is still no basic agreement on the nature of a nursing diagnosis or on how it is derived from the assessment data.

Some generalities can be drawn, however. Unlike its medical predecessor, the nursing diagnosis seldom is captured in a single, summative term. For example, many symptoms may lead the physician to a single diagnosis: myocardial infarction. In contrast, a nursing diagnosis for the same patient (depending on the classification scheme selected) might have several, not one, nursing diagnoses (e.g., pain, fear for life and future, resentment of dependent role) —not to mention the physiologic diagnoses.

As with the medical diagnosis, these nursing diagnoses serve as conclusions based on assessments, and they lead to the next stage of goal setting. A few nurse authors deny the existence of nursing diagnoses separate from medical diagnoses. For these nurses, there is a single class of diagnoses used by both professions.

Goal Setting

Goal setting in nursing can be loosely equated with prognosis from the medical model.

Both are similar in that they represent anticipated patient outcomes. The nature of these outcomes is quite different, however. Medical prognosis is a practiced guess at the statistically likely health outcome for the patient. In those rare systems in which the term *nursing prognosis* is used, it has a similar meaning (statistically likely health outcome).

Goal setting in nursing differs from the statistical approach to outcomes. Long-term nursing goals define the *desired* patient outcome, given the realities of the patient's impairment. Although prognosis aims at the statistical average, long-term goals aim at the highest level of health outcome that can be realistically anticipated, given optimal health return. This realistic goal setting requires both knowledge of the usual health outcome for a given illness and the ability to estimate the patient's motivation, opportunities, and capacities. Thus, statistical and unique individual factors are combined in setting long-term nursing goals.

In the medical model, the prognosis is not further compartmentalized, although it may change as the patient's condition alters. Goal setting in nursing has a different nature. It would be more accurate to talk about goals setting (plural) or nursing prognoses. Because nursing diagnosis typically produces a series of discrete factors rather than a unified entity, it is not surprising that multiple factors appear in the goal setting and in nursing prognosis, too.

Not only does goal setting involve multiplicity in content, but each goal is further broken down into goal stages. A good care plan indicates immediate goals and shows how each immediate goal is related to one or more long-term goals. For example, the following immediate goals might appear at one time or another on the way to the long-term goal of return to normal ambulation: (1) increase strength of arm and shoulder muscles for use of crutches, (2) ambulate safely on crutches without weight bearing on injured side, and (3) ambulate safely on crutches with graded weight bearing.

In evaluating the adequacy of goal-setting activities, one should be aware of several sources for error in both long-term and immediate goal decisions: an inappropriate goal, omission of a needed goal, and setting an appropriate goal but for the wrong time.

Therapy Planning

Goal setting is translated into action by conversion of immediate goals into nursing orders for therapies most effective in reaching those goals. Nursing orders are the ongoing plans for nursing care, and a nursing care plan represents the conformation of such orders on any one particular day.

Conceptual Problems

To make a judgment about nursing care on the basis of one day's nursing care plan is as limited a perspective as trying to judge the adequacy of a course of medical treatment by viewing the medical orders in effect on any one day of illness. Such a process totally ignores the need for longitudinal data that record permanently the nursing orders and the progression of changes in those orders. Nursing orders need to be kept as a permanent record to compare them with permanent records of patient progress. Only in this way will nursing be able to research and evaluate its own process and its effect on health outcome.

Therapy planning is more complex than its medical counterpart, prescription, because it must combine and coordinate nursing orders and physician orders. This summation usually takes the form of the nursing care plan. The effective care plan should be organized to show the relation between each immediate goal and its associated nursing and/or physician orders. It is important that the relation between goals and ordered-care activities be documented, for the sake of future nursing research. Many traditional nursing activities are assumed to be appropriate means for reaching certain goals on very little documented evidence. Only research can cure this problem.

Some institutions still have difficulty getting nursing therapy plans written, although accreditation standards serve as a not-so-gentle prod. Obviously, care plans are essential because

1. Nursing as a profession must identify its own content above and beyond the carrying out of medical orders.
2. Consensus in nursing approach requires a written plan of care.
3. Continuity in nursing approach (over three shifts) requires a written plan of care.
4. Formulation of a written plan will help the nurse to clarify and solidify her nursing goals.
5. Identifying precise components of nursing care is necessary to have a check against care omissions.
6. Nonprofessional personnel need to have well-communicated nursing directives.

One reason for resistance to committing a plan to paper is that the nurse is frequently educated to think that there is a right answer for every nursing problem. The nurse is taught that she is a scientist and must plan her clinical care on scientific principles. She comes to expect that if she makes the correct decision, she can expect the desired outcome.

Yet, clinical practice is not so simple. A good teaching program, for example, does not guarantee the requisite learning. The uncertainty of patient outcomes is one reason some nurses dislike committing plans to records. The nurse tends to judge herself on patient outcomes rather than on the inherent worth of the proposed plan of care itself.

Instead, patient outcomes should be used nonjudgmentally, as checks on care designs. As in strategic management, when a plan does not work, it should be changed without incurring defensiveness. One deals with empirical evidence rather than judging the inherent value and logic in a proposed nursing action.

Too often, the nurse is taught to ignore the distinctive character of practical activity, which is *uncertainty*. Individual situations are unique and never duplicated. No complete assurance of outcome is possible; the nursing plan is not the sole determinant of the patient outcome. Overt action cannot avoid risk. Certainly, it is the aim of nursing planning to decrease the number of variables that will negatively affect patient out-

comes, but it is not possible to establish complete control over these variables.

Nursing, for example, involves more numerous acts of uncertain consequence than medicine. If the culture and sensitivity shows that an organism is sensitive to penicillin, the physician has little reason to doubt the outcome of this drug selection. If the nurse plans a strategy to encourage a disturbed new mother to accept her newborn, she has far less security in her selected strategy.

The more one has to deal with the behavioral and social sciences, the less predictable are the outcomes. A behavioral response can never be predicted in the same manner as can a physiologic response.

For most nursing situations, many different plans might be evolved to meet the same nursing needs. Indeed, one plan might be just as likely to lead to the desired patient outcome as another. As resource-driven care emphasizes, many different methods can lead to the same patient outcome. The nurse must not feel responsible for finding the one plan that suits her superiors; she is responsible only for determining a plan that seems to have a high probability of success in the given circumstances.

Care plans represent conclusions, but usually they fail to show the lines of reasoning behind those conclusions. In this respect, they are like physician's orders. Thus, the nurse often wishes she had a written way to justify her written plan. Indeed, certain nursing orders (strategies) may actually work better and be better enforced if the care supplier understands the aim of the strategy. For example, the nurse may have a valid reason for requiring that a patient do a difficult dressing change himself, but if her strategy is not immediately obvious to the rest of the staff, they may hesitate to follow the plan.

In establishing a system for recording nursing orders, one needs to consider the nurse's need to explain her judgments and strategies. If such an option is not available, she may hesitate to write nursing orders that have complex derivations.

Operational Problems

Operational problems exist in instituting written care plans. A care plan is really a set of nursing orders. It is useful to contrast nursing orders with physician's orders. With the physician's orders, one physician has overriding responsibility and authority. Even when physicians work in teams, they have an established pecking order. No intern countermands the attending physician's orders simply because he would like to see the case managed in a different way.

Unless the nursing system assigns a primary nurse to each patient, there is a danger of having too many cooks spoil the broth. If any nurse on duty can alter the nursing care plan, a simple management problem arises: If it is everyone's job to write care plans, it is really no one's job. Unless a particular person is held responsible for each care plan, there is no way to ensure that each care plan will be formulated.

Another problematic practice in care planning is that of permitting licensed practical nurses and nursing assistants to write on the nursing care plan. This allows lower-level personnel to determine the nursing orders for a patient. Although it is essential that such staff members have an input system to the registered nurse, it is difficult to substantiate the need for professional decision making if anyone can do the care planning.

The following principles may help the nurse leader in avoiding the obstacles discussed here:

1. Evaluate each care plan on its inherent worth as well as on patient outcomes.
2. Be supportive of nursing care plans that are thoughtfully and logically developed even if one would personally have selected other strategies.
3. Provide some means for the nurse to explain and communicate the reasoning behind her nursing care plans to other staff members.
4. Assign responsibility for a care plan to one particular nurse, over a sustained period of time.
5. Derive a system for staff input to the planning nurse.
6. Provide a system for review of care plans and of guidance to the planning nurses by a selected nurse expert.

Care Implementation

Care implementation is the stage comparable with therapy in the medical mode. Again, the nursing therapy has a complex structure because it involves implementing both nursing regimens and medical regimens. The routine nurses' charting is a legal document that validates the care given, including medications, treatments, diagnostic examinations, teaching/learning, baths, and hygiene. These records primarily certify that prescribed care was given.

Of equal importance is the nursing progress notes. Some institutions use one set of progress notes for both nurses and physicians; others use separate notes for each professional group. Either system is acceptable so long as it meets the objectives of the institution. It is important that nursing progress notes be just that, professional judgments of patient response to the related nursing and medical therapy. Nursing progress notes should be separated from the routine nurses' charting, allowing the nurse to find quickly the clinically relevant materials that she needs for decision making.

Care Plan Evaluation

There are at least two discrete parts to care plan evaluation. The first part evaluates the plan itself (and its implementation), and the second part evaluates changes (outcomes) that occur in the patient and are contiguous in time with the nursing process.

Evaluating the nursing process involves a step-by-step analysis of the decisions made for each phase in the nursing model. Evaluation is needed for (1) the accuracy of the patient assessment, (2) the logic of the selected nursing diagnoses, (3) the fitness of the goals selected, (4) the adequacy of the therapy planning, and (5) the skill demonstrated in applying that therapy.

When a resource-driven model is used, additional evaluation is required concerning (1) accuracy in assessment of resources, (2) numbers of goals selected, (3) priorities established among goals, (4) efficiency of methods selected in the light of available resources, and (5) general cost-effectiveness.

For research purposes, evaluation requires various techniques: (1) cross-sectional sampling of multiple individuals who are in various phases of health care ranging from initial phases to rehabilitation phases, (2) longitudinal study of selected individual cases to evaluate complete courses of nursing therapy, and (3) comparisons of therapies across different resource/environmental conditions.

There must be a systematic method for outcome evaluation. In group data, patient outcomes need to be evaluated at various stages of the recovery process. Some illnesses or conditions present clearly defined stages; others require arbitrary definition of stages for evaluation purposes. An evaluation of patient outcomes requires the setting of patient outcome standards, with outcomes established in criteria that can be measured.

Relating patient outcomes to nursing therapies is an important step in care plan evaluation. Clearly, it is the area that offers promise for establishment of new and validated nursing practices.

Evaluation of the individual case is as important as the analysis of group data, and ongoing evaluation is one of the main tasks of the primary nurse, the case manager, and/or the head nurse.

Outcomes Management

More and more, the nursing process model is combined with some form of outcomes management. This model is in keeping with the resource-driven model because outcomes are managed within the boundaries of the resources.

Outcomes management may extend beyond the division of nursing to become a truly interdisciplinary process involving all the patient caregivers. Case management often provides the incentive for this interdisciplinary approach. As outcomes research becomes more available, the outcomes identified, as well as a general outcomes orientation, will be an important model for the future.

As fewer dollars become available to the health care system, facilities are being forced to take a hard look at redundancies in the system and barriers that impede caregivers from delivering care. Untold dollars are wasted in the health care system because of variation between clinicians, the units, and the procedures provided for patients. Outcomes management is a method to map out the expectations for care through pathways that define clinical and financial outcomes. This provides health caregivers with a road map to use in guiding the care for the patient.

When care is directed toward the outcomes as stated, a continuous learning process and continuous quality improvement occur. In these models, variations are analyzed and a plan is put in place to eliminate the variations that reduce the expected level of quality or financial performance.

By determining the "best practice" at a facility, paths that guide patient care can be developed around this best practice. This entails knowing what procedures prevent side effects and learning which physicians, which nurses, and which units can achieve the stated outcomes with the most cost-effective level of resource consumption. For example, in outcomes management, if it were determined that the cost of an instrument tray for a vaginal hysterectomy varied by physician preference from $200 to $800 a tray, the next question would be: Which tray produces the best outcomes, and how can other physicians be encouraged to adopt similar preferences?

One of the side effects of outcomes management is a real push to engineer processes and to make process improvements throughout the facility. By re-engineering, redundancies can be eliminated and the patient will not be faced with multiple duplications.

SUMMARY

Determining the model for practice is very important for a nursing division. Models provide the necessary structure as well as clear information for clinical and financial decision making. By using one overall model, waste can be eliminated. Effective nursing care is greatly enhanced by selection of a model for nursing practice that fits the other choices, goals, and values in the nursing system.

SUGGESTED READINGS

Andersen, J.E., and L.L. Briggs. 1988. Nursing diagnosis: A study of quality and supportive evidence. *Image* 20, no.3:141–144.

Dennison, P.D., and A.W. Keeling. 1989. Clinical support for eliminating the nursing diagnosis of knowledge deficit. *Image* 21, no.3:142–144.

Gebbie, K.M., and M.A. Lavin, eds. 1975. *Classification of nursing diagnoses.* St. Louis: C.V. Mosby Co.

Geissler, E.M. 1991. Transcultural nursing and nursing diagnoses. *Nursing and Health Care* 12, no.4:109–192, 203.

Gordon, M. 1987. *Nursing diagnosis: Process and application,* 2nd ed. New York: McGraw-Hill Publishing Co.

Jenny, J. 1989. Classifying nursing diagnoses: A self-care approach. *Nursing and Health Care,* 10, no.2:83–88.

Johnson, M., et al. 1991. The Iowa model: A proposed model for nursing administration. *Nursing Economics* 9, no.4:255–262.

Kleffel, D. 1991. Rethinking the environment as a domain of nursing knowledge. *Advances in Nursing Science* 14, no.1:40–51.

Kobert, L., and M. Folan. 1990. Coming of age in nursing: Rethinking the philosophies behind holism and nursing process. *Nursing and Health Care* 11, no.6:308–312.

Levin, R.F., et al. 1989. Diagnostic content validity of nursing diagnosis. *Image* 21, no.1:40–44.

Mitchell, G.J. 1991. Nursing diagnosis: An ethical analysis. *Image* 23, no.2:99–103.

Scahill, L. 1991. Nursing diagnosis vs goal-oriented treatment planning in inpatient child psychiatry. *Image* 23, no.2:95–97.

Shiber, S., and E. Larson. 1991. Evaluating the quality of caring: Structure, process, and outcome. *Holistic Nursing Practice* 5, no.3:57–66.

Vincent, K.G., and M.S. Coler. 1990. A unified nursing diagnostic model. *Image* 22, no.2:93–95.

Weber, G. 1991. Making nursing diagnosis work for you and your client: A step-by-step approach. *Nursing and Health Care* 12, no.8:424–430.

6

Nursing Division Philosophy

The nursing division philosophy captures the values and beliefs that influence the practice of nursing in a particular institution. The written form of the philosophy may either incorporate the theory of nursing or complement that document. In institutions that have a single document, the philosophy expresses the beliefs about nursing that would appear in a more formulated theory of nursing were one adopted. The discussion of philosophy to follow assumes that a specific theory of nursing has been chosen because that is the more common practice.

The philosophy of a nursing division is considered from two perspectives. First, the dominant nursing ethos of an institution can be recognized in the *practices* of its members. This is philosophy in action. Second, a philosophy is captured in a written document that guides nursing practice.

ON WRITING DOCUMENTS

Seldom will the real philosophy and the written document of philosophy correspond exactly. This is because the reality is in flux, whereas a document is only revised periodically. This is a problem for any document that purports to represent the extant situation. The same problem occurs for documents stating purposes, objec-

tives, functions, assignments, evaluations, or any other structures that organize a nursing service division.

The nurse executive will want to have his documents as current as possible so that they reflect the present situation. But documents not only *reflect,* they *direct.* Hence he will also want documents that lead to the envisioned future. A document serves a dual purpose: (1) It reflects the present with some accuracy—otherwise it is misleading—and (2) it indicates the immediate future toward which the organization is heading.

In composing a statement of philosophy, the greatest outcome is not the document itself but the interaction among managers that takes place while they thresh out its content. Indeed, this interchange and examination of values is so critical that the philosophy should be re-examined each time there is a major turnover in managerial staff or when there is a major change in the way an organization operates.

Another purpose served by the philosophy is orientation of new members. Furthermore, it serves as a descriptive document to inform trustees, accrediting agencies, and others within the health care institution. Other operating documents share in these functions. For an operational document to fulfill its functions, it must meet three criteria: (1) The document must be clear, precise, and meaningful, (2) the content must reflect the reality of the nursing practice, and (3) the document must give direction toward desired practice. Too often, operational documents are seen merely as paper to have on file for needed occasions.

The practical problem that a nurse executive has in composing any operational document occurs when he assumes that the task is one of editing rather than of expressing ideas. A typical scene is one in which the nurse executive decides to review a certain operational document (e.g., the philosophy). He calls for a meeting of his top management staff and gives each member a copy of the current document. Starting with the first sentence, the group reviews the document, making grammatical and content alterations until the entire document has been revised. This process usually involves several meetings as wording sentences is a complex task. Finally, a new document is produced, and the task is completed until the next revision.

What is wrong with this way of operating? First, it is a composition job, not a management operation. Worse, starting with the old document puts the management staff into a mind-set dictated by the old form. This mind-set is reinforced by a line-by-line revision, a practice ensuring that no attention will be given to the document as a whole or to its implications for practice.

What would be a better approach to producing a viable document? The nurse executive calls a meeting of his top management staff. He requests that any copies of the prior document be put aside. After appointing a recorder (ideally the person who will compose the final document), he asks for discussion of the philosophy reflected in the group's present nursing practice. When this topic is exhausted, he turns the group's direction to the philosophy they would wish to have. Instead of working with composition, the group works with ideas. The nurse executive tries to achieve consensus or majority approval on ideas, not wording of sentences.

Once the ideas have been sorted, approved, or rejected, the person assigned to draft the document begins composition. This duty is assigned to an individual with writing ability. At a later meeting, the draft of the document is reviewed

to see if it accurately reflects the meaning of the discussion. If not, the author revises it again. At no time does the group focus on composition; their job is to produce ideas that relate to managing the division. The same procedure pertains for revising any operating documents. On a job description, for example, the group would discuss the job as reflected in present practice and the job as it ought to be.

In this way, the documents produced convey the desired criteria: description and direction. By grounding the discussion in actual practice, one ensures that the final document will not be some utopian vision, unattainable in the concrete work environment. By analyzing what the operation *ought* to do, one projects the needed future practice and ensures that irrelevant traditions will not be continued. Decisions produced in this way are realistic resolutions of the conflict between idealistic aims and the constraints of a concrete situation.

CONTENT OF A PHILOSOPHY STATEMENT

Unless there is a theory of nursing, the philosophy is often the first operational document of a nursing division, a belief statement that characterizes the nursing practice in the institution. Too often, the nursing philosophy is thought of as a general statement; on the contrary, it should be a specific statement representing a particular institution uniquely.

One does not need to be a philosopher to write a statement about nursing practice. The philosophy statement represents the central beliefs and values of the division relative to nursing and nursing practice as well as its reflections on the general health care situation or institutional circumstances.

Philosophy statements are not right or wrong; they reflect beliefs accurately or inaccurately. Their content may vary from institution to institution, depending on what values are dominant to nursing in a given setting. It is, however, difficult to write a nursing philosophy without talking about what nursing is perceived to be and how nursing relates to the patient and to the particular organization.

Typical Subject Matter

The following content areas are found in most comprehensive nursing philosophies. If the division has no strong values concerning a given content area, the area may be omitted in the philosophy statement.

1. a specific nursing theory, incorporated or given by reference to another document
2. nursing practice values, which may or may not include commitments to various practice models and assignment systems
3. nursing education values, with respect either to staff education, to education of students, or both
4. nursing research values, with respect to active research programs, to the application of research findings of others, or both
5. relationship of nursing practice to nursing administration or institutional administration
6. relationship of nursing or the nursing division to the client (or patient)
7. perceived rights of clients and significant others in relation to patient care and health-related choices
8. values related to human rights and other beliefs about patients/people
9. relationship of nursing to patient outcomes, their achievement and measurement
10. relationship of nursing to the rest of the organization, which may include reference to its modes of operation
11. relationship of nursing staff with other health professionals or to other nurse professionals not among the nursing staff
12. relationship to the goals of other departments (e.g., to research goals of medicine or placement goals of social service)
13. relationship to other value systems (e.g., religious beliefs or societal preferences)
14. nursing management values (may include commitments to particular modes of management, e.g., participative management)
15. relationship of the nursing division (or its members) to professional nursing—organizational or conceptual
16. relationships of nursing to other institutions of health care (coordinative and cooperative relationships)
17. relationship of nursing to the extended client world (e.g., the community or the society)
18. values related to employee rights or concepts of professional and occupational growth and development
19. values related to promotions, retentions, and transfers within the organization
20. values related to ethical conflicts and related nurse decision making

Usually a nursing division philosophy does not repeat value statements found in the institutional philosophy statement unless it is making a point of solidarity. It is important, of course, that the nursing philosophy not only be compatible with the institutional philosophy but embody it.

The nursing philosophy statement may be written from several perspectives. From the nursing administration perspective, a statement might sound like this: "We believe that each staff member should be provided with the in-service education needed to optimize his or her capabilities." Here, the assumed entity responsible for the "providing" mentioned in the belief is nursing administration.

An alternate perspective is that of the staff: "We believe it is our individual responsibility to maintain and update knowledge of professional nursing." Here the "we" is the staff, not the administration. Other perspectives are possible: Some philosophies are written from the perspective of the patient, others from the perspective of the total organization.

If the document of philosophic statement is to have internal consistency and coherency, it is important that the perspective not fluctuate. One should be able to determine who—what group or entity—is making the statement.

Unit/Department Philosophies

A single statement of philosophy typically is used for the entire nursing division. Occasionally, a nursing department may feel the need to express its own philosophy. Some acquired immune deficiency syndrome (AIDS) units, for example, compose a statement of philosophy. Such a subordinate philosophy would need to be consistent with the divisional philosophy, but it could characterize the nursing care within a particular department. A brief sample of a subordinate philosophy for a psychiatric nursing department follows:

- We concur with the philosophy of the Nursing Division and support its beliefs and values. The philosophy of this department is based on a belief that nursing can help patients improve the quality of their lives by assisting them to reflect on the pattern and organization of their behavior as well as its underlying assumptions.
- We believe in an interdisciplinary approach, working closely with physicians, psychologists, social workers, and other health care professionals.
- We believe the nurse should be skilled in various psychological treatment modalities so that he may support the therapy prescribed for each patient by his respective physician.
- We believe that each nurse in this unit should be familiar with Peplau's theory of psychiatric nursing as a basic foundation for practice.
- We believe that the nurse is an independent professional who establishes therapeutic relationships with patients.
- We are committed to the development of psychiatric nursing research by use of the longitudinal case study method. We recognize that data must be kept to correlate nursing strategies with patient outcomes.

This philosophy does not repeat generalities that might be found in the divisional philosophy. Instead, it focuses on what is unique within the context of the department.

Philosophies may be more or less sophisticated, depending on the capabilities and needs of a given nursing division or department. Even an unsophisticated document constructed by those who use it is better than a sophisticated one imposed from above or created externally by an expert.

RELATIONSHIP OF PHILOSOPHY TO DIVISION MISSION, PURPOSE, AND OBJECTIVES

The philosophy of the division has a unique relationship to the mission and goal statements of the division. The philosophy itself is not so much a goal as a statement of the value structure through which the mission and objectives are achieved. Suppose, for example, that a given philosophy has a strong commitment to the human rights of patients. This does not mean that preservation of human rights becomes a major objective of the division. Instead, one would expect to see human rights considered and respected in all the workings of the division.

Seldom is an aspect of philosophy directly repeated in the organization's objectives; however, the linkages are obvious. Suppose, for example, that a given organization has a real commitment to placing ultimate accountability for each patient with a single professional. One might find this philosophic value reflected in an administrative objective to implement case management on all nursing units within the next calendar year.

The philosophy tells what values will be respected while achieving organizational objectives. Hence, it is possible that two organizations might have very similar objectives but achieve them through very different philosophies. Conversely, it would be possible for two organizations with similar philosophies to apply them in the achievement of very different objectives.

Some authors take a rigid position concerning which document is written (or conceptualized) first, the philosophy or the division's purpose. This is a moot issue. The purposes that one selects are influenced by the philosophy, whether it has been captured on paper or not. One's purposes emerge from the context of one's value system. Similarly, any given philosophy is compatible with certain purposes and incompatible with others. Whichever document is composed first, the two are irreconcilably interwoven.

PHILOSOPHIC IMPLICATIONS IN METHODS OF NURSING PRACTICE AND EDUCATION

Many nursing acts, events, or strategies (methods of one sort or another) have implications for philosophy, even if they are beyond the scope of the typical statement of philosophy. The nurse executive should develop a sensitivity to these philosophic issues so that he will not use methods inconsistent with his announced philosophy.

As demonstration models, two such philosophic structures, the logistic method and the problem-solving method, are discussed in this chapter. For purposes of contrast, other philosophic methods are briefly mentioned. It is necessary that the nurse executive be analytical in his approach to nursing and nursing management to achieve the desired consistency.

Logistic Method

The first example, the logistic method, is easy to understand and recognize in nursing practice. This method might be viewed as a systems model, with each component of nursing understood by its place in reference to the other components in the system. The so-called nursing process typifies this sort of thinking, as does the creation of a critical pathway to plan the movement of patients in a disaster. The focus of a logistic system is on the parts and their relationships.

Logistic components tend to be clearly distinguishable from each other rather than global or overlapping. Not surprising, the logistic design is found in computerized systems in which they share three common components: (1) some form of input, (2) central processing, and (3) output. The parts relate to each other in a precise order and in specific, predictable ways.

In each case, data are processed in the same fashion.

An apnea alarm mattress is a simple example of such a system. The input is the displacement of air in the mattress caused by respiratory movements of an infant. The central processing is a comparison of the rate of displacement with a preprogrammed minimum. (Many systems have both minimum and maximum criteria.) The output is the notifying alarm that sounds should the input fail to remain within the programmed limits of respiratory rate.

The systems models have greatly affected the concept of nursing. All such models define nursing as a series of components put together in an invariable way. Each uses a critical-pathways approach in which arrows show the movements of the process and the lines of feedback. The important factor in these systems is the clear, prescribed relationship of parts to each other. Typified by the nursing process, these models and their parts remain stable, with unchanging relationships, regardless of the nursing situation in which the models are applied.

Computerized monitoring/regulating systems (such as intravenous pumps and cardiac monitors) are logistic systems. In a logistic system, not only do the components have univocal meanings, but each nurse applying such a system supposedly should use it in the same fashion.

Problem-Solving Method

The problem-solving mode, in contrast to what some nurse theorists say, is not a logistic system. We will compare the nursing process/nursing diagnosis model with problem solving to demonstrate the uniqueness of each method.

In problem solving, it is acceptable if different nurses identify different patient problems or alternate solutions. In a problem-solving mode, more than one alternative may be appropriate, or the right alternative for one person (practitioner or patient) may be wrong for another.

A problem-solving approach is a convenient viewpoint for nursing. Although the steps of problem solving may be presented in different ways, they generally follow the steps identified by John Dewey (1966): (1) perplexity in which one is involved in an incomplete situation, (2) conjectural anticipation (i.e., a tentative interpretation of the situation), (3) careful survey and exploration, (4) elaboration of tentative hypotheses, and (5) taking a stand on an hypothesis as a plan of action for testing.

The steps in problem solving differ from those in a logistic system because they are not as neat. There is back-and-forth interaction, with the nurse moving from one step to another, possibly an "earlier" step based on her findings. For example, a careful survey might lead her to reframe her tentative interpretation of the situation.

Remembering this flexibility and "folding back," one might elaborate on Dewey's components to create the following series:

- Recognizing that a problem exists
  1. lacking the means to a desirable goal
  2. identifying the character of a situation with difficulty
  3. lacking ability to explain unexpected events
- Understanding the problem
  1. delimiting
  2. defining
- Collecting data concerning the problem
  1. evaluating possible sources of information
  2. attaining adequate data for solution
- Formulating one or more hypotheses
  1. determining what, if anything, one might do about the problem
  2. planning action based on one or more assumptions about the facts
- Testing the hypothesis
  1. choosing the most likely hypothesis for testing
  2. reasoning deductively the consequences of the selected hypothesis (if H, then C)
  3. determining a method that will test for evidence of whether the consequences do occur
  4. evaluating testing results and modifying hypothesis accordingly

Appropriate clinical tools can greatly reinforce the problem-solving process. The nursing care plan, for example, can be structured to encourage the nurse in problem-solving thinking. The differences in the modes of thought required to fill out the sample care plans shown in Exhibits 6–1 and 6–2 contrast logistic and problematic formats.

The performance appraisal form can also encourage or discourage problem solving. Exhibit 6–3 clearly addresses the nursing process, and Exhibit 6–4 reinforces problem solving.

Just as the evaluation format and the care plan can support either nursing process or problem solving, so can every other clinical tool if appropriately structured. For example, a supervisor's bimonthly report could take the problematic form shown in Exhibit 6–5.

A problem-solving philosophy can be instituted in nursing service by carefully designed routine forms. Education in the problem-solv-

Exhibit 6–1 Logistic Care Plan

Patient Name: _____

Room Number: _____

1. Assessment Completed
   __ Patient History
   __ Physical Assessment
2. Nursing Diagnoses
   a. _____
   b. _____
   c. _____
3. Goals for Each Diagnosis
   a. _____
   b. _____
   c. _____
4. Nursing Interventions for Each Goal
   a. _____
   b. _____
   c. _____
5. Evaluation for Each Intervention
   a. _____
   b. _____
   c. _____

Note: Care plan is based on a logistic system (the nursing process).

Exhibit 6–2 Problematic Nursing Care Plan

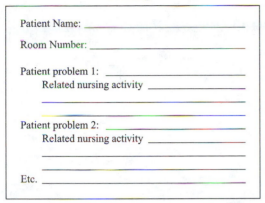

```
Patient Name: _____

Room Number: _____

Patient problem 1: _____
    Related nursing activity _____
    _____
    _____
Patient problem 2: _____
    Related nursing activity _____
    _____
    _____
Etc. _____
```

ing process, of course, would assist staff members in using such materials, but even without special education the forms themselves promote problem-solving processes of thought among staff.

The problem-solving method enjoyed a short popularity in nursing when the problem-oriented medical record was introduced (Hurst and Walker 1962), but it was soon eclipsed by the logistic nursing process model. Still, a significant number of agencies have elected to stay with the problematic method. When applied to nursing, the problematic method requires that the nurse identify specific patient problems and relate each nursing action and observation to the appropriate problem when he charts. Requiring

that all charting relate to identified problems enforces use of the problem-solving process far more effectively than occurs with any number of lectures about problem solving.

Operational Philosophies in Nursing

In contrast to logistic problem-solving forms, an operational philosophy has a different effect on nursing behaviors. In this concept, the focus is on choosing one set of behaviors over another. Often, the operations to be performed belong to the nurse rather than on the recipient of those actions. Hospitals that classify patients into self-care, minimal care, intermediate care, and acute care units are following an operational mode.

This division does not depend on anything about the patient per se (his physiologic systems, his problems). Instead, it is related to the kinds of activities to be performed for him. In one unit, for example, the nurses may specialize in actions maintaining life support systems; in another unit, the consistent work may be patient teaching.

Some health maintenance organizations (HMOs) make divisions on the basis of activities to be performed. Patients are separated into groups for well-care and health education,

Exhibit 6–3 Performance Appraisal Record

Employee: _____		Nursing Unit: _____	
	Satisfactory	Unsatisfactory	Not Observed
Patient Assessment Effectiveness			
1. History taking			
a. Accuracy			
b. Comprehensiveness			
2. Physical assessment			
a. Accuracy			
b. Comprehensiveness			
Nursing Diagnosis Effectiveness			
a. Accuracy			
b. Comprehensiveness			
Intervention Effectiveness			
a. Appropriate selection			
b. Application skills			

Note: Employee appraisal is based on nursing process.

Exhibit 6–4 Problematic Performance Record

CLINICAL EVALUATION			
	Satisfactory	Unsatisfactory	Supportive Anecdotes
Recognizes and identifies patient problems			
Formulates realistic nursing solution			
Identifies nursing activities which contribute to the solution			

Exhibit 6–5 Problematic Supervisor's Report

SUPERVISOR'S REPORT

Supervisor _____ Date _____

Present Problems	Related Solutions	Present Status of Problem Resolution	Planned Strategies for Future Resolution

chronic maintenance care, and acute episodic ill-care. Again, the division is based on the work to be performed, not on some holistic concept of the patient. The patient, over a period of time, is likely to move through several different sectors, each sector performing different functions for him.

Because HMOs have evolved partly in response to economic costs of health care delivery, it is not surprising that they have an operational form. Clearly, the focus is on how to facilitate things for optimal efficiency for the operators.

The only major nursing theory with an operational design is Orem's (1985) self-care model. Here, the agent may be either nurse or patient, but self-care itself is an activity, divided in subcategories from which the nurse chooses one or many but seldom all. Orem identified content domains of (1) air, water, and food, (2) excrements, (3) rest and activity, and so forth. The specific forms for self-care differ with each content item. For example, she speaks of maintenance (process) of sufficient intake of air, water, and food (content), or provision of care (process) associated with eliminative processes and excrements (content).

In another section of her book, Orem (1985) classified these processes according to the method of giving assistance:

1. acting for or doing for another
2. guiding another
3. supporting another (physically or psychologically)
4. providing an environment that promotes personal development in relation to becoming able to meet present or future demands for action
5. teaching another

Holistic theories of nursing are also popular today, and these face the most difficult questions of method. Simply put, no matter how holistic one's concept of a patient, one still does specific acts that must arise from some principle of segregation. Methods of phenomenology and hermeneutics are often suggested as appropriate, but a discussion of this extensive subject is not possible here. Those interested may refer to Barnum (1994).

Logistic, problem-solving, operational, and holistic philosophies are all evident in today's nursing. It is not important that the nurse administrator be able to apply some philosophic term to each nursing system he uses, but he should be able to support his choices with reasoned arguments. Put simply, it is important that his choices be appropriate for his nursing objectives. Philosophic methodologies have important implications for nursing theory and for nursing action.

SUMMARY

The nurse executive needs to consider philosophy in two discrete ways: first, as a reflection of the values of the division; second, as a representational and directive document describing what is unique about his organization.

He should be concerned that the explicit values and beliefs of the nursing organization are expressed for the benefit of staff and various other reviewers. Next, he needs to be cognizant of the philosophic underpinnings of the methodologies and systems of care used in the division. Ideally, he will strive for conformity and complementarity among the explicit and implicit philosophic positions.

Although the philosophy of a nursing division is not itself a goal, it colors what goals will be selected and how these goals will be enacted. Philosophy interacts with divisional mission, purpose, and objectives. These documents that direct activities of the division and the philosophy are mutually interactive.

REFERENCES

Barnum, B.J.S. 1994. *Nursing theory: Analysis, application, evaluation,* 4th ed. Philadelphia: J.B. Lippincott Co.

Dewey, J. 1966. *Democracy and education.* New York: The Free Press.

Hurst, J.W., and H.K. Walker, eds. 1962. *The problem-oriented system.* New York: Med Com Press.

Orem, D.E. 1985. *Nursing: Concepts of practice,* 3rd ed. New York: McGraw-Hill Publishing Co.

SUGGESTED READINGS

Abdellah, F.G., et al. 1960. *Patient-centered approaches to nursing.* New York: Macmillan Publishing Co., Inc.

Arndt, C., and L. Huckabay. 1980. *Nursing administration: Theory for practice with a systems approach,* 2nd ed. St. Louis: C.V. Mosby Co.

Caramanica, L., and J. Thibodeau. 1987. Staff involvement in developing a nursing philosophy and the selection of a model for practice. *Nursing Management* 18, no.10:71.

Henderson, V. 1990. Excellence in nursing. *American Journal of Nursing* 90, no.4:76–77.

Johns, C. 1990. Nursing practice: Developing a philosophy. *Nursing Practice* 3, no.2:2–6.

Johnson, M., et al. 1970. *Problem-solving in nursing practice.* Dubuque, Iowa: Wm. C. Brown Publishers.

Kershaw, B. 1990. Nursing models as philosophies of care. *Nursing Practice* 4, no.1:25–27.

Kim, H.S. 1989. Theoretical thinking in nursing: Problems and prospects. *Recent Advances in Nursing* 24:106–122.

Mawdsley, D. 1991. Who needs nursing philosophies? *Professional Nurse* 7, no.2:78–80, 82.

Nyatanga, L. 1991. Nursing and the philosophy of science. *Nursing Education Today* 11, no.1:13–18.

Riehl, J.P., and C. Roy, Sr., eds. 1980. *Conceptual models for nursing practice,* 2nd ed. New York: Appleton-Century-Crofts.

Sandman, P.O., et al. 1992. Nursing philosophy as starting point for change activities in surgical, medical, neurological and psychogeriatric care. *Vard I Norden* 12, no.3–4:34–39.

Watson, J. 1988. *Nursing: Human science and human care: A theory of nursing.* New York: National League for Nursing.

7

Nursing Division's Mission and Objectives

The divisional mission and objectives are the major goal statements of a nursing division. Other goal statements flow from these. Purpose and objectives are reviewed separately, tracing their relation to each other.

DIVISIONAL MISSION

The divisional mission, sometimes called the statement of purpose, gives the reason that a particular nursing division exists, the intent that it serves. The term *mission* has become popular because it sounds more future-directed than does the term *purpose*. The goal orientation is the same whatever terminology is used.

Usually a mission statement is broad in nature, listing only major purposes of the nursing division. The mission may be limited to one, the delivery of care to patients, or it may be multiple, possibly incorporating service and education. Some nursing service divisions display nursing research as a major mission. In the mission statement, these broad basic goals are usually qualified in a manner that reflects the character of the individual nursing organization.

The mission of a nursing division is constrained by several factors. First, the purpose must be compatible with and advance the mission of the institution of which it is a part. Usually, the nurse executive has the authority to de-

termine the manner in which the nursing division mission will be enacted. Although the nursing division's purpose must conform to the institutional mission, there is usually considerable room for freedom within that guideline.

Another constraint on the nursing division purpose is that imposed by law. A division's purpose cannot deviate from the constrictions imposed by the nursing practice act of the state in which the institution is located. The main issue is always one of scope of nursing practice; the nursing division cannot assume a purpose beyond the bounds of legal nursing practice within a given state without jeopardy. As use of nurse practitioners becomes commonplace nationwide, often including admitting privileges for nurses, the nurse executive must be cognizant of *de jure* and *de facto* practices in her state.

Further constraints on divisional purpose may be offered by credentialing and accrediting bodies. Although these do not hold the force of law, the desirability of accreditation or credentialing (for purposes of financial, contractual, or status benefits) effectively controls one's mission.

Writing a Division Mission

Most mission statements for nursing divisions are short (a paragraph or two) and concise and will usually deal with one or more of the following topics: delivery of patient care, provision or support of teaching programs, and provision or support of research efforts.

A statement of mission may be worded from several different perspectives: that of the nursing division itself, that of the nursing process, or that of patient outcome. A statement from the perspective of the nursing division describes the desired *structure* that provides for and controls nursing services, for example, "The mission of this nursing division is to provide professional nursing services for all patients admitted to the institution."

A second option is to word the mission to describe the *process* of nursing desired. In this case, the purpose envisions a particular concept of nursing as its goal: "The purpose of this nursing division is to provide problem-centered nursing care for each patient."

Other statements are worded in terms of desired patient *outcomes*: "The mission of this nursing division is to ensure that each patient attain an addiction-free physiologic status along with new coping abilities designed to avert recidivism." Some statements of mission include all these perspectives: structure, process, and outcome.

Departmental Purposes

Although the divisional statement of mission gives the general goal of the nursing organization, that purpose at times is broken down into subpurposes by department. Several examples of departmental purpose follow:

- *Operating Room*: The purpose of the Operating Room is to organize, direct, and deliver those specialized nursing services that effectively contribute to meeting consumer health needs during the entire perioperative experience.
- *Intensive Care*: The purpose of the Department of Intensive Care is to provide continuous and comprehensive nursing care to the critically and seriously ill patient, preserving life and maintaining function during the critical episode.

- *Consumer Education*: The purpose of the Department of Consumer Education is to promote enhanced health and healthful life-style choices through providing for informed consumer decision making.

Clearly, the subordinate statements of purpose must conform to the mission of the nursing division, but as with departmental statements of philosophy, the clarification of departmental purpose may be a useful device for shaping goals.

NURSING DIVISION OBJECTIVES

Even though a division's objectives flow from the divisional mission, many different combinations of objectives could have been selected to enact any purpose. Hence objectives often are statements in which the individuality of the nursing division becomes even more apparent.

The nursing division mission is elaborated into two specific kinds of objectives: permanent and temporary. Where subpurposes have been derived by departments, they are complementary sources of objectives. Permanent objectives represent those ongoing goals that must be achieved continuously, over and over again. Thus, they remain objectives, even though they may be successfully achieved at any given time. A typical list of permanent objectives might contain statements such as the following:

1. Advance the practice of clinical nursing within the division.
2. Implement useful new research findings in clinical nursing.
3. Provide adequate resources for implementation of nursing care to meet patient care standards.
4. Foster an environment that encourages research, creativity, inquiry, and personal growth in staff members.
5. Retain a staff that is up to date in knowledge, application, and conceptualization of nursing practice.
6. Maintain productive relationships with other divisions and departments of the institution.

7. Contribute productively to interdisciplinary research and education as well as to patient care.

These objectives are permanent in that they demand ongoing achievement, require continual monitoring, and demand ongoing efforts. Although the nursing division will review its permanent objectives at frequent intervals, there tends to be a relative stability in these selected goals.

The temporary objectives (often called the strategic plan at the divisional level) use the principle of focus: Certain objectives are selected for special attention in a given year or other time period. Objectives to be emphasized usually are selected based on the present state of the nursing division or institution. They are selected for the purpose of bolstering known weak spots, enhancing strengths, or responding to critical changes in the organization's environment. Some examples follow:

1. Improve quality control scores by 10 percent.
2. Implement a system of head nurse accountability for unit costs.
3. Reorganize the nursing office for achieving greater managerial efficiency with fewer personnel.

Typically, focus objectives are one-time events, supplanted by other needs once they have been achieved.

Divisional objectives are distributed downward through the nursing organization. Some departments may be responsible for achieving some part of a given divisional objective, whereas others (or other levels of the organization) may be responsible for other components or subcomponents of the objective. This downward branching allows for objectives to be achieved at various levels (divisional, departmental, unit) in totality or in part. The nurse executive, then, may construct a schema of accountability for achievement of objectives throughout her division.

Often, downward distribution of objectives is combined with an upward branching. In the up-

ward branching, the lower managerial level or nursing staff identify objectives of importance to them—objectives that reflect goals specific to the managerial unit, goals that may not have been included in the conception of the divisional goals.

A few authors recommend only an upward flow of objectives, in which management (at least top management) becomes the recipient of ideas and decisions from below rather than the directing force for subordinate workers. In reality, a combination of these two methodologies probably produces the best results.

In the upward format, a supervisor of the operating rooms may have certain ecologic objectives that are unique to her area. Objectives of this sort are negotiated upward with the management and the subordinate agreeing on a list that combines downward- and upward-oriented goals.

Permanent objectives tend to be set in the traditional management by objectives (MBO) format, whereas temporary objectives often arise from strategic planning. This is not to say that one-time-only objectives might not also arise from the MBO model.

Differentiating Educational and Managerial Objectives

Because of a focus on teaching in nursing, objectives sometimes are mishandled as if they were educational objectives. Yet, managerial and educational objectives serve different purposes.

Educational and management objectives both set goals, but they differ in a least one important aspect. Attainment of educational objectives involves a change in behavior on the part of the learner. Successful acquisition of an educational objective increases the learner's repertoire of possible responses in relevant situations. The management objective, however, directs staff behavior by selecting among multiple, potentially available behavioral responses. Educational objectives provide the learner with new options; management objectives point out the preferred option for a given staff in a given institution.

When educational objectives are met, certain ignorances are removed. But removing ignorance may or may not be a requisite part of a managerial objective. Bad staff practices, for example, often have more to do with personal inconvenience or lack of motivation than with ignorance of how things should be done.

Sometimes this educational paradigm gets in the way of good nursing management. When the nurse executive or subordinate manager assumes that everyone will do what they have learned, management may suffer from this naivete. Ideally, the educational model should hold for professional behavior, but even here there is slippage, requiring managerial supervision as much as education. Managers can not rely on education to remove problems of motivation or issues of values conflict.

Selecting Objectives

Selecting managerial objectives is a creative valuing process that structures the rest of the nursing program. Granted, the selected objectives must be consistent with the philosophy and purpose, but they cannot be inferred from those documents. Selection of objectives is not a case of sorting out, in which objectives consistent with the stated philosophy are selected and those inconsistent with it are rejected.

Instead, the process is one of selecting a reasonable number of the right sort of attainable objectives from an infinite number of possible and philosophically consistent ones. The constraint of philosophic and organizational consistency may be of some help in eliminating ill-fitting objectives, but it is of little guidance in selecting among the potential appropriate ones, objectives from which the character of the whole program will flow.

In selecting objectives, some groups have difficulty rejecting any worthy objectives. This unwillingness leads to two problems: selecting more objectives than any program can reasonably attain, and selecting objectives that are mutually incompatible. If a program tries to do everything it sees as worthy, diffusion of effort and lack of direction result.

In management, the objectives follow the natural hierarchical work divisions: organization objectives, nursing division objectives, department objectives, and unit objectives. At each level, there is both constraint and freedom. The constraint is to carry out the higher-level objectives that are applicable at the level, and the freedom is in the manner in which those higher-level objectives are converted into lower-level goals.

For successful translation of objectives into concrete actions, it is necessary to show how objectives at each level are distributed through objectives at the next lower level. Otherwise, objectives may be defined but never put into effect. Most attainment of objectives actually occurs at the lowest level: action on the patient units. If the nurse administrator cannot trace the extension of higher-level objectives done into lower-level programs, then she has no assurance that work is being performed to attain them.

Objectives serve several purposes: (1) They tell why a program has been created, (2) they clarify its purposes, and (3) they serve to direct the responsible individual in the selection of appropriate activities.

Writing Objectives

Objectives are used throughout the nursing division for everything from top management to individual care to the patient. In this section, examples are drawn from all levels to illustrate how such objectives are constructed.

Focus for Objectives

Three common foci for objectives relate to the *structure*, the *process*, and the *outcome*. *Structure objectives* most often relate to the structures designed to deliver care or management. Some examples follow:

1. to ensure that each patient unit is under the management of a registered nurse at all times
2. to provide a program for continuous quality improvement for patient care
3. to establish teaching protocols for all common patient education needs

Process objectives focus on how the work is processed. Some examples of process objectives follow:

1. to recognize abnormalities in electrocardiograph patterns
2. to provide active and passive exercise for the patient with a cardiovascular accident
3. to apply participative management in all department meetings

Process objectives focus on what the agent should do. Frequently, they relate to hands-on care, but as the last example illustrates, they may deal with managerial processes as well.

Outcome objectives define the desired goals for the client, the nurse, or the institution. Some outcome objectives follow:

1. to regain use of the weakened extremity
2. to become certified as a nurse practitioner within the first 6 months of employment
3. to open the new birthing room by November

Patient-centered outcome objectives are commonly found in nursing care plan goals and in patients' Bill of Rights statements. Quality control forms also use this type of outcome objective.

There are obvious relationships among the three types of objectives. What ultimately counts is the outcome (as the Joint Commission on the Accreditation of Healthcare Organizations has stressed). If outcome objectives are attained, then success is ensured. If, however, the outcome is not achieved, one must ask why the goals (outcome) were not accomplished. One might seek the flaw in the processes used to achieve the desired outcome. If the processes seemed satisfactory, one might question the structural influences. Has the organization made if difficult to exercise proper processes? Hence objectives form a logical series; outcome can be affected by process, and process can be affected by structure.

Further, in today's economy, effective outcome is usually one-half the game. One must also ask, Could the same effective outcome be achieved at less cost? Less use of resources?

One problem with outcome objectives is that if they are not reached, they do not tell what went wrong. It takes an investigation to decide the relationship of an outcome to ongoing processes and structure.

Reference Sources for Objectives

It is impossible to talk about objectives without considering how their attainment or degree of attainment is measured. One common reference against which objectives are measured is an internalized standard. A nurse might determine a patient's degree of wound healing, for example, by comparing him with other patients she has observed.

Such norms are not always written, but they still exist. The nurse who determines that a new surgical patient is ready to ambulate has used a norm of readiness indicated by the patient's muscle strength, pulse status, and toleration of upright positioning. Similarly, the nurse executive may know when the time is right to implement case management based on certain organizational signals. In nursing management and practice, norms are learned primarily by experience.

A second reference source for objectives is comprised of formalized statements of outcome (e.g., a criterion-referenced set of patient standards). In this case, norms and intuited signals are not used, but an absolute standard of performance or a desired state of being is determined. In a criterion-referenced system, it would be possible, for example, for all employees in a group to reach the same criteria or for them all to fail to do so. There is no normal distribution: Evaluation depends on individual achievement in relation to the standards.

Quality management systems are usually criterion-referenced. When a determined criterion for the nursing unit is that no patient develop decubitus ulcers, this criterion becomes the measure of the quality of nursing care. The nurse who remarks that it is normal for an obese, paralyzed patient with poor circulation to have bedsores misses the point of the criterion-referenced objective.

A third source for objectives is individual growth. Here, a patient might be evaluated on rate of change, amount of added knowledge, or some established criterion that relates his present status to his own past status. A nursing executive who compares the general level of her staff's education this year with last year's level is using organizational growth in the same fashion.

SUMMARY

In addition to setting goals that direct her division, the nurse leader is also an executive of the institution or corporation. In this role, she is involved in the long-range and strategic planning for the parent body. More than was the case in the past, the directions set at the corporate level have an effect on the nursing division.

Every organization is more and more subject to external demands—legislative, fiscal, and societal. No division of a modern corporation is free from these influences nor can any division act in isolation. Nor can the nurse executive set her mission and objectives apart from her obligation to contribute to the achievement of the organizational mission.

Within that context, the mission statement of a nursing division represents the first concrete document delineating goals. Typically, this general purpose is elaborated into several objectives that, taken together, are assumed to be capable of achieving the mission. These objectives may be permanent or strategic and subject to change.

The objectives usually are distributed through subobjectives over the entire nursing division. In this manner, responsibility for achievement may be spread through the different organizational levels and structures according to a logical plan. Departments and/or units may contribute additional, more specific objectives incurred locally by the special functions that they mediate. Taken together, the mission statement and the elaborated divisional objectives represent the main goal statements of a nursing organization.

SUGGESTED READINGS

Anvaripour, P., et al. 1990. A nursing department can and should plan for the future. *Nursing and Health Care* 11, no.4:207–209.

Marquis, B.L., and C.J. Huston. 1992. *Leadership roles and management functions in nursing.* Philadelphia: J.B. Lippincott Co.

Marquis, B.L., and C.J. Huston. 1994. *Management decision making for nurses: 118 case studies,* 2nd ed. Philadelphia: J.B. Lippincott Co.

Porter-O'Grady, T. 1989. *Reorganization of nursing practice: Creating the corporate venture.* Gaithersburg, Md.: Aspen Publishers, Inc.

Reilly, D.E., and M.H. Oermann. 1990. *Behavioral objectives: Evaluation in nursing,* 3rd ed. New York: National League for Nursing.

Swansburg, R.C. 1990. Mission, philosophy, objectives, and management plans. In *Management and leadership for nurse managers,* ed. R.C. Swansburg, 46–60. Boston: Jones and Bartlett Publishers.

8

Nursing Goals and Management Goals

Nursing administration is a synthesis of nursing and management in which both disciplines are altered because of their interplay. The nature of this interplay is especially important in relation to goals. The goals of nursing remain primary; that is, they remain the chief ends toward which the nursing division strives. Toward that end, the goals of management are secondary and instrumental.

Yet, management goals may themselves be equally important in determining whether an organization remains viable in today's tough, competitive environment. Economy is the chief managerial goal imposed on today's nursing division. Effective management is measured in efficiency and productivity.

As with the nation in general, there was a time when most nursing administrations could look to an expanding and ever-improving situation. Twenty years ago, nurse executives saw their resources grow: more clinical specialists, better prepared generalists, more patient care programs. Moreover, they had no reason to think the enhancement would not continue.

Today, few organizations can afford continued growth as the model. If it is a model, it is to gain economies of scale rather than to extend more and more resources to its various departments. Instead, the national press to reduce the cost of health care has been unceasing. Most

nurse executives must now cope with limited, not ideal, resources. In such an environment, the goals of management take on special significance; if management goals (efficiency, economy) are achieved, then the nursing care goals can be achieved in greater quantity and quality.

There is, then, a need to blend the visions of efficient management and effective nursing. And that starts with the nurse executive who simultaneously fills the two roles: nursing leader and corporate manager. In addition to these institution-bound roles, the nurse executive assumes another role, that of professional leader and spokesperson for nursing as a discipline. These three visions, then, intermingle in the nursing product of an organization. The institutional nursing goals—formal and informal—are derived from the interplay of all these factors:

1. the nurse executive's vision of vanguard clinical practice, his idea of where nursing as a profession is heading
2. the situational context in which the given nursing division finds itself (i.e., the nature of its environment and the nature and level of nursing practice at the time)
3. the efficacy with which management goals, values, and techniques may be applied in moving the nursing division toward vanguard clinical practice

PROFESSIONAL NURSING GOALS

The nurse executive must be clear about his vision of nursing, where nursing is going, and what future should be carved out for it. He must be able to identify and communicate his vision both within and outside of the institution. His professional goals for nursing are important whatever the immediate state of the art in his own organization. The communication of this projective vision is a critical motivator. The nurse executive sets the tone of a nursing division, and part of that tone has to do with how he envisions and enacts professional nursing. His perception of vanguard clinical practice is important, whether or not the division is able to practice at that level.

It is hoped that the executive's vision of vanguard clinical practice will arise out of a personal philosophy and value system that are shared by staff. Ideally, that vision will be one that conceives of nursing as a legitimate discipline, with its own unique domain for scientific inquiry. Because he is working in and through a health care organization, the executive will have a concept of vanguard clinical practice that is consistent with the notion of the organized delivery of nursing care.

NURSING GOALS FOR THE DIVISION

The nursing goals for a division (mission, purpose, objectives, and strategic plans) may or may not coincide with the executive's concept of vanguard practice, depending on the stage of development of the division. It is unrealistic to think that all institutions will be practicing on the frontier of advanced practice. Nevertheless, it is important for the executive to convey how his goals link to that vision of practice, how his goals move the division in the right direction.

At any one time, different divisions may select different methods of reaching the same clinical goals, and different divisions may be at various levels of development toward those clinical practice goals. Nor can the nurse executive

be judged by an absolute standard of nursing care produced. A director who takes a substandard division and elevates it to the level at which it is providing good, safe nursing care actually may be more effective than his counterpart who inherits a nursing division with a higher level of nursing care and does nothing to advance it.

Any two effective nurse leaders are likely to share certain professional values and objectives. They both will desire to implement the best possible nursing care, given the nature of their staff, their resources, and the patient populations to be served. Both will have a clear concept of what constitutes a safe level of nursing care, and neither will tolerate forces that serve to undermine safe practice. Further, both will seek to upgrade the level of nursing practice in their respective institutions whatever the level of care already given.

Because they share professional values and knowledge, nurse executives share in setting the boundaries for nursing practice: They determine the baseline beneath which practice should not fall, and they determine the level of practice toward which the nursing division should aspire.

Both vision and managerial instrumentality enter into determining the institution's nursing goals. The nurse executive uses his nursing vision and managerial skills to get the best possible nursing care given the contextual situation in which he finds himself. Certain elements of the context are not within the nurse executive's control. He cannot, for example, have a significant effect on the clinical quality of the physicians' care as it affects nursing's domain. Nor can he increase the funds that will be reimbursed under dominant insurance carriers. These and other situational constraints must be taken into account in determining nursing goals for a division.

Even in a difficult situation, an effective nurse executive provides an environment in which nurses are challenged to improve their practice and to respect professional nursing values. The nurse executive sets the tone, cultivating the vision, ambition, and insight of his staff. His vision of nursing—if he is respected—filters down through the nursing organization.

As was said in discussing the resource-driven model, such a vision of nursing is separate from the vision of nursing under ideal circumstances. If nursing can occur only in the ideal, then nursing hardly exists. Every time a nurse says, "We were too busy to practice professionally today," he is contributing to the demise of nursing as a discipline. The vision of nursing conveyed by the executive deals with the nature of nursing, with its primary characteristics, not with some ideal practice setting.

Although care delivery goals dominate in nursing, many institutions have related goals for nursing research, theory development, and education. Without achievement of these complementary goals, the discipline will remain static. Too often, these goals are perceived as the prerogatives of separate institutions (i.e., schools of nursing, university hospitals). This misperception has led to the slow development of nursing as a discipline.

Clinical nursing research cannot take place apart from the care delivery settings. Research at the bedside is the source of nursing theory development as well as the advancement of practice. Even if a nursing division is not able to support its own research programs, it should be cognizant of the need to retain nursing data that may be of use in future research. It is critical that all significant nursing data be kept as a permanent part of the patient's record. Nor is the retention of nursing interventions adequate without a correlative record of the nursing goals and patient responses.

Research can be seen as a natural practice activity. Nurses can be encouraged to view their practice as a search for relationships among variables, as an exploration for new variables that have an effect on patient care. Even simple field studies foster a research mentality. Quality management data are another source of research activity. If certain goals are not achieved, they should become targets of practical research. If a nursing division is experiencing too many postoperative infections, for example, this might provide impetus to test different methods of wound care.

Most nursing divisions need to set goals concerning the use of their facilities and patient populations by outside nurse researchers. Certainly, one must establish the means of evaluating research proposals, but control should facilitate nursing research rather than frustrate it. The nurse executive needs to ensure that nursing research projects receive fair consideration in institutional research review boards.

Goals for education are important, too. The executive needs to consider a diversity of elements: patient education, staff education, and responsibility for offering educational opportunities to students in health careers. Patient and staff education programs often are developed as a matter of course. However, an institution may hesitate to make opportunities for education open to local students. There is little doubt that today's student is more burden than help for the average nursing staff, but a nurse executive with vision accepts the obligation to help educate future generations of health careerists.

In particular, nurse executives have much to gain by exchanges with schools of nursing. Trading services may be the best way for all institutions to achieve their goals. Clarity in one's own goals is the first step for mutual explorations. Today's exchanges are creative. Some involve fees where the relationship is one-sided. Often barter arrangements take place instead. For example, it is common practice for qualified staff to be given faculty appointments in exchange for student precepting. Or faculty may provide inservice education hours as recompense for use of facilities. Alternately, faculty may assume responsibility for a caseload of patients requiring care. On the other side of the equation, qualified nurse experts in practice may agree to lecture in a school of nursing as part of a reciprocal agreement.

MANAGEMENT GOALS

Table 8–1 contrasts the typical work world ideologies of management and nursing. If the nurse executive is sensitive to the differences in these paradigms, he will be better able to make appropriate applications (or modifications) of principles from the management discipline. Equally important, in his role as corporate exec-

Table 8–1 Comparison of Typical Management and Nursing Ideologies of Work

Subject	Management Ideology	Nursing Ideology
Raw materials (Entering client)	Uniform, with predictable reactions to processing	Diverse, not alike in all responses to processing
Process of production (Nursing)	Known, easily prescribed for each product	Some nursing acts known; many still being researched with relation to product unsure
Product (Exiting client)	Limited number of uniform products	Extensive number and classes of products, with each unit somewhat unique
Workers	Interchangeable; most do programmed tasks	Not interchangeable; many levels, few programmed tasks
Goals	Determined and directive of production	Under exploration, changing; negotiated between the ideal and the feasible
Time frame	Nine-to-five mentality; time to plan ahead as the norm	24-hour, continuous present; often crises with no advance planning time
Interaction with environment	Planned, controlled, based on production needs	Unplanned, uncontrolled, based on environmental needs (of patients and physicians), pressured
Decision making	Few key decisions yearly, usually made at the top	Critical and continuous decision making at all times, multilevel
Evaluation	Regulative, prescribed quality control procedures and systems	Problematic as evaluation techniques are complex, often yet to be created; must evaluate complex phenomena

utive, a knowledge of these ideological differences will help him understand the orientation of his corporate peer non-nurse managers, the kinds of questions that concern them, and the kinds of expectations they hold.

Even experienced nurse executives must carefully consider conceptual and ideological differences between the two models before they judge the application of a managerial principle or technique to be appropriate for nursing. In a sense, the nurse executive is blending two worlds where his corporate peers are seldom concerned with both management and a clinical service.

Even the chief of medicine, who is most comparable with the nurse executive's work, seldom holds the same sort of corporate responsibility. Like his peer managers, the nurse executive must be concerned with output and quality of a product. Yet, the product of nursing care is far more complex to define than most other institutional products.

Because of the world we live in, the trend is to give more weight to managerial goals. We can no longer assume that health care will (or should) receive all that is necessary to do the best job possible. Indeed, our technological capacity has outstripped our ability to pay for it.

The following sections look at some basic managerial principles (control, effectiveness, economy, and efficiency), considering how they appear in the typical managerial ideology and in the nursing care context.

Control

Control is a principle that specifies management's ability to monitor and adjust the work process. If one does not have control of the processes of production, one cannot be held accountable for or effective in achieving one's goals. Similarly, control is important for nursing as a discipline. No discipline can research and advance its practices unless it controls those practices and inquiry processes.

Control can be a problem in the nursing context for several reasons. First, nursing takes place in complex organizations in which it must negotiate with other power groups that traditionally have influenced nursing practice. Furthermore, the nursing division, as the hub of patient-related activity and as the custodian of the patient, is likely to be affected by anyone or any group that interacts with the patient. Indeed, to a great degree functions of others (e.g., the medical staff) dictate specific work functions that fall to nursing. At best, interface with other individuals and units of the organization requires ongoing negotiation concerning who is responsible for what.

Sometimes, nursing has difficulty in asserting control of its own domain of practice because its clients are perceived as belonging to the physicians. In some organizations, if a physician objects to certain independent nursing functions or to certain nursing research designs, he may withdraw "his" patient from the treatment. Such intervention, if supported at higher levels, can do irreparable damage to nursing research as well as impair the consistent use of preferred nursing strategies.

Nor is it possible to ignore the power of the economic dollar. The nursing division that is able to substantiate its fiscal contribution to the organization will inevitably have more say in controlling its practice. A nursing division must view prospective patients as potential customers of nursing. Individual nursing divisions need to establish mechanisms whereby they can market profitable services to customers.

Control, then, involves having enough power to impose one's decisions for nursing on the organization. Second, the nurse executive must devise systems that determine where control (in the form of altering the status quo) is required.

Effectiveness

Effectiveness, as a managerial goal, is the satisfactory achievement of one's objectives. In nursing, there are many measures of effectiveness:

1. Quality management tools and systems measure the statistical effectiveness of nursing care in reaching defined or selected patient care goals.
2. Performance appraisal tools and systems measure the effectiveness of performance of the individual worker.

3. The evaluation component of the nursing care plan determines the success or failure in the individual patient care.
4. External review standards, such as those of the Joint Commission on Accreditation of Healthcare Organizations, and internally derived standards and objectives serve to supply criteria for evaluating nursing division operational effectiveness.

Whatever criteria are used for measurement, it is the responsibility of the nurse executive to see that measures of effectiveness are determined for all nursing and management goals of significance. These measures give concrete data on which to judge the overall effectiveness of the nursing division. They also provide a basis on which one makes decisions concerning needs for alterations in the methods and resources. A failure in effectiveness indicates the need for a different delivery system for that particular element of the nursing system.

Effectiveness, then, is the achievement of one's goals. Determination of effectiveness is a requisite for all major objectives. Nursing has had some long-standing systems for measuring effectiveness, namely, staff performance appraisal and quality management of patient outcomes. The setting of standards for achievement of managerial objectives is fast becoming a part of every nursing organization.

Economy

The principle of economy dictates that the nurse executive get the most for his investments be they financial, material, or human. He must derive systems that monitor for economy, and he must impart a philosophy of economy to the nursing staff. Economic achievement is measured through productivity indices. One traditional productivity index relates a unit's staffing to its patient acuity figures. Comparing man-hours worked with numbers of clients seen in a given clinic illustrates this same point. Similarly, one might compare the use of supplies with patient census. Ratios of this sort prevent complaints that nursing uses "too many" supplies when, in fact, the increase is supported in increased patient activities (i.e., activities resulting in increased income to the organization).

One important principle of economy is the opportunity cost. Here, the nurse executive recognizes that resources put to one purpose are withdrawn from other potential benefits. For example, if a committee has five more members than it needs to achieve its charge, then the committee time of the five excess members represents a lost opportunity. The opportunity cost is benefit that might have been achieved were those hours devoted to some other purpose than the meeting. Committees often are a great source of opportunity costs.

Similarly, if evaluative activities are carried out to no end (reports prepared but not used to change practice), then a great opportunity cost is suffered. The nurse executive must learn to regard staff time as his most precious resource. Investments of staff time at all levels must be closely monitored in a labor-intensive field such as nursing.

Efficiency

The managerial principle of efficiency is a combination of effectiveness and economy: meeting one's objectives with the least outlay of resources. Efficiency often is captured in some index of units produced per time period. The following indices of productivity represent the economy side of efficiency but fail to contain the effectiveness element: (1) obstetrical deliveries per shift, (2) surgical cases per operating room per day, (3) nursing hours per patient day.

These indices may be combined with a measure of effectiveness for a true measure of efficiency. For example, one could devise an efficiency index that relates staff man-hours to quality assurance outcomes on a given unit.

Efficiency is an open-ended concept in a sense, for even if one improves one's efficiency, it is still possible to ask, Could the objective be achieved even more economically? Is the achievement of the objective worth the cost? Might alternate but related objectives be achieved more economically?

SUMMARY

Nursing goals and management goals intermix in several ways at the nurse executive level. The nurse executive's vision of the professional goals of nursing care affects and is affected by his managerial goals. Goals cannot be set apart from the context in which care is to be delivered. Today, that health care context typically is characterized by limitations on resources.

The constraints of the environment are important to consider in enacting professional nursing, but they should not be seen as detrimental to setting goals that represent a professional orientation. Indeed, a difficult circumstance may pose a case for more, not less, application of professional nursing. The nurse executive must have a clear vision of nursing and of the care delivery to be achieved in his organization. He also must consider related goals for education, research, and theory application.

Management of a nursing division and participation in the overall management of the larger institution requires careful and considered interplay among nursing and management goals and ideologies. The nurse executive must appreciate the management ideology espoused by the nonprofessional managers in his organization. He must be able to communicate in both languages: nursing and management. He must use management and his knowledge of it to educate others as to the significance of nursing care and its values for the client. The nurse executive role calls for a delicate synthesis of management and nursing.

SUGGESTED READINGS

Berger, M.S., et al., eds. 1980. *Management for nurses: A multi-disciplinary approach.* St. Louis: C.V. Mosby Co.

Bower, J.L. 1983. Managing for efficiency, managing for equity. *Harvard Business Review* 61, no.4:82–90.

Fralic, M.F. 1992. Nursing administration: The next decade. In *Nursing administration: A micro/macro approach for effective nurse executives,* ed. P.J. Decker et al., 3–22. Norwalk, Conn.: Appleton & Lange.

Knopf, L. 1982. Applying cost-analysis techniques to nursing. *Nursing and Health Care* 3, no.8:427–430.

Kovner, A.R., and D. Neuhauser. 1990. *Health services management readings and commentary,* 2nd ed. Ann Arbor: Health Administration Press.

Kudzma, E.C. 1982. Patterns for effective nursing actions within health bureaucracies. *Nursing and Health Care* 3, no.2:68–72.

Maritz, D.G. 1980. Management principles and nursing: The inefficiency of efficiency. *Supervisor Nurse* 11, no.3:40–41.

Marszalek-Gaucher, E., and R.J. Coffey. 1990. *Transforming healthcare organizations: How to achieve and sustain organizational excellence.* San Francisco: Jossey-Bass Publishers.

O'Brien, B.L. 1993. Nursing leadership and healthcare reform. Part III: Nurse executive role in a reformed healthcare system. *Journal of Nursing Administration* 18, no.12:6–9.

Porter-O'Grady, T. 1992. The future of nursing administration. In *Nursing administration: A micro/macro approach for effective nurse executives*, ed. P.J. Decker et al., 647–663. Norwalk, Conn.: Appleton & Lange.

Reddy, J., and A. Berger. 1983. Three essentials of product quality. *Harvard Business Review* 61, no.4:153–159.

Relman, A. 1993. Medical practice under the Clinton reforms—Avoiding domination by business. *New England Journal of Medicine* 329, no.21:1574–1575.

Shostack, G.L. 1984. Designing services that deliver. *Harvard Business Review* 62, no.1:133–139.

Sommers, J.B. 1993. The struggle for the soul of health insurance. *Journal of Health Politics, Policy and Law* 18, no.2: 287–317.

Taunton, R.L., and D.K. Boyle. 1992. Institutionalizing research in nursing service. In *Nursing administration: A micro/macro approach for effective nurse executives*, ed. P.J. Decker et al., 613–626. Norwalk, Conn.: Appleton & Lange.

Weil, T., and M. Stack. 1993. Health reform—Its potential impact on hospital nursing service. *Nursing Economics* 11, no.4:200–207.

Part III
Building the Structure

There are many tools and tactics that a nurse executive uses to build an organization. In Parts I and II, we looked primarily at scanning the environment, getting a hold on one's context, and then setting directions and determining goals. But goals have to be enacted through an organization, through its people, and through its values. Part III looks at the task of building the organizational structure to best accommodate the people and the goals.

What are the executive's tasks in structuring the nursing division? In relating it to the rest of the organization and its various communities? The ideas and goals discussed in Part II must be captured in how people are organized to do the work.

Simply put, some structures and approaches work better than others. Yet, what works depends on the environment and the sort of organization in which the nursing division exists. Chapters 9 through 11 look at the organizational structures by which work and decision making are distributed within the nursing organization, namely, how the division is governed, how nursing fits into the institutional organization chart, and, in turn, how its own nursing departments are organized, as well as how committees are used to get the work done.

Chapters 12 and 13 look at two contemporary modes of organizing the work: restructured practice and use of case management. These modes affect the work at the level of bedside care as well as having an impact on the total organization and its use of resources. Part III, then, takes the goals discussed in Part II, looks at the environment discussed in Part I, and begins to lay out the organizational structure required to achieve the goals.

9

Governance Structures

An important link in implementing the strategic mission and vision of an organization or division thereof is that of choosing the most appropriate governance structures. Governance structures are the vehicle by which work gets done in the organization. They are selected based on the opportunities and constraints in the environment, the sophistication or lack of sophistication of the staff, and the operating framework of the facility.

INSTITUTIONAL ARRANGEMENTS

One factor to consider in making a decision to accept a nurse executive position is the placement of that position in the total organization. The placement can be viewed from at least two perspectives: (1) where it falls on the table of organization and (2) the powers vested in the position. Normally, one assumes that the higher the position, the greater the powers, but that is not always the case. The assumption must be tested in each case.

There are two levels of nurse executives in many organizations today: (1) the institutional executive and (2) the corporate nurse officer. There are complexities related to both these positions.

Institutional Nurse Executive

The nurse executive in a single institution (freestanding or in a corporation) needs to consider her placement on the table of organization. Ideally, she will prefer to report to the chief executive officer (CEO). Whatever that person's title—CEO, President, or other—CEO will be used here to indicate the top hired official with accountability to a board or to a central corporation officer in a multi-institution corporation. It is preferable in most cases that chief nurse executive officer (CNEO) report to this person in her facility.

At one stage, the pattern of having the CNEO report to the top executive was almost routine, but with growing complexities in the health care industry, some major institutions have redesigned to have the CNEO report to the second administrative officer, here titled chief operating officer (COO) although the titles may vary.

When the institution is very large, there may be some justification for having the CNEO reporting to the second officer. For example, in places where the institutional CEO focuses on external relations—raising funds, promoting the institution's visibility, negotiating with related university programs, and promoting community relations—the "inside" role of managing the institution may fall to the COO.

In such circumstances, it might be appropriate for a nurse executive to report at this level. If, however, reporting to a COO actually means that nursing is seen as merely one operational center among others, then the candidate should be concerned about the placement. The issue is, What does the organizational placement of the CNEO say about how nursing is perceived by the organization?

In the multi-institution corporation, the CNEO may have a dual reporting relationship whereby she reports to both an institutional CEO and a corporate nurse executive. A matrix design of this sort is common today, and the important need is for clarity concerning the nurse executive's accountability to each boss. Is her position in a hierarchical line reporting arrangement to both superiors? Or is the relationship to a corporate nurse executive a coordinative (staff) relationship? Or are both relationships that of line authority, with the content of accountability different to each superior?

The answers to these questions may be complex; the issue is whether the nurse executive knows what product is required by each boss. Further, she will want to be assured that she has the authority requisite to deliver on those expectations.

Nor should the CNEO assume that the organization chart tells the whole tale concerning her authority. It is important to ask whether any nursing practice in the institution falls outside the bounds of her authority. If so, how will she deal with that issue?

And it is important to know whether she has the full confidence of her boss, that he will not make "end runs" around her authority. Such end runs may not be blatant but take forms such as allowing a personnel director to override a CNEO policy, allowing a financial officer to arbitrarily change a CNEO budget plan, or keeping the CNEO out of important policy-setting administrative groups.

In looking at such power issues, the CNEO will get a sense of how seriously her role is taken. One certainty is that if she allows incursions into her authority, they will only increase. When a new CNEO replaces a weak nursing officer, there may be patterns of practice in place that ignore her organizational authority. Changing such defeating practices may involve much effort and require an excellent interpersonal relationship with the CEO and other important players.

Corporate Nursing Officer

If the nurse executive is seeking a corporate position, the question of authority becomes even more important. If she is responsible for CNEOs who also report to institutional CEOs, what is her power to enforce her directives for these nurse executives? Has the organization developed ways to resolve conflicts if, for example, a corporate directive of hers conflicts with orders given to the institutional CNEOs by their respective CEOs?

Lines of relationship and power are complex today, but when there are no institutional paths for resolution of conflict, one may predict difficulties ahead. One mitigating force, of course, is one's ability to foster positive interpersonal relationships. But that skill alone will not suffice for the nurse executive who finds herself in a highly competitive environment with other executives who care more about building kingdoms than fostering cooperation.

This is not to say that all corporate nurse positions must have direct-line authority to work. Instead, the point is that everyone needs a clear understanding of who is accountable to whom for what functions and responsibilities.

NURSING DIVISION GOVERNANCE

As the nurse executive develops the program and the overall mission as well as the vision of where the division of nursing ought to be, these projections must be constantly checked with the environment to determine (1) what is possible and (2) how to implement the changes within a particular setting. Analyzing the environment to determine the best way to develop governance structures is critical.

Although the nurse executive might be biased in favor of one form of governance, it is entirely possible that within a particular setting, this governance structure is not feasible. Often, the constraints of the environment force a nurse executive to work within a governance structure that is not her first choice but the one most workable.

There are two central issues in governance. The first concerns the actual relationships among units, departments, and jobs. This is the organization question. The second issue is that of power and decision-making authority. Often, but not always, these two factors are interwoven.

Organizational Arrangements in Governance

Historically, hospitals and their divisions of nursing came from a bureaucratic and militaristic model of governance. Although bureaucratic organizations are not as highly thought of in today's world as they were formerly, they do serve a purpose and in some organizations are the most feasible form of governance structure. Bureaucracies traditionally have been hierarchical organizations with highly articulated rules and procedures to direct the operations of the organization.

Specialization of the staff into single or limited purpose jobs is common, typically with differentiated staff who only do administration, discrete components of clinical care, or education. Typically, administrative and staff positions are segregated in the bureaucratic model, and there may be many layers of supervisors. Staff participation in managerial decision making and operating of the unit is not usually a part of their job.

Although a range of bureaucracies exist from highly specialized and bureaucratic to more open and participative, they remain a common form of governance in hospitals. Even when the nurse executive would like to move to a more participative format, this model is often familiar and ingrained in people's way of getting the work done. Many nurses have been socialized into this model in both school and the workplace.

Today, many organizations that were once highly bureaucratized are more decentralized (i.e., self-contained units are created within the division, accountable for all their own functions and goals). Chapter 10 gives more details concerning the structural differences between a hierarchy and a decentralized model. In essence, in decentralization accountability is pushed downward in the chain of command, with individual departments being more autonomous.

By contrast, the way that professionals organize themselves is often different from either a highly bureaucratized format or a decentralized one. In professional models, one often sees forms of matrix management in which the work is organized around projects as the operational units of the organization. Project management may involve a team that organizes, completes, and evaluates a project, as well as maintains its ongoing operations. All or part of the work of an organization may be distributed according to projects.

In the matrix model, the bureaucratic rule of one man–one boss becomes blurred. People can have responsibilities in diverse project teams, filling different roles in each of these project teams as the work flow demands. The same person might be in charge of one project while reporting to someone else in another project. In a project design, the role of the nurse executive becomes that of a coordinator, facilitator, and integrator, as well as tracker of projects.

In a professional model, there is less supervision because it is assumed that professionals supervise themselves and that they need minimal direction from administrative staff not actually participating in the work of the professional on a daily basis. It is assumed that professionals can take on more accountability and can govern and evaluate themselves through the process of peer review. After all, professionals have the expertise to do this.

Authority Structures

As well as looking at how an organization is distributed on an organizational chart, one can trace the authority structure. Participative management and shared governance structures have become popular in nursing. The term *participative management structure* refers to an organizational arrangement whereby the staff participates in the decision-making process but is not delegated authority for ultimate decision making.

Shared governance structures, in contrast, actually delegate authority, although the amount of authority (and for what aspects of the operation) may vary from minimal to extensive. In mature shared governance structures, one sees a high degree of decision making among staff and extensive decentralization of authority.

Although it is more common for shared governance structures to reflect a matrix or highly decentralized organizational model, it is not a prerequisite. Shared governance structures range from highly centralized bureaucratic structures to highly decentralized ones. A bureaucratic structure in which staff nurses and a central management core do the work of the organization can still provide for staff governance. Similarly, a highly decentralized structure might delegate much authority to the staff nurse at the bedside through unit-based shared governance systems.

The most successful examples of shared governance usually are those that have matured as the staff and executive both learn how the group best functions. Shared governance can be implemented in a step-by-step fashion in which various functions can be brought in line as the staff develops competence.

Shared governance structures can be centralized with the work being done through central staff committees. It can also be conceptualized as a unit-based system. In a unit-based structure, the governance group is responsible for taking issues that they cannot resolve or that have implication for more than one unit to the larger staff council for discussion decisions.

The two models differ primarily in the flow of information. In a centralized model, the information flows from the central shared governance structure to the units; in the unit-based system, the flow is reversed.

As the staff becomes more familiar with their roles, the shared governance structure often undergoes movement from a highly centralized structure in which few staff nurses participate in decision making to a decentralized structure in place on individual units in which a high degree of participation and accountability is accepted by all the nursing staff.

Although most nurses see shared governance as important for a truly professional practice, it is not accepted as essential by all nurses. With the acceptance of authority comes greater responsibility, and one must be willing to be held accountable. Not all nurses are prepared to accept this level of authority and responsibility.

Staff nurses who want to expand their practice and take on more authority, those who envision achieving a "professional" status, find shared governance structures appealing. Other staff nurses by contrast may prefer simply to provide good patient care and not be bothered by the responsibilities of a fuller professional role.

The difference in perspective may reflect many different factors, one's education, one's notion of professionalism, and one's other commitments at the time. Some nurses who are in school, involved with young families, or into many activities outside of nursing might prefer just delivering good patient care. At another time in their lives, these same nurses might be ready for more accountability and willing to become involved in more shared governance activities.

SUMMARY

Determining the best structure to carry out the mission, vision, and goals of the nursing program depends on assessing weaknesses and strengths of the staff, the environment in which the nursing division has to relate and integrate, and the overall mission and philosophy of the organization. In some organizations, the nurse executive will not have the opportunity of choosing a governance structure. In others, choosing an appropriate governance structure will be an expectation.

If the nurse executive matches the governance structures to the goals with the division and the organization, then higher levels of quality and productivity will be obtained. One strives for congruence between where the organization needs to go and the structures that can best get it there, within the parameters of the environment.

SUGGESTED READINGS

Curran, C. 1991. An interview with Karlene M. Kerfoot. *Nursing Economics* 9, no.3:141–147.

Flarey, D.L. 1991. The nurse executive and the governing body: Synergy for a new era. *Journal of Nursing Administration* 21, no.12:11–17.

Havens, D.S. 1992. Nursing involvement in hospital governance: 1990–1995. *Nursing Economics* 10, no.5:331–335.

Jenkins, J. 1988. A nursing governance and practice model: What are the costs? *Nursing Economics* 6, no.6:302–311.

Jenkins, J.E. 1991. Professional governance: The missing link. *Nursing Management* 22, no.8:26–30.

Jones, C.B., et al. 1993. Shared governance and the nursing practice environment. *Nursing Economics* 11, no.4:208–214.

Lachman, V. 1993. What is shared governance? *ASLTCN Journal* 4, no.2:4–5, 19.

McMahon, J.M. 1992. Shared governance: The leadership challenge. *Nursing Administration Quarterly* 17, no.1:55–59.

Porter-O'Grady, T. 1992. *Implementing shared governance: Creating a professional organization*. St. Louis: Mosby Yearbook.

Scott, V.L., and N.W. Totten. 1993. Living the dream: Shared governance in the role of nurse executive. *Journal of Nursing Administration* 23, no.12:44–48.

Snowdon, A.W., and D. Rajacich. 1993. The challenge of accountability in nursing. *Nursing Forum* 28, no.1:5–11.

10

Organization and Departmentalization

As indicated in the last chapter, the responsibility for meeting goals is distributed over organizational units such as departments or patient units. The nurse executive often determines both the divisional functions and organizational units simultaneously because of their vital interaction.

Departmentalization is the allocation of functions and responsibilities designed to achieve goals through a formalized arrangement of human and material resources in organizational units. Most health organizations still use some bureaucratic structures, even when a high degree of decentralization has taken place.

Nursing divisions tend to follow this hierarchical pattern, although extensive decentralization is common. In many organizations, head nurses (by whatever title) report directly to the chief nurse executive officer (CNEO) or, in larger organizations, to department chiefs. The layer that has been limited or sacrificed in the popular move toward decentralization tends to be the supervisors. Even in the most decentralized institution, there are at least two levels of nursing management: head nurse (first-line) and director (nurse executive level).

Most nursing divisions can be described by Weber's (1978) traditional description for a bureaucracy: (1) Regular activities are assigned to fixed, official areas; (2) there are hierarchical

layers and levels of authority such that higher levels control and supervise lower levels; (3) all important administrative directives are reduced to written statements; (4) people are selected and assigned to tasks on the basis of specialization; and (5) there is policy guidance for all activities of the organization.

ORGANIZATION CHARTS

The organization chart is a graphic representation of the departmentalization process. Most organization charts are positional; that is, they are organized by title and rank, as in Figure 10–1.

Position and function need not necessarily coincide. It is possible, therefore, to construct an organization chart based on function rather than position, as in Figure 10–2. Unless function and position are closely tied, it usually is not possible to show both of these organizing principles in one chart.

Whether an organization chart is positional or functional, there are several common patterns for the distribution and relation of its components. The line pattern is strictly hierarchical, as shown in Figure 10–3. The line-staff pattern usually occurs when an organization is large

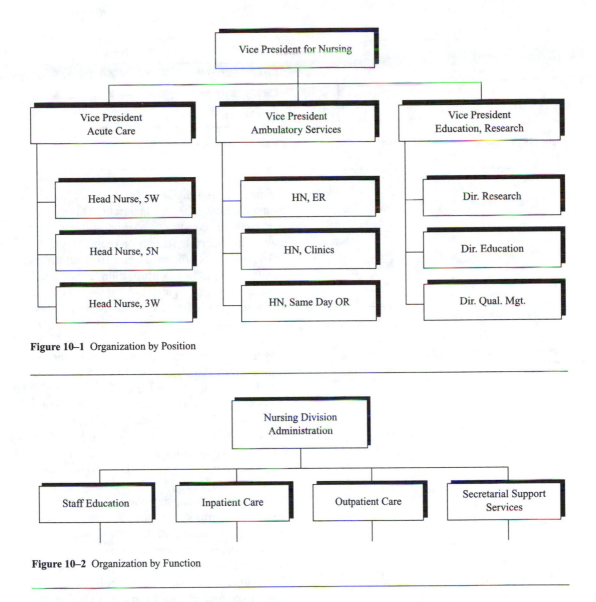

Figure 10–1 Organization by Position

Figure 10–2 Organization by Function

and needs specialized functions (Figure 10–4). In this example the two staff positions, or functions, are advisory extensions of the chief executive; they do not have responsibility down the line of command. Such staff positions are likely to be staff education, personnel work, accounting, or other functions that require special education or expertise. With the line-staff pattern, line people are relieved of a function that is better handled from a centralized position.

The third organizational pattern is typical of the institution that divides duties by function rather than by spatial congruence. This functional pattern is shown in Figure 10–5. Here, for example, C might be in charge of nursing care for units D, E, and F, and B might be in charge of general administration and materials management on those same units. This form of management uses a matrix design in which different managers are responsible for different functions within the same geographic location.

The fourth organization pattern is one in which committee structures are the vehicles for management (Figure 10–6). This pattern of organization, based on committee power, is more common in nursing education than in nursing

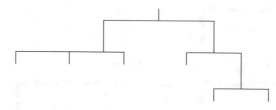

Figure 10–3 Organization by Line Pattern

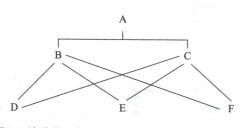

Figure 10–4 Organization by Line-Staff Pattern

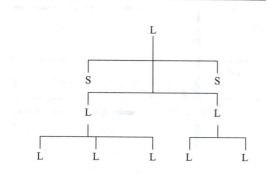

Figure 10–5 Functional Pattern

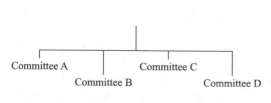

Figure 10–6 Committee Pattern

	Head Nurse A	Head Nurse B	Head Nurse C
Case Manager A	X	X	X
Case Manager B	X	X	X
Case Manager C	X	X	X

Figure 10–7 Matrix Organization

Some nursing divisions are organized totally by matrix rather than by hierarchy. This pattern is a complex construct in which an employee may be responsible to two or more bosses for different aspects of work. Figure 10–7 illustrates a matrix design. In this illustration, a staff nurse stationed on a given patient unit is responsible to the head nurse of that unit but also to a case manager who oversees the clinical progress of her patients.

Potential problems with the matrix-type organization can easily be discerned. If, for example, the head nurse and the case manager give conflicting orders to the staff nurse, the job may be untenable. Or a manipulative staff nurse may play his two bosses off against each other. When a matrix organization is used, there must be clear decision rules and, it is hoped, good interpersonal relationships. The employee must know which boss has the final word when he receives conflicting orders or conflicting demands concerning work priorities.

Clear decision points will assist the employee, but to apply them still requires good will and cooperation. Suppose the rule is that, in case of conflict, the staff nurse is to follow the head nurse's orders. An uncooperative head nurse can make the case manager's role very difficult if he so chooses; he can undermine his fellow manager by contriving to give countermanding orders until the case manager loses credibility with the staff nurse.

Nevertheless, a matrix organization is productive when clear rules are established and when good will predominates among peer managers. A sense of give and take and the ability to cope with a negotiated-order management model will enable all the managers in this organization to develop viable and productive roles.

services. Its use as a mode of management in nursing service, however, is increasing as nursing services seek more and different ways to distribute nursing responsibilities. In some matrix designs, this design might apply to projects rather than committees.

24-HOUR OPERATIONS

Departmentalization of nursing is complicated by 24-hour-a-day operations. Often, an institution has a different organization chart for each shift. The organization may need to be different because the functions of each shift vary.

This situation is further confounded if certain units or staff work 8-, 10-, or 12-hour shifts, respectively, or when different organization patterns pertain during different shifts. The authority and responsibility of all organizational units over the 24-hour period must be clarified.

At one stage, only the CNEO had 24-hour responsibility for nursing operations. Now, that responsibility often is placed at the head nurse level. To complicate this further, some institutions maintain off-shift supervisors with shift authority that must be coordinated with the head nurse's 24-hour accountability. Role clarity is essential in such situations. Who is responsible for what? What authority does the single-shift manager have when on duty? How accessible is the 24-hour officer if the authority of the shift manager is limited?

As if this were not enough complexity, the off-shift nursing supervisors often have responsibility for institutional administration, whether or not this responsibility is made evident in organizational documents. Although this arrangement is not necessarily bad, the role needs to be built into the corporate organization plan so that the nurse officer is accorded salary and rank commensurate with his administrative assignment.

Usually a 24-hour role is involved with long-term planning and design of operations, although a shift-only role is primarily involved with immediate operations. All too often, there is an attempt to blend these roles by having a 24-hour officer also responsible for one 8-hour shift per day. If the 24-hour role is tied to managing the day shift, then it is difficult to say that the manager has real 24-hour authority.

The 24-hour officer should be free to plan his own hours within the 24 hours based on the requirements of his job description. For example, if the 24-hour officer is expected to evaluate staff on all shifts, then he must be present on all shifts to observe the staff performance. The real

problems usually arise when role authorities and responsibilities are not defined well in a system or when a system is trying to pay one person to do two jobs simultaneously.

NURSE EXECUTIVE IN MULTI-INSTITUTION RELATIONSHIPS

A matrix model often is found in multi-institutional corporations in which the CNEO in each institution reports to an institutional chief executive officer (CEO) as well as to a corporate-level vice president for nursing. The complexities of multi-institutional corporations inevitably involve matrices, dual reporting relationships, or both. Also, one may find a matrix incorporating a committee structure.

In a corporation of many institutions, it is most important that nursing be represented at the corporate level. Nursing can be disenfranchised if not represented in corporate strategic planning. Corporate nursing roles are designed in many different ways, but two general patterns dominate:

1. The corporate nurse officer has line authority over the nurse executives of the separate institutions within.
2. The corporate nurse officer has a staff relationship with the nurse executives of the separate institutions.

Both patterns are workable, although the second may present problems if the nurse executives are not supportive of the corporate nurse officer. Such a situation, of course, has the danger of removing nursing *de facto* from the seat of action and decision making.

In a multi-institution corporation, it is critical that the institutional nurse executives relate to each other, whether or not a formal matrix plan requires it. The multi-institution presents great opportunities for sharing, economies of scale, and mutual research. Sharing of managerial processes and tools across diverse institutions provides an exceptional opportunity for the advancement of nursing management as well as of clinical care.

When at all feasible, nurse executives in the same corporation should try to find mutually shared methods for staffing, patient classification and acuity systems, performance appraisal, quality management, and recording/reporting. If the operational systems of the institutions are shared, everyone gains. Research is enhanced, communications are simplified, and interinstitutional sharing of resources promotes economies of scale.

The matrix or dual reporting structure of such multi-institution corporations requires new ways of operating in the institutional nurse executive role. In the single organization, the nurse executive is used to making decisions on his own and simply implementing them. In the multi-institution corporation, he finds it essential to keep a well-functioning communications network with his peer nurse executives.

In such a complex organization, the independent decision of a nurse executive in one setting may affect executives and institutions other than his own. One soon learns that sharing should take place before any decision of significance is made in any one institution of a corporation. A consultative model arises in which the institutional nurse executives (and the corporate-level nurse officer) act as a steering committee, with a clearinghouse function to review and regulate any necessary diversity in operations.

Whatever the corporate form, the nurse executive in an institution that is part of a corporation will find his role more focused on upward and lateral relations than in the past. In a complex organization, nurse executives at both corporate and institutional levels play full executive roles. They must function as executives of the total organization; they cannot afford simply to focus on the discrete functions of the nursing division.

Unification Model

Another complex organizational pattern arises when the nursing practice component of a corporation is joined with a nursing educational component (a school or college program, not simply staff inservice education). This model,

the unification model, attempts to overcome traditional gaps between service and education through creating roles that span both sides of nursing. Obviously, such joint roles have much to offer to the role incumbent as well as to practice and education. When, for example, faculty members carry active patient practices, they are not likely to become clinically obsolete. And when a staff nurse has a group of students for clinical education, he develops a sensitivity to the problems inherent in the teaching role.

The unifying roles may be administrative, staff, or both; they may occur at various levels in the organization chart. Unification at the highest level occurs when the same nurse executive is both chief officer of nursing service and the dean of the school of nursing. Sometimes, this is the only link, with the nurse executive having associates who are responsible respectively for the educational and service components. In other settings, many roles are combined. For example, one might see the chairman of an educational medical-surgical department simultaneously holding the associate directorship for service management of medical-surgical units. Some illustrations of such mixed roles follow:

1. a nursing executive with his own group of students in a specialty track
2. a head nurse with a group of clinical students assigned to her
3. an inservice educator with an appointment to teach in the school of nursing
4. a supervisor of service who is also chairman of a nursing education specialty program
5. a staff nurse who teaches geriatric nursing in the school of nursing
6. a dean who manages a well-care clinic
7. a faculty member who works as a staff nurse 2 days a week

The linkages that have been made are more numerous than can be identified here. The chief variables are

1. Both roles may be staff positions (e.g., a faculty member/staff nurse); both roles

may be administrative (e.g., a head nurse/ department chairman); or staff and administrative roles may be mixed (e.g., a staff nurse/dean).

2. One role may be more prominent than the other (e.g., a dean with a patient case-load); both roles may be equal in status (e.g., vice president of nursing service/ dean).

3. Time may be equally distributed between the two roles, or one role may be the more extensive (e.g., a 70 percent faculty load, with a 30 percent clinic care assignment). Time may also be episodic (e.g., a faculty member with a patient care assignment between school terms and for summers, with full-time teaching responsibilities at other times).

Such roles, although beneficial to the incumbents and the profession, present many practical problems for an institution. For example, if one job is lower on a pay scale, how is that handled? Is the dean's salary reduced for the time in which he does clinical staff nursing? How do benefits accrue when the two jobs are at different levels? What happens if the two institutions (school and service) have different personnel policies?

Role-specific problems also arise. For example, does it make sense for a nurse executive to leave a critical budget meeting to teach his clinical students? Can a head nurse really manage a clinical contingent of students without lessening her attention to the head nurse role demands?

Faculty members have their own role problems, chief among them the reward system in academia. Academics are rewarded more for scholarship and research in most institutions than for clinical practice. Does the faculty member threaten his position by using discretionary time for nursing practice?

No two institutions solve these problems in the same way, but the solutions should be determined before the joint roles are filled. The answers for nursing are more complex than for medicine, because medicine may be practiced in an episodic fashion (e.g., the physician may do most of his patient contact in short-term visits).

Nursing, however, involves sustained patient contact, making the commitment to other intervening activities more complex to arrange.

Because the problems of interface are complex, joint roles often arise as informal trade-offs. A faculty member, for example, may simply take on clinic care tasks without changing his official role and salary structure. In exchange, a clinic nurse might reciprocate by giving equivalent time to student education needs. Although the reciprocities may be difficult to work out, such barter arrangements may be the easiest solution in many settings.

Joint role arrangements are even more complex when they occur between two unrelated institutions. This might occur if geographically close hospitals and schools determine to create mixed roles. Here, a participant might have much to lose if his job were half funded by one institution and half by another. For example, the incumbent might lose the sick days and retirement rights of a full-time employee. Barter, again, often allows such roles to be created. As complexity becomes the rule in modern organizational life, one may assume that even more diverse mixed nursing roles will arise.

WHAT DEPARTMENTS IN A DIVISION?

Many nurse executives take their departments as a given. Indeed, it may be difficult to make changes in an entrenched pattern. Nevertheless, it is worth some reflection to determine if the departmentalization scheme really best serves the institution.

Criteria for Partitioning of Nursing Divisional Units

Many criteria may be applied as the basis for forming organizational units. A nursing division usually combines several of the following criteria.

- *Function.* The nursing division itself is an example of an organizational unit based on a function (nursing care). Within the nursing division, departments organized around function might include an inservice department and an emergency department. In some instances, the functions that determine the organizational units are managerial (e.g., a nursing office or an accounting department). In other instances, the functions are based on nursing rather than managerial processes (e.g., an operating room suite or a coronary care unit).

- *Customer.* An emergency care department, for example, might provide different services for different customers. It might differentiate between patients having real emergencies and those using the emergency department in lieu of a family physician. Similarly, an obstetric department might be seen as serving a specific clientele. In this case, one could argue the presence of two criteria: customer and function.

   Some facilities have certain departments designed to provide consumer-intensive services for the patient who can afford such extra services. In these cases, additional hotel-type services may be added as an inducement for the well-off customer to select this institution over its competition.

- *Objectives.* Even when functions and customers differ in many respects, the criterion of desired outcome or objective may determine organizational units. For example, patients on a rehabilitation unit may exhibit many different impairments requiring diverse nursing therapies. Yet, these patients may be gathered on a single unit because the staff shares a single objective for them all—optimal return to independent living.

- *Geography.* Often a nursing department is created out of physically adjoining nursing units. Hence, a supervisor's department may be comprised of 3 West, 3 East, and 3 North, not because of similarities in patients, functions, or objectives, but because of their physical proximity. Geography almost always is a criterion for a head nurse's unit of responsibility, but even here, there may be exceptions. For example, a

head nurse might be responsible for two patient care units that are geographically remote.

- *Logistics.* Using this criterion, patients or subordinate units are joined under a single department if heavy interaction among units (or patients) is anticipated. Hence, postpartum mothers and newborn infants will be found in the same department even though they require different care. Similarly, preoperative, operative, and postoperative units often are grouped under a single managerial department because they are linked by the sequential passage of patients through all three units.

Factors Affecting Decisions about Departmentalization

In nursing management, it is important to examine the control question concerning departmentalization. Who makes the departmentalization decisions? Often, nursing is expected to form its units according to criteria that better suit medicine than nursing. When medical groupings consist of persons who need similar nursing care (e.g., a genitourinary unit), this may not present a problem.

However, a medically determined neuropsychiatric unit may present the nursing department with diverse clients having diverse nursing needs. Because nursing provides a 24-hour ongoing service, it ought to have control over its own departmentalization decisions rather than having control in the hands of medicine, a service that provides intermittent practice.

Several other factors affect decisions about departmentalization, namely, span of control, number of hierarchical levels, centralization versus decentralization, line versus staff, and unity of command. These are briefly reviewed.

Span of Control

No nurse executive can manage effectively if too many persons report directly to him. An ideal (if abstract) span of control might consist of eight reporting persons. The nurse executive who has 20 head nurses reporting directly to him with no intervening management layer probably has exceeded a practical span of control. Of course, this span might be acceptable if the head nurses already were expert managers needing little day-to-day supervision or guidance.

In contrast, an individual with fewer than four persons reporting to him may not really be needed. For example, an organization that has 10 head nurses reporting to five supervisors probably should reduce its supervisors. Professional organizations, however, tend to use smaller spans of control when the consultative process is frequent and necessary between superior and subordinate.

One of the most common distortions in span of control occurs when various specialists are hired with the status privilege of reporting to the chief nurse executive. In the past, clinical specialists often demanded this right; today, it might be an off-shift supervisor who resents reporting to 24-hour head nurses.

The organization should be planned to make sense in distribution of the tasks and responsibilities rather than distorted to please hard-to-hire workers. Ironically, the clinical specialist who once could set such demands is now much less in demand. In many cases, recent shifts in supply and demand have corrected such misplacements.

Hierarchical Levels

The organization that has more than five, or at the most seven, levels of workers from the top person to the lowest-level employee is probably top heavy. The organization should aim for the least number of levels that can exist given the appropriate spans of control. The fewer the levels, the less distortion between management goals and the actual work done. The larger the organization, the more hierarchical levels it tends to have.

Of necessity, there is an important interplay between span of control and number of hierarchical levels. When one increases, the other decreases. For example, if the nurse executive decides to eliminate the supervisory layer (a decrease in the number of hierarchical levels), then, instead of having four supervisors reporting directly to him, he will have 20 head nurses

reporting directly to him (an increase in span of control).

Centralization versus Decentralization

A division is highly centralized if major decision-making power and responsibility for key functions are concentrated in the top levels of that division. A division is highly decentralized if decision making and responsibility for key functions are delegated to the lowest possible managerial level in the division. Thus, a centralized nursing division might have major decisions made by a council of the nurse executive and his associate directors. Such a division would be likely to have many major functions (e.g., budgeting, staff education, quality assurance, and nursing research) in separate departments reporting directly to the nurse executive or his associates.

In contrast, a decentralized division might place most decision making at the head nurse level, with each head nurse running her unit independent of the decisions of her peer head nurses. Unlike a head nurse in a centralized division, the head nurse in a decentralized division would provide for budgeting, staff education, quality assurance, nursing research, and staffing of his unit with his own personnel and unit resources.

Nursing organizations vary greatly in their degree of centralization. The degree may differ for different tasks and responsibilities. There are general advantages and limitations to each mode of departmentalization. A highly centralized division, for example, usually commands considerable power, achieves economies of scale, and develops expertise in the specialized functions that are served by discrete departments. A limitation of a highly centralized operation is that it may not attract ambitious first-line and middle managers who are looking for authority and control over their own units.

A highly decentralized division has the advantage of placing the decision making near the action; it also allows for diverse responses from managerial unit to managerial unit. Limitations of the decentralized form are that it loses economies of scale and that it sometimes shifts responsibility and authority to managers unprepared for them. For example, a head nurse who is responsible for providing inservice education for his own staff may not have the educational expertise required for the job.

Today, most nursing services claim to be decentralized because it is highly recommended by the experts. But one must look closely to see what is actually decentralized and what is not. In some cases, decentralization becomes a ploy for weakening and breaking a united nursing service. If a strong nurse leader gives up his centralized role to become a staff consultant to decentralized subordinates, those subordinates (each weaker than the centralized leader) may be vulnerable to separate power plays.

Decentralization has another limitation when functions are decentralized to the level of incompetency. Here, a unit is given responsibility for a function it is unprepared to carry out. Usually that function falls through the cracks and is forgotten. The nurse executive must always ensure that a unit develops competency in the functions that are being decentralized before this reorganization takes place.

The nurse executive cannot delegate to someone who is unprepared to handle the function. Therefore, it is imperative that he not decentralize functions until competency has been established and the function can be performed at the appropriate level of quality.

Decentralization also is an error if too many tasks and responsibilities are decentralized to someone already suffering from role overload. This is a frequent occurrence in today's cost-conscious management. Functions and responsibilities must be sent down the line to persons prepared to do them and having enough time to absorb them into their role functions.

Because decentralization is seen generally as a good thing and centralization as suspect, most errors are made in decentralizing rather than centralizing. Decentralization is often a risky tactic in an environment in which the nursing division is under threat from powerful, competitive organizational components.

Line versus Staff

A line position is one in which a person has responsibility for subordinates. Here, one can trace the line from one's superior, through oneself, down to one's subordinates. A vice president of nursing, for example, may trace the major line for patient care from vice president to assistant director to head nurse to staff nurse.

Staff positions are jobs that lack direct authority over others. For example, the CNEO may have a staffing officer who rearranges daily staffing patterns based on patient acuity reports and unforeseen contingencies. This person is not the superordinate or subordinate of the head nurses, even though he may adjust the staffing on their floors. His power comes through the CNEO, who is his direct boss.

A role may have both staff and line elements. For example, the director of staff education is staff to the nursing supervisors but line to her group of educators. The line or staff designation is determined by the organization chart, not by the job's high or low placement on the organizational chart. Hence, it is not the case than any registered nurse has line authority over a nursing aide on her unit. Only the head nurse would have such authority.

Staff positions, because they are not backed by official authority, often require incumbents skilled in interpersonal relationships. For example, if a clinical specialist in a staff position is to make substantial changes in the quality of nursing care, he must win the good will of the staff who must change practice patterns. The person in a staff position has to be an expert at getting the job done by being influential and by understanding the difference in leading by influence and leading by power.

Bellman (1992) discussed such concepts as using the 10-step consulting process, understanding cross-functional work, and building solid relationships as examples of skills that are important in staff positions. In matrix organizations, more staff relationships exist than in hierarchical organizations. Hence, the principles of staff work become key in these organizations.

Unity of Command

According to this principle, each employee should report to one and only one boss. It is not fair, states the principle, that a person be responsible to more than one boss, for to do so may expose him to conflicting demands. Of course, this principle is broken every day in the matrix organization.

A head nurse, for example, might be responsible to the director of quality management for the quality of care on his unit and at the same time be responsible to an associate director for the general running of the unit. As the complexity of health care organizations increases, this principle will be more and more stretched.

Unity of command can be approached, however, if job descriptions and lines of authority are clarified. If a person is responsible to more than one boss, he should know his responsibilities to each manager. Even with clarity of responsibility, there can still be problems. Suppose, for example, that there is no overlap in required functions, and no conflict in goals for a given position, yet both supervisors envision that they have claim to 60 percent of the employee's time. Reasoned negotiation becomes a major necessity when unity of command is sacrificed.

Sometimes, the nurse executive finds that he has problems with other division chiefs or department heads assuming that they can issue orders to the nursing staff. Suppose, for example, that the chief dietitian puts out a policy concerning what nurses will do in relation to tray delivery. Nursing staff need to understand the line of command and to recognize that such an order is not legitimate unless cosigned by the nurse executive. Not infrequently, others make intentional or unintentional incursions into the nursing domain.

Other Relations within Organizations

In addition to considering departmentalization within the nursing division and changes that link education and service departmentally, it is important to view the departmentalization of nursing in relation to the non-nursing components of an organization. Here, issues of control and equity arise.

Some nurse executives, for example, find that they do not control all nursing practice in the organization. It is still not unusual to find that nurses of an emergency department, a psychiatric unit, a research unit, or some other specialized unit report to some manager other than the nurse executive. When this pattern exists, it should be the nurse executive's highest priority to gain control of all nursing practice within his institution.

When all nurses do not report to the nursing division, the quality of nursing care varies, and resources may be managed in ways that favor some units over others. More importantly, unless nurses can share a common vision and work under the same standards and policies, poor quality of care may be the result. As a first step in gaining authority for all nursing practice, the nurse executive needs to negotiate accountability for the quality of the nursing care provided by the nursing staff and departments that do not report to him.

This can be realized by having the nursing functions outside the division of nursing report to the quality management committee in the nursing division and through other committees such as the recruitment and retention committee as well. This also makes these nurses feel they are a part of the nursing community.

Nurses in other parts of the facility that do not report to the division of nursing should feel that they have the same responsibilities and accountabilities as those working in the division of nursing. Without this kind of interface, it is impossible to achieve consistency of quality outcomes throughout the facility.

Sometimes, the problem arises not on the department level but in relation to certain nursing roles. For example, nurse practitioners may be reporting to a physician instead of to the nursing management line. It is critical that such roles be instated within the nursing division even if their role incumbents coordinate closely with medicine. Otherwise, such practitioners may lose their nursing identity.

Another matter is the status of nurse managers compared with non-nurses with equivalent or fewer responsibilities. The issue of equity is always sensitive and often appears at the head nurse level. For example, the head nurse clearly has responsibility equal to or greater than that of a purchasing manager. The head nurse has more staff, probably a larger unit budget, a 24-hour commitment, and certainly more responsibility for clients.

Most institutions accord head nurses the status as department heads. If this is not the case, it should be a goal of the nurse executive. Nor is holding of the title alone adequate. Head nurses should have the same organizational privileges and responsibilities as do their peer non-nurse department heads.

Nurse Executive Advancement

Today, many nurse executives see two paths to increased responsibility. Within the parent institution, however, options may be limited. In a corporation, an institutional nurse executive may try for an open corporate nurse position but such a job is not open every day. Two other options involve becoming a CEO or taking on more functions within his present role.

Taking on other divisions or departments need not impair one's commitment to nursing. Because virtually all organizational functions support the nursing activities, it is not difficult to justify such an extended role. Activities as diverse as laboratory, pharmacy, or management information systems can easily be seen as supportive to the nursing function.

Ironically, until recently many nurses gave up much power in the name of getting rid of non-nursing functions. Although it may not make good sense to have a nurse doing something that can be equally well done by a lower-level employee, nurses failed to differentiate between *doing* and *managing*. The nurse manager who gave up the transportation function because it was non-nursing, ultimately decreased the power of the nursing division. All too often, freeing nurses to do nursing was interpreted as the divestment of power over support services at the managerial level.

A recent reorganization movement in hospitals has been reversing this trend. In patient-focused redesign, functions that were taken off the unit and assigned to a centralized department such as transportation and phlebotomy are now being moved back to the patient care unit under the direction of the nurse manager. Staff on the unit are cross-trained to pick up many of these functions. And people from these departments move to a unit-based assignment.

The motivation for this program is to reduce the time that such specialty staff spend waiting for someone to call them to do their job and to decrease the numbers of contacts that patients have over the course of a day. With this movement, the nurse executive automatically adds support services to his division, perhaps without the same obvious turf-building as occurs when new departments appear on the revised organization chart.

Other nurses seek a CEO position as a career move. This is a credible goal, and nurses should be grateful when a committed nurse brings her professional perspective to managing an institution or corporation.

Nurses should be highly supportive to nurses who achieve high-power positions by either tactic discussed here. Indeed, nurse executives should be prime candidates for CEO positions if they so desire. However, those who do not want to give up the special and unique function of managing a professional service should not be criticized if they refuse a CEO role.

Another pattern appreciative of nursing's role is developing in some socialist countries. In one such organization in New Zealand, the hospital administrator, the chief of the medical staff, and the nursing director form a triumvirate for institutional rule. The three roles were cast as equal. Clearly, this is a complex managerial strategy, but it does give nursing appropriate recognition. This pattern also is described in the literature in this country (Schulz and Johnson 1976), so some instances may be evident here.

In this era, we are likely to see many new forms of organization in health care. The corporate models will vary, and the horizontal linkages of similar organizations (e.g., numbers of acute care hospitals) and vertical linkages of different purpose institutions (e.g., acute care plus long-term care facilities) will call for experiments in organizational arrangements. Our objective in all cases is to see that nursing achieves the recognition in organization design required for it to achieve its necessary goals in the organization.

SUMMARY

Departmentalization is one mechanism by which the nurse executive distributes the functions of his department and contributes to the larger organization. There is always some degree of freedom in determining the departmentalization schema, no matter what the past practices.

Some constraints exist on the selection of departments, more particularly on the patient groupings desired by medical staff. Further constraints may be imposed by the specifics of architectural space and geographic location of various institutional resources. Past practices of the nursing division also contribute to departmentalization decisions.

Other constraints may be present in the form of resources. For example, if the nurse executive lacked experienced head nurses, he would be foolish to decentralize his division to the unprepared level of managers.

There is no single right way to organize a nursing department. Each nurse executive must determine the best functions and best departments for his division, given the unique characteristics of his setting and his institution.

REFERENCES

Bellman, T.M. 1992. *Getting things done when you are not in charge*. San Francisco: Berrett-Koehler.

Schulz, R., and A.C. Johnson. 1976. *Management of hospitals*. New York: McGraw-Hill Publishing Co.

Weber, M. 1978. Bureaucracy. In *Classics of organization theory*, ed. J.M. Shafritz and P.H. Whitbeck, 37–42. Oak Park, Ill.: Moore Publishing.

SUGGESTED READINGS

Appenzeller, L.M. 1993. Merging nursing departments: An experience. *Journal of Nursing Administration* 23, no.12:55–60.

Grohar-Murray, M.E., and H.R. DiCroce. 1992. *Leadership and management in nursing.* Norwalk, Conn.: Appleton & Lange.

Jones-Schenk, J., and P. Hartley. 1993. Organizing for communication and integration. *Journal of Nursing Administration* 23, no.10:30–33.

Marquis, B.L., and C.J. Huston. 1994. *Management decision making for nurses: 118 case studies,* 2nd ed. Philadelphia: J.B. Lippincott Co.

Pabst, M.K. 1993. Span of control on nursing inpatient units. *Nursing Economics* 11, no.2:87–90.

Porter-O'Grady, T. 1991. Shared governance and new organizational models. In *Issues in nursing administration*, ed. M.J. Ward and S.A. Price, 315–321. St. Louis: Mosby Yearbook.

Smeltzer, C.H., et al. 1993. Work restructuring: The process of decision making. *Nursing Economics* 11, no.4:215–222.

Swansburg, R.C. 1990. Organizing nursing services. In *Management and leadership for nurse managers*, ed. R.C. Swansburg, 263–297. Boston: Jones and Bartlett Publishers.

11

Committee Structure

The nurse executive's committee structure offers her another mechanism for distributing functions in addition to the departmentalization plan. The committee structure may be used for those functions that necessarily cross department lines. Except in the case of the rare organization that uses committees as the mode for departmentalization, the nurse executive must be aware of a major difference between departments and committees. Departments have mechanisms for distributing functions downward to groups and individuals in the chain of command. Committees, however, usually function by group activity across traditional lines.

There are different kinds of committees and groups, including the following: (1) standing committees, (2) design groups (or task forces), (3) groups based on organizational position and job function, (4) interdivisional committees, and (5) institutional or corporate committees.

STANDING COMMITTEES

The nurse executive reveals her operational definition of nursing in the selection of *standing committees*, for these committees represent the focal point of action in providing nursing services. The following demonstration model compares the standing committees of two hypothetical directors of nursing services to illustrate how standing committees reflect the concept of nursing. Analysis is limited to the three primary standing committees for each director (Table 11–1).

A comparison of the committee structures of the two hypothetical directors will show some clear differences. Executive A divides operations into products (things), procedures (actions), and patients (people). This is certainly a valid approach and tends to be rather comprehensive. In this approach, each sector is treated as a separate entity. In each case, the committee has a specific output that clearly belongs to it (e.g., a new product, a new procedure, a new care plan).

There is little if any confusion about committee tasks; the job of each group is clearly delineated. This is one of the greatest strengths of a division into things, actions, and people. Under this committee structure, a change by any one committee can produce the necessity for a change by another committee. A new product, for example, might require a new procedure, but each committee is still very clear as to its own particular function. The committee structure gives a view of nursing as being composed of a series of separate parts that, when added together, form the totality of nursing.

Table 11–1 Comparison of Committee Structures

Executive A	*Executive B*

I. Procedure Committee
  A. Evaluates ongoing nursing practices
  B. Reviews and updates the procedure manual
  C. Composes new procedures as needed to accommodate new equipment, new supplies, or advances in nursing
	I. Patient Care Evaluation Committee
	  A. Establishes criteria for evaluation of patient care
	  B. Conducts quality control checks of patient care
	  C. Conducts periodic nursing chart audits
	  D. Provides for feedback to the nursing units and to nursing administration

II. New Products Committee
  A. Assumes responsibility for keeping up to date on advances in equipment and supplies
  B. Arranges for demonstration of interesting new products
  C. Evaluates utility and cost of each new product and recommends acceptance or rejection
  D. Implements purchase of selected new products and introduces the products to appropriate staff members
	II. Patient Care Improvement Committee
	  A. Uses feedback from Patient Care Evaluation Committee, accident reports, and other available data as a basis for instituting changes in patient care
	  B. Identifies recurrent problems in patient care and seeks means of solving these problems
	    1. Identifies the care problem
	    2. Decides the appropriate avenues for solution
	    3. Institutes change
	  C. Serves as an advisory group to the nursing staff education section

III. Patient Care Committee
  A. Evaluates ongoing patient care
  B. Recommends changes in nursing care practices
  C. Evaluates and promotes patient safety
    1. Reviews accident/error reports
    2. Promotes safe working practices
    3. Promotes a biologically and physically safe environment
  D. Recommends needed educational programs
  E. Develops new tools for use in patient care
    1. Patient data forms
    2. Nursing care processing forms
	III. Nursing Systems Improvement Committee
	  A. Identifies problems in nursing delivery systems (examples: means of giving patient reports, means of assigning staff, means of distributing drugs)
	  B. Proposes solutions to delivery problems by modifying old systems or creating new ones
	  C. Plans and coordinates changes in nursing systems within the institution

Executive B has a different concept of nursing. She tends to view nursing as a process rather than as consisting of parts. Her committees seem to flow from each other; work of the Care Evaluation Committee naturally leads to the work of the Care Improvement Committee. Similarly, improving patient care will call for changes by the Nursing Systems Improvement Committee. All three of these committees may involve things, actions, and people. All three focus on processes. Some of the items that were *ends* for Executive A (products and procedures) here become *means* to the goals of Executive B.

For Executive A, two of three primary committees (new products and procedures) focus primarily on tasks. Her concept of nursing is that of a series of activities to be performed. For Executive B, however, two of three primary committees focus on the patient. Her concept of nursing reflects a need-oriented approach. Executive B starts with patient needs, whereas Executive A starts with nursing tasks.

This difference can be illustrated by comparing the approach to a new product that each chief nursing executive officer (CNEO) might take. For Executive A, a product is considered simply because it exists and has come to someone's attention; that is enough reason to evaluate it. Executive B, however, does not approach products this way. When a particular patient need is identified, she then has a criterion for a products search if a product is required to meet the need. In one system, the movement is from the product to the patient; in the other, it is reversed, from the patient to the product.

No one division of standing committees is right or wrong. There can be as many possible organizations of standing committees as there are different executives to think of them. The real question is whether the selected committee structure accurately mirrors the philosophy of nursing of the organization and provides for effective management. For example, an administrator who desires to implement a needs-oriented philosophy of nursing will have difficulty accomplishing this through a task-oriented committee system. Internal consistency among nursing concepts, divisional goals, and committee structure will simplify the work of the division.

DESIGN GROUPS

The *design group*, sometimes called the task force or project team, is a temporary committee, brought into existence to investigate and to propose solutions for a specific problem. The design group is a problem-solving, problem-oriented unit that ceases to exist once its problem is satisfactorily solved. Design groups tackle many different kinds of problems: administrative, procedural, interdepartmental, and patient-oriented. Indeed, they may be used for any problem that best can be solved by a select, informed group.

In some instances, a design group does not take a problem-solving approach but instead is appointed to enact a decision or strategy decided on at a higher level. Although the efforts of this group are controlled by the objective, the function is similar to that of a problem-oriented group.

The composition of the design group is dictated by the problem or goal itself. Those persons who have the most knowledge and experience to bring to bear on the subject are appointed to the committee. For example, a staff nurse with broad experience in restructured practice might be chairman of a committee investigating that system. Head nurses and supervisors might be among the committee members.

Because the goal of the design group is to apply the organization's best talents to a particular problem, no two task forces are likely to have a similar composition. Some design groups draw on resource people outside the nursing division or even the institution.

GROUPS BASED ON ORGANIZATIONAL POSITION AND JOB FUNCTION

Groups based on organizational position and function exist in most nursing divisions. A *head nurse group* and a *steering committee* of nurse managers are examples. In determining whether such groups should be formally designated, the nurse executive needs to evaluate the desirability of providing a vehicle for group cohesion and power. For example, a nursing executive might want her supervisors to meet regularly to promote problem solving. However, she might not want a committee of nursing assistants if she suspects it would provide a nucleus for unionization. Even if the power of a group is limited, its very existence as a formal body serves as a nucleus for demands and actions.

It is the prerogative of the nurse executive to decide what groups will exist and what amount of authority will be granted to them. A group is formally recognized when on-duty time is granted for its meetings and its proceedings are recorded as part of the division's permanent file.

Most nurse executives find it useful to create an administrative council to provide a source of communication and participative management. A few factors, however, should be considered in selecting the membership for this council:

1. Any group much larger than 10 or 12 in number seldom works as a single unit. Larger groups tend to break down into factions.

2. A group can comfortably combine persons with different functions if they share similar objectives.

3. The advantages of representation from nonmanagement groups against the efficacy of administrative privilege must be

weighed if the council is to be a group that will make administrative decisions and recommendations.

As with other committees, groups based on organizational position should exist only if they serve a useful purpose. For example, that an organization has always had a head nurse committee is not a good enough reason for maintaining one.

The functions of groups based on organizational position differ from the functions of regular committees. These ongoing groups typically monitor and respond to the changing work environment. They tend to be responsive to immediate administrative problems of diverse kinds and function to grease the wheels of the day-to-day operations. The content with which they deal varies greatly over time.

One function of groups whose members hold comparable jobs is the support, education, and role training of individual members. The output of such groups may be measured in the improved performance of individual members as well as in relation to specific group projects.

Evaluation of the group must take into account the assistance that it offers to individual members. Functions of information sharing, mutual support, and member education are seldom evidenced in minutes of such groups, so benefits for individual members must be assessed in other ways. One good evaluation method is surveying members or the nurse executive may periodically attend the meetings.

As discussed in Chapter 9, in many institutions the nursing staff forms a group for a shared governance model by creating a staff organization, operating with bylaws and other trappings of formal groups (e.g., rules and procedures). Sometimes, the formation of such a body becomes an issue when negotiating staff employment contracts. Nurse executives hold different positions on such groups. Some fear them as adversarial; others welcome them as a means for professionalizing nursing practice.

Typically, such staff organizations take on goals related to standards of nursing care. Sometimes they become self-policing bodies, decreasing the sources of unprofessional behavior. Indeed, many nurse executives encourage the creation of such a body when one does not exist.

In shared governance structures, it is important for the staff to know what they share and what they do not share. One of the greatest stumbling blocks in steering the staff through shared governance is to help the group understand its accountability.

INTERDIVISIONAL COMMITTEES

Nursing's participation in committees that cross divisional lines is critical. Usually interdivisional committees result when the following conditions arise: (1) when coordination of goals and activities is necessary, such as between service and education or among divisions working toward a common strategic plan, and (2) when recurrent problems occur because of conflicting goals or systems, as may occur between nursing and human resource departments.

Situational problems between two divisions can best be ironed out if members in interdivisional committees have first-hand experience with the problems. A head nurse can offer more insight on a proposed plan for altering tray service than can a nurse executive, for example.

In addition to the assigning of appropriate level personnel to interdivisional committees, the nurse executive must always consider that the division needs to put its best foot forward in interdivisional work. A committee member must be one who will impressively contribute and represent the best nursing has to offer.

The nurse executive also needs a certain sense of the political in appointing members to interdivisional meetings. If, for example, her organizational peers are members of a given committee, then it may be in her interest to represent nursing herself in that group. Similarly, if all non-nurse members are drawn from lower levels in the organization, it may be inappropriate for a nursing executive to fill the slot herself.

Nevertheless, there is no ironclad rule. Some issues may hold more importance for nursing, some less. The questions to be answered include: Who can best represent nursing? What is the importance of the issue? What are the powers and influence of the committee?

In joining an interdivisional committee, it is important that the executive consider the structure and power of the committee. Seldom will she want to bind herself to the decisions of such committees without qualification. Committee power to recommend is usually a safer policy.

INSTITUTIONAL OR CORPORATE COMMITTEES

The nurse executive must be assertive in seeing that the nursing division is represented on all the important decision-making committees of the institution or corporation. Sometimes, she will meet resistance to suggestions that nursing join such committees. Sometimes such membership may be negotiated by the executive when she assumes her position. In other instances, membership may be won by proving that nursing (and its informational input) is essential to the effective performance of the committee in question.

The nurse executive must be critical in her selection of members for such committees. They must be persons who will do their homework, representing nursing while maintaining the corporate perspective. The visibility of nursing on such committees can be a major factor in how others come to view nursing in the organization.

Sometimes, achievement of full committee rights is won step by step. It is better to have attending rights than no rights at all. Once nursing's presence is taken for granted, the executive is in a better position to press for more committee power. Attendance at medical committees and major administrative committees is essential, as is access to the institution's board. At the worst case, the nurse executive can expect to make several presentations to the board yearly. At best, the nurse executive may be a voting board member. Often, the reality falls between—with attendance without vote as a satisfactory compromise.

If the nurse executive has good relations with the chief executive officer, she will know that her position is only enhanced, not threatened, by invitation to be part of such critical meetings.

COMMITTEE EFFECTIVENESS

One common problem in committees is failure of members to acquire the necessary commitment. Committees are seen by some as add-on functions, not as critical as their day-to-day work. Leaders of committees must be given clear charges so that they understand their responsibility. Further, they must be able to communicate this sense of purpose to members. Reviewing committee achievements and requiring that the chairman submits reports of progress in addition to mere minutes is one administrative tool to keep a committee on target.

Sometimes, in attempting to give equal consideration to various factions, a dual leadership is created with cochairmen. But a committee that is the responsibility of more than one person may not be perceived as the responsibility of anyone in the long run. Usually, it is better to alternate chairmen than to split the chairmanship.

In addition to placing responsibility and holding leaders accountable, the executive needs to provide for effectiveness in the committee process. Simply put, leaders should be taught how to run an effective meeting. Many sources are available on how to run a meeting; every committee leader should be held responsible for learning the basics. In the best of all situations, the leader and all the members will be familiar with how groups work.

SUMMARY

Committee organization is one mechanism by which the nurse executive distributes the necessary activities of her division and contributes to the larger organization. Care is needed in selecting a system of committee work. The executive needs to keep committees productive and on target.

She also needs to understand the political implications of nursing's presence or absence on interdivisional and corporate committees. The performance of nursing in such committees has a major effect on how nursing is viewed in the rest of the organization.

SUGGESTED READINGS

Decker, P.J., and E.J. Sullivan, eds. 1992. *Nursing administration: A micro/macro approach for effective nurse executives.* Norwalk, Conn.: Appleton & Lange.

Grohar-Murray, M.E., and H.R. DiCroce. 1992. *Leadership and management in nursing.* Norwalk, Conn.: Appleton & Lange.

Jenkins, J.E. 1994. Professional governance: The missing link. In *Contemporary leadership behavior: Selected readings,* ed. E.G. Hein and M.J. Nicholson, 363–369. Philadelphia: J.B. Lippincott Co.

Marquis, B.L., and C.J. Huston. 1992. *Leadership roles and management functions in nursing.* Philadelphia: J.B. Lippincott Co.

Marquis, B.L., and C.J. Huston. 1994. *Management decision making for nurses: 118 case studies,* 2nd ed. Philadelphia: J.B. Lippincott Co.

Swansburg, R.C. 1990. Committees. In *Management and leadership for nurse managers,* ed. R.C. Swansburg, 298–322. Boston: Jones and Bartlett Publishers.

12

Restructured Practice

Virtually every major health delivery institution is restructuring its care delivery to meet today's environmental constraints. When a whole institution is not involved in a unified program of restructuring, most nursing divisions are restructuring on their own. No two institutions are restructuring in just the same pattern.

Just as the resource-driven model of care and strategic planning represent adaptations to today's environmental presses, so does restructured practice. The goal of this activity, as with the other two designs, is improved patient care capacity given the resources at hand.

Indeed, restructured practice represents one very special way of enacting a resource-driven model. Restructured practice evolved as nurse executives sought ways to keep quality of care high while getting optimal use from scarce resources. Although restructured practice typically begins in nursing, its effectiveness can be enhanced as other departments and divisions are brought into the plan.

One of the early factors forcing a change of care delivery models was a shortage of registered nurses (RNs) relative to the constantly increasing demand for their services. The shortage raised nursing salaries as supply-and-demand forces took over.

The final result was not anticipated by everyone. RN salaries rose precipitously just when the overall financial resources available to health care institutions were shrinking. The result was that institutions could no longer afford to maintain an ever-increasing number of RNs on staff. Indeed, the opposite happened. Many nurses were laid off, often replaced with less-expensive, less-prepared nonprofessional staff. The nation had moved from a real shortage of RNs available for hire to a shortage caused by the institution's inability to afford all those that it could effectively use.

What are the common threads in the restructuring of care? Almost all the restructuring plans involve a careful analysis of the tasks that must be accomplished to achieve the desired care goals and an equally careful assessment of who is able to do the requisite tasks.

Often, the decision concerning who can do what involves creating new jobs with new constellations of skills and educational requirements. The decisions involve looking anew at prior practices that reserved certain tasks for certain advanced levels of workers. In many cases, restructured practice involves adding one or more levels of workers to the lower end of the ladder of care personnel.

The chief principle underlying the restructuring tactic is not to use overqualified personnel for tasks that can be performed by lesser-skilled personnel. In many instances, this is achieved by combining tasks that may not have been combined formerly in the same role. When each task is looked at anew, the decision concerning who should do it has often been radically different than in the past.

RESTRUCTURED PRACTICE IN HISTORICAL CONTEXT

The easiest way to understand restructured practice is to contrast it with other nursing assignment systems as they have emerged over time. In the history of nursing, every new system has been offered as a solution to the limitations of its predecessor. After an initial flurry of enthusiasm for the newer system, its own flaws inevitably begin to emerge. A third design then is proposed to address these defects, and so the pattern continues.

Private Duty Model

From an historical perspective, nursing—even in hospitals—began with a private duty model. The old private duty nurse had exclusive responsibility for planning for and doing for one patient. In this sense, private duty was a highly patient-oriented system.

The duties of the nurse typically included around-the-clock care. Sometimes, the nurse slept on a cot in the patient's room. The pattern in the hospital and the private home were similar: one nurse, one patient. The patient orientation prevailed, not unlike private duty care in today's hospitals. This one-on-one pattern lasted until it proved dysfunctional during World War II. The war drew off large numbers of nurses to tend the troops, creating a subsequent civilian shortage of nurses.

Functional Model

To counteract the civilian nursing shortage, so-called functional nursing was conceived. As expected, it was the antithesis of the private duty model. What was the flaw in private duty? Why

did it no longer mesh with its environment? The homefront nursing shortage created a need for efficiency, a requirement that the few available nurses stretch further. It was achieved by shifting from a patient-oriented system to a task-oriented one.

At the time, functional nursing was hailed as a great invention. As enacted then, functional nursing was a simple form of task division. Instead of each nurse doing everything for one patient, tasks for patients on a unit were divided up. A medicine nurse could distribute pills to a whole floor of patients with greater efficiency than could 20 nurses separately setting up medications for their individual patients.

The functional model was the factory model. The system evolved roles such as medicine nurse, treatment nurse, bath giver, and bedmaker. The head nurse in this system was the linch pin that made the wheels move. He knew what everyone was doing and served to pass on new orders and to coordinate activities of the unit.

Eventually, several major flaws in the functional nursing system became evident, chief among them the fact that patient problems not fitting the categories (medicines, treatments, baths) tended to fall through the cracks. Also, some theorists proposed that patients suffered from personnel overload: Too many people came and went performing too many different tasks.

Another problem, some claimed, was that the nurse never had a sense of a finished product. He had tasks, not patients. It was not surprising when a new system arose to replace functional nursing.

Team Nursing Model

Team nursing was touted as the solution to all the flaws of the functional nursing system. With team nursing, nurses would have distinct products: patients (not unlike the old private duty model). The whole patient in his personhood, with all his needs, would be considered. He would no longer be a product on an assembly line. All this would take place because he would be exposed to fewer workers who know him better: the team.

With all its attempts to correct the flaws of functional nursing, team nursing did not escape the task-oriented design. Instead, a role shift occurred. Now, it was the team leader instead of the head nurse designating who would do what tasks.

The role of the head nurse in team nursing changed radically. Instead of being the coordinator of the unit, he turned into a consultant for clinical care and a management educator for team leaders. Most of the time, he worked through a subordinate managerial layer instead of directly with his staff.

In time, the flaws of team nursing were discovered, most of them related to the managerial and coordinating functions. Management had been pushed down the line from an experienced head nurse to a less experienced team leader, often a nurse not used to organizing people as a work team and not used to giving orders.

Although fewer personnel saw each patient, the coordinating activities actually increased because several people were involved with each patient without their roles and responsibilities being as clearly defined as they were in the old functional system. Hence the team leader was eternally deciding anew who would do what on any given day.

Coordination problems with other groups increased because team leaders often changed from day to day. Physicians, for example, never knew with whom to discuss patient orders. Questions from physicians, various technicians, and nurses themselves often were frustrated by the answer, "I don't know; he's not on my team."

Primary Nursing Model

It was inevitable that a new system would arise to replace team nursing. Primary nursing tried to resolve the coordination and management problems by returning to a patient-oriented rather than task-oriented work design. Namely, if a single nurse were responsible for a patient's care, then coordinating and assigning problems would be eliminated or radically decreased.

Primary nursing was accompanied by a thrust toward professional staffing as an ideal resolution to the task distribution problem. If only one nurse were responsible for a patient and he were educationally prepared for all care needs, then coordination needs fell away. Further, the problem of inexpert team leaders was resolved: They no longer existed; primary nurses reported directly to the head nurse.

In one sense, primary nursing was a return to the old private duty model, but that was only partially true. The old private duty nurse had sole responsibility for planning for and doing for her one patient. In contrast, the primary nurse had responsibility for a group of patients, and she shared the actual delivery of care with other staff. An average primary nurse was only present on the care unit for 40 or fewer hours of 158 per week. The realities forced the primary nursing model to shift from a care delivery model to a care planning and accountability model. Accountability and planning, not caregiving, remained her exclusive domains.

From a managerial perspective, the head nurse role shifted to a highly consultative model. Accurate assessment of the abilities of each primary nurse was essential because the system was only as good as were the primary nurses. The head nurse became arbiter for those systems where some RNs became second-class citizens (i.e., helpers instead of primary nurses with their own patient caseloads).

The primary nursing care model had a shorter pre-eminence than team nursing. Its flaws became evident rapidly when demands for fiscal constraint grew. The stage was set for change when today's nursing shortage brought about a crisis. Today's restructured practice—differentiated practice as some prefer to call it—was born.

Restructured Practice Model

Restructured practice returns to the task orientation of functional nursing. It does this for the sake of producing efficiency in a time of scarcity of resources. Given abundant resources, nurses always prefer a patient-oriented system. Only circumstances of privation bring about a retreat to a task-oriented system.

Yet, today's restructured practice tries to compensate for the task orientation by superimposing a patient-oriented system on top of the task design. The case manager or, in some cases, a primary nurse is responsible for keeping a sharp eye on assigned patients' outcomes. Hence the better restructured practice models of today are a blend of the two orientations: the patient and the task.

In all cases, restructured practice, like other resource-driven models, has involved a look at the interface between quality and quantity, a nitty-gritty estimate of what needs to be done. Yet, more than in any prior system, what needs to be done is determined by the desired results and performance.

And—more than in any prior system—the decisions concerning who will do what are up for reassessment. Finally, there is work concerning what decisions (and what sort of decisions) should be made by the various levels of workers.

Although restructured practice focuses on the nuts and bolts, it is the closest we have ever come to a system that balances outcomes (quality) and work load (quantity). It is also the most complicated system of care we have ever had—the most complicated for the staff nurse, for the head nurse, and for the nurse executive.

TODAY'S RESTRUCTURED MODELS

Two terms are often applied to today's care delivery revisions: *differentiated practice* and *restructured practice*. Although not everyone agrees on what these terms mean, many people use the terms interchangeably. Where people use the terms distinctively, they tend to use differentiated practice to refer to separate roles among RNs of different educational preparation and restructured practice to refer to patterns of practice that include other lower-level helper roles in addition to RNs.

The use of the term *differentiated practice* began as a label for a movement to reserve so-called professional nursing for the baccalaureate-prepared nurse. The differentiation envisioned was primarily between the Bachelor of

Science in Nursing (BSN) and the Associate Degree in Nursing (ADN)/diploma nurse. Advocates of this pattern desired to differentiate the work requirements of the two groups as a device to upgrade the professional standing of the BSN.

The call for differentiation was heard, but the practice was extended to the differences between what an RN and various aides and technicians could do. The term *restructured practice* grew in popularity to refer to this downward differentiation.

Whether one differentiates between these two terms (restructured practice and differentiated practice) or not, the principle remains the same: Assignments are made on the basis of the qualifications of the people who will do them. The higher the preparation, the more difficult the assigned tasks. The principle is one of safeguarding precious resources; in this case—as was true in functional nursing—the resource that is most husbanded is the time of the professional nurse.

Notice that in eras when nurses earn comparatively low wages and there is not a critical shortage, there is a tendency to use nurses as all-purpose workers. After all, they tend to have a good work ethic and they are self-monitoring. If they are not paid too well, they make great all-purpose workers—as Aiken (1990) has always asserted. The trend toward professional staffing pushed this strategy to the hilt and was successful just as long as nurses were plentiful enough to have their wages suppressed. With today's higher RN salaries, it no longer makes sense to pay them to do tasks requiring lower levels of knowledge and expertise.

Devising New Roles

The modes of restructured practice across this nation are diverse, interesting, and even, some would say, exciting. One of the most unique aspects is the way the pie of work is being sliced. In the old functional design, every institution had a similar division: a medicine nurse, a treatment nurse, and so forth. In restructured practice, each institution designs its own roles with its own tasks and skills. One of the things making for different patterns this time is nursing specialty practice, not merely differences in education but differences in practice patterns as well.

At one time in our history, a supervisor could pull a nurse from obstetrics and send her to a critical care unit, for example. The nurse might need a little guidance, but she would already have the essential skills. Today, that nurse would stare at the equipment, not knowing what to do with it. Specialism has occurred *de facto*.

From a managerial perspective, this means that nurses are not as flexible as they once were; their tasks are naturally segregated by specialism. If they cannot be used as interchangeable units, then there is nothing to be lost in defining them by their specialized work patterns.

Further, it was soon discovered that the less-prepared personnel who worked closely with nurses in specialized units could be taught tasks that were not appropriate for lower-level workers in a generalized practice setting. In essence, when tasks were examined anew, it was clear that some tasks previously seen as complex were not all that difficult in some limited settings.

While preventing standardization in practice and limiting the flexible use of staff, specialism has the charm of encouraging individual units to assess their unique practices to differentiate unit practice effectively. Indeed, when this individual analysis and work design are allowed, no two units may end up doing exactly the same thing in their practice scheme.

Many institutions are creating new classifications of workers, called everything from patient care technicians to environmental health workers. Every title imaginable is used except registered care technician, thanks to the fact that physicians proposed just such a role. Many of the positions are modified aide positions, often themselves reflecting specialism.

These technicians work directly for the head nurse in some units, for the staff nurse in others. In many institutions, there are two or more levels of technicians or, more common, different technician specialists for different units or services.

Many places, whether with RN-technician teams or with RN-licensed practical nurse (LPN) teams, use a variant of Manthey's (1988) paired-partners concept. The adaptations vary. *Paired partners* sometimes is used to mean that an RN has a permanent partner, LPN or nursing assistant, who invariably works with him. In other places, the partnership is between a senior nurse (BSN-prepared) and a junior nurse (ADN or diploma-prepared.) Where the luxury exists, the senior nurse may have a say in selecting his own partner. At the system's best, the permanent work team shares the same duty schedules. Other places apply *paired partners* more loosely, meaning that two people are assigned to work together on a given day.

Where the partnership is sustained, the RN is able to train the lower-level worker in what she wants done and how she wants it done, moving the concept of specialism to the lowest level. In this restructuring, certain tasks once seen as strictly professional can be performed safely by lower-level personnel if the number of such tasks is delimited and the training is carefully monitored.

Many factors are involved in deciding what tasks may be passed down. The complexity of the task is one. Yet, even a complex task may be passed along if it has little deviation from one patient to the next, providing the trainee is given adequate supervised experience with the procedure. One must also consider whether a procedure (or its interpretation in the case of a test) is likely to do harm if inexact.

Another question to be answered is whether the procedure is likely to require decision making or reorganizing during the procedure. In other words, are there intervening variables that may complicate the performance or interpretation of the procedure? Many procedures once seen as status granting, on further consideration, are seen to be repetitive and transferable to lower-level workers.

Sometimes differentiated practice occurs among different RN roles (e.g., an institution may differentiate what 2- and 3-year prepared nurses can do from what a 4-year baccalaureate nurse can do in clinical care). These institutions have enacted the original differentiated practice model.

In yet another application of differentiated practice and paired partners, a physician and an

RN are paired in specialty practice. Sometimes, this is called an advanced practice model. In the advanced practice model, the nurse member functions quite independently, with protocols negotiated and signed by her physician partner. The chief difference between this nurse and a primary nurse practitioner is that she functions in primary and secondary care but only in conjunction with one physician. The partnership is not unlike the RN-LPN or RN-technician partnerships in which the helper has an RN mentor. Typically, nurses in advanced practice with physicians have BSNs and 5 to 10 years of experience. In most places, they must have master's preparation, often with a nurse practitioner certification.

Imposing Outcomes Management

A more common differentiation in roles is between the clinical care nurse and the case manager. In this design, a case manager, usually a nurse, is responsible for seeing that all the patients in her caseload stay on recovery trajectories predetermined for their particular conditions. In effect, the case manager's job is to view the patient from the perspective of achieving his desired health outcomes. It becomes the case manager's role to intervene anywhere in the care process if these health outcomes are not being achieved.

A secondary function of the case manager is to make sure that the patient progresses as rapidly as possible. The recovery trajectories are determined with that goal in mind. Outcomes management, then, recognizes the fact that the most cost-effective management moves any given patient in and out of the system as rapidly as possible. Even if the diagnosis-related groups (DRGs) are replaced by other reimbursement schemes, the chief lesson learned under DRGs has been that length of stay is the most important variable in determining what it costs an institution to care for a patient.

Fortunately, the two aims of case management fit together nicely, namely, getting a patient well and achieving it as quickly as possible. That plan suits most patients, too.

In terms of structure, the case management role is usually but not always separate from both the direct care function and the utilization review function. The case manager uses critical pathways involving prescribed outcomes to be achieved for each patient within given time parameters. The case manager role is such an interesting new nursing role that it is examined in detail in Chapter 13.

Unless the case manager also is the direct caregiver, his presence on the unit means that there are two people, two chains of command, responsible for the same patient. Hence today's nursing unit functions in a matrix design. Matrix management requires management sensitivity and know-how far beyond the skills needed in a traditional hierarchical design.

Involving Others in Restructured Practice

Nor is the nursing department always isolated in the renewed task analysis and reassignment. Departments from pharmacy to social work to housekeeping and dietary services often participate in role reorganization.

In the prior era of professional staffing, many institutions paid for the costly privilege by eliminating various supportive personnel in non-nursing departments. Now, many of those roles (or modified ones) are being recreated.

In some cases, the functions of these support roles are being blended along with other tasks into nurse technician roles. In other cases, the roles may be restructured while remaining in a support service outside the nursing division.

SUMMARY

Whether just in the nursing division or institutionwide, the *greatest reorganization* taking place in restructured practice is *skill mix reassessment*. The new designs assume a long-term shortage of nurses and aim to preserve the limited time of all registered nurses, freeing them for complex direct care and essential decision making. In most care settings, this means creating new and different subordinate roles.

Restructured practice arises primarily as a response to scarce resources. The chief scarcity is that of professional nurse time, a scarcity created by the increasing wages of nurses and nurse specialists more often than by the inability of an organization to recruit nurses. Simply put, institutions that can only afford a limited number of high-priced professionals learn to develop less-educated levels of workers.

Nursing's ideologies, interestingly, have always changed to fit the times. Indeed, we have been remarkably flexible: changing our patterns of practice to get the most that is possible out of any given era. Restructured care is today's answer. Tomorrow's care designs will be the result of the circumstances that pertain in tomorrow's world.

REFERENCES

Aiken, Linda H. 1990. Charting the future of hospital nursing. *Image* 22, no.2: 72–78.

Manthey, M. 1988. Primary practice partners: A nurse extender system. *Nursing Management* 19, no.3:58–59.

SUGGESTED READINGS

Anderson, R. 1993. Nursing leadership and healthcare reform. Part III: Nurse executive role in a reformed healthcare system. *Journal of Nursing Administration* 23, no.12:8–9.

Bolster, C.J. 1991. Work redesign: More than rearranging furniture on the Titanic! *Aspen's Advisor for Nurse Executives* 6, no.11:4–7.

Bostrum, J., and J. Zimmerman. 1993. Restructuring nursing for a competitive health care environment. *Nursing Economics* 11, no.1:35–41.

Brett, J.L.L., and M.C. Tonges. 1990. Restructured patient care delivery: Evaluation of the ProACT model. *Nursing Economics* 8, no.1:36–44.

Bunkers, S. 1992. The healing web: A transformative model for nursing. *Nursing and Health Care* 13, no.2:68–73.

Curran, C. 1991. An interview with Karlene M. Kerfoot. *Nursing Economics* 9, no.3:141–147.

Dienimann, J., and T. Gessner. 1992. Restructuring nursing care delivery systems. *Nursing Economics* 10, no.4:253–258.

Goertzen, I.E., ed. 1990. *Differentiating nursing practice into the twenty-first century.* Kansas City, Mo.: American Academy of Nursing.

Hastings, C., et al. 1992. Professional practice partnerships: A new approach to creating high performance nursing organizations. *Nursing Administration Quarterly* 17, no.1:45–54.

Jones-Schenk, J., and P. Hartley. 1993. Organizing for communication and integration. *Journal of Nursing Administration* 23, no.10:30–33.

Kovner, C.T., et al. 1993. Changing the delivery of nursing care: Implementation issues and qualitative findings. *Journal of Nursing Administration* 23, no.11:24–34.

Larson, J. 1992. The healing web—A transformative model: Part II. *Nursing and Health Care* 13, no.5:246–252.

Lengacher, C.A., et al. 1993. Redesigning nursing practice: The partners in patient care model. *Journal of Nursing Administration* 23, no.12:31–37.

Smith, P., et al. 1994. Planning for patient care redesign: Success through continuing quality improvement. *Journal of Nursing Care Quality* 8, no.2:73–80.

Sovie, M. 1992. Care and service teams: A new imperative. *Nursing Economics* 10, no.2:94–100.

Tonges, M.C. 1989. Redesigning hospital nursing practice: The professionally advanced care team (ProACT) model, Part 1. *Journal of Nursing Administration* 19, no.7:31–38.

Tonges, M.C. 1989. Redesigning hospital nursing practice: The professionally advanced care team (ProACT) model, Part 2. *Journal of Nursing Administration* 19, no.9:19–22.

Tonges, M.C., and E. Lawrenz. 1993. Reengineering: The work redesign-technology link. *Journal of Nursing Administration* 23, no.10:15–22.

Yancer, D. 1990. Redesigning the work. *Aspen's Advisor for Nurse Executives* 5, no.8:4–5.

13

Case Management

Case management, the newest role to develop in nursing, is a series of structural strategies designed to control health care costs and decrease length of stay while preserving quality of care. Indeed, many would argue that case management can greatly improve care while achieving substantial cost savings.

Case management usually is comprised of the care of an individual through the duration of an illness. It is a system in which a patient's case is managed and coordinated for the entire health episode by a single person, usually a nurse, who is accountable for his pattern of care and its outcome.

In some health delivery systems, patients with chronic health conditions or known high risk for given health problems may be case-managed for a lifetime.

Case management aims to

1. allow for collaborative practice and planning among all health care professionals involved in a patient's case
2. focus on outcomes achievement
3. foster early discharge from health care facilities and programs
4. increase efficient use of health care resources
5. improve professional satisfaction with practice

CASE MANAGER ROLE

Case managers are typically, but not exclusively, registered nurses. In some models, social workers (or social work aides) fill the role. In other models, physicians are case managers. However, the vast majority of case managers are nurses for very practical reasons.

First, it is easier for nurses to incorporate into their knowledge the additional elements of case management than it is for other role players to do so. For example, a nurse can learn available community resources quicker than a social worker can learn the pathology and care elements already known by physicians and nurses. And physicians often are ill-prepared by their education to incorporate social/social work aspects of care.

Further, few physicians are interested in becoming case managers because these are organizational roles rather than independent practice, not to mention the economic considerations. Institutions, of course, want effective case managers at the lowest cost possible.

The nurse, then, is an ideal candidate for case management, and most find it a rewarding role, calling on all their nursing knowledge and skills. Most case managers, whether or not their roles involve hands-on care, believe that they are actively practicing nursing in their case management role.

CHANGES FOSTERING DEVELOPMENT OF CASE MANAGEMENT

Case management grew out of a series of separate but related changes in the nature of health care management, namely, the increased use of outcome measures, use of diagnosis-related groups (DRGs), growth of managed care, and initiation of restructured practice. Although it is difficult to separate these influences, we do so for purposes of discussion, beginning with outcome measures.

Outcome Measures

Nursing's quality control systems have always been among the best in health care. Although the Joint Commission on Accreditation of Healthcare Organizations (JCAHO) and most boards of health were still using structure standards (mostly focused on aspects of how a health care institution was organized), nursing already had moved into use of process standards (especially standards dealing with what the nurse did to, for, and with the patient).

The next logical step after process standards was to develop outcome standards, especially those specifying the interim and final outcome states desired in the patient. Many nursing settings had begun to incorporate outcome standards into their quality assurance tools long before these standards became popular with other constituencies. Case management simply carries forth on this outcomes focus, that is, organizing a patient's care with an eye on his eventual health status.

Diagnosis-Related Groups

The reimbursement system using DRGs focused on controlling costs and created an economic incentive for hospitals and other health care providers. Providers soon discovered that the most effective way to cut costs in any given case, whatever its DRG classification, was to decrease the patient's length of stay (LOS). This fact will continue to influence system operations even when (and if) the DRG system is replaced (as is already happening in some locations).

LOS is dependent on the patient's recovery or recuperation—and the related ability of the institution to pass the patient along to a step-down care facility or home care. Each agency, in turn, profits by moving the patient to a lower level of care (elsewhere) if it receives a set fee for a case irrespective of the length of stay. LOS and costs are shortened, therefore, if a patient's outcome, his achievement of a desired level of recuperation, occurs at the earliest possible time.

Although the system aims to push the patient through each facility (acute, long-term, or skilled care) rapidly, this also benefits the patient by enhancing the overall pace of his recovery. Decreased LOS suits everyone: providers, payers, and patients. Case management, by considering how each day contributes to the patient's ultimate recuperation and discharge, serves this goal.

When DRGs were first put in place, some institutions made inappropriate early discharges, resulting in patients' readmittance. Subsequently, penalties were put in place to correct for these poor judgment calls, preventing an institution from collecting twice by readmitting a patient who should never have been discharged. Case management looks to an early, but not premature, discharge.

Managed Care

DRGs and a cost-controlled health care system forced organizations to rethink the way care was delivered. In this burst of rethinking, many new systems were designed. Most of the new structures used some form of managed care. Sometimes, the notions of case management and managed care get confused. Managed care is the larger concept of which case management is often one strategy.

Managed care is a collection of strategies used by insurers and providers to influence health care decisions. It helps people know when they need care, helps them get that care, and controls the care. The most common forms include health maintenance organizations (HMOs), preferred provider organizations (PPOs), and independent practice associations (IPAs). In all these arrangements, price is controlled by contract arrangements and discounts or by strategies that keep the subscribers healthier (i.e., less likely to require costly acute care). Chapter 1 provided a brief orientation to various managed care forms.

Even when providers are not prescribed by the patient's coverage, more insurance carriers are limiting the amount they will pay for a given condition. In effect, the insurance policy exerts great influence on the patient's choice of provider. If, for example, the insurer will not pay for a hip replacement performed in Hospital X because the institution's rates are deemed too high, then the patient's choice is limited: to bear part of or all his own costs or go to an institution approved by the insurance carrier. The same principle may apply to which physicians are approved for what procedures under what policies.

Managed care is a series of strategies designed to control and constrain costs for payers as well as to protect the quality of care. Managed care usually is initiated by insurers and employers to get better care for the dollar in the light of constantly increasing health care costs. Managed care has several objectives:

1. less loss of work time by the employee
2. fewer and shorter hospitalizations
3. less costly health care

Some aspects of managed care may resemble what used to be called occupational health—with health education, routine exercise, weight and stress reduction, smoking cessation, and other health maintenance programs in the workplace. Other aspects look like public health nursing—with case finding and monitoring, especially for employees or subscribers who have the conditions known to be costly to treat in their acute manifestations. Many case managers within the industrial work world focus on pre-crisis care in their managed care plans.

Companies enter managed care because it pays. Insurers, at one time hand-in-glove with the medical community, have changed their tune in today's economy. Now, payers seek less costly ways of providing care if they are available. This has worked to nursing's advantage. In managed care, one now sees direct payment for nurses operating in traditional institutions and nurse-run agencies such as nursing homes, hospice care, and home care facilities. Alternate settings, alternate providers, and less costly preventive care have great appeal to insurers under economic restraints.

In essence, managed care interposes a third party between the physician and the patient in deciding what will be done. Decisions are reached only after considering prevention, lifetime health care management, and total costs.

Restructured Practice

The most important factor fostering the growth of case management is its intrinsic part in restructured practice. The reader is referred to Chapter 12 for a discussion of restructured practice. Restructured practice is a task-oriented delegation system in which assignment of duties is distributed according to the level of preparation and special training of each involved worker. The plan may be limited to a nursing department or extended to include workers in other departments.

Inevitably, restructured practice involves looking anew at the work to be done, and that in turn results in creation of new roles with unique task constellations. The roles are designed to get the job done most efficiently. Restructured practice has been nursing's response to the continued demands for economic stringency combined with decreased numbers of professional nurses being hired.

Given today's technology, the complexity of a task-oriented system begged for a unifying thread to connect the pieces together, and this was provided by the case management concept.

However the role is devised (and there are many different plans), the case manager superimposes a patient orientation on top of the system's inherent task orientation, making sure the patient does not get lost among the many activities assigned to diverse workers. Case management becomes the glue that holds restructured practice together.

FORMS OF CASE MANAGEMENT

Case management takes place under many structural arrangements. Providers for case management include

1. a separate business selling case management services
2. a subsidiary of a corporation whose business is not health
3. a subsidiary or department of an insurance company
4. a subsidiary of a health care organization that manages total patient care (e.g., HMOs and PPOs)
5. a separate department in an acute care hospital or other health care facility
6. a separate department within nursing
7. regular, decentralized departments of a nursing division that have assumed the case management function
8. nursing units with one or more case managers per patient unit
9. a bedside nurse who is expected to perform case management functions within her care role

Case management started in many nursing organizations as a nursing strategy to improve quality of care. Some organizations reported use of the role even before DRGs and restructured practice came on the scene. In these organizations, case management arose as a natural part of an outcomes management focus.

More recently, case management has grown as a payer response to expensive health care. Companies (business employers and health insurers) discovered that certain employees/policy holders accounted for a substantial portion of the health service given. These patients, if case managed, incurred less costly care.

Companies such as American Telephone and Telegraph and Chrysler, as well as insurers such as Kaiser Permanente, got into the case management business early on.

Systems using case management now are found nationwide, including such organizations as New York Hospital, Robert Wood Johnson Hospital, Tucson Medical Center, Pacifi Care in Southern California (an HMO), Alcoa of Tennessee (nonhealth business), and the Center for Nursing Case Management, New England Medical Center, Massachusetts (a separate for-profit subsidiary).

Although case management systems differ in their statistical data, often the patients identified as most likely to incur extra costs are those with acquired immunodeficiency syndrome (AIDS) and the elderly population (Cohen and Cesta 1993). Those with circulatory problems and genitourinary infections, as well as those subject to substance abuse and psychiatric problems, are frequently cited also.

Whatever the high-cost groups, with case management, they can be monitored continuously (e.g., receive routine blood pressure checks or urine testing for drug usage). With appropriate preventive measures, expensive acute episodes can be avoided. Many systems also include education and motivation plans as essential parts of prevention as well as ongoing monitoring.

Many businesses with a managed care system use a case management approach. Which employees, clients, or patients get case managed, of course, depends on the system and the circumstances. From a payer's perspective, both the high-risk employee and the employer benefit from the ongoing case tracking and management.

Who gets case managed may vary even in the traditional setting of the acute care hospital. Some hospitals case manage every patient. Often institutions initiate case management condition by condition, starting with health care problems that are easily plotted on recovery trajectories, that is, conditions (diagnoses and/or treatments) in which there is little variance in treatment and recuperation patterns among patients.

Other institutions only case manage patients with health problems that are long and involve expensive regimens of care. Patients with conditions not ordinarily insured may be another target of case management, as may be patients with conditions that ultimately require interface with other organizations (e.g., home care services or nursing homes).

Some institutions do not put a patient on case management until a protocol for care has been established (a path for recovery expectations designed by critical pathways or other mapping devices). In other institutions, patients with conditions lacking standardized case management plans are placed on individualized plans derived by the case manager, often with input from various professionals.

PROCESS OF CREATING CASE TRAJECTORIES

In the best situations, recovery trajectories are determined by the various professions working together. In the collaborative practice model, at the very least nursing, medicine, and social work are involved in determining case maps or pathways.

In a joint committee, often under the leadership of a director of case management, each participant defines the current practices of his profession and examines the outcomes and practices leading to them. Obviously, these outcomes may vary from institution to institution and from community to community, in the light of the local situation and standards of practice. The identified patient outcomes become part of the map or trajectory for the case management protocol.

When necessary, trajectories can be individualized and modified for each patient, but the normative patterns guide outcomes management. It is up to the case manager to ensure that the patient stays on the path as his case progresses.

Group consensus in creating the case trajectories promotes productive communications among disciplines. In most cases, initial resistance to case management is overcome when the professionals see better results for patients.

The initial work of the director of case management is to get the cooperation required to produce the case trajectories. That established, periodic reviews will keep the trajectories updated.

After such groundwork has been laid, the function of the case manager becomes continuous monitoring of assigned patients for deviances from their plotted recuperation trajectories. When a deviance occurs, the case manager seeks out the causes, discusses it with the appropriate professionals, seeks solutions to obstacles, and alters the plan of care to achieve the desired outcomes.

Critical pathways are the most common way in which case trajectories are displayed. Each day of an illness or a given condition is marked with the key events of care and the expected levels of recuperation. Patient outcome statements are usually correlated with the expected professional interventions. Some institutions prefer to develop their care trajectories in grids or maps. However the case management details are displayed, they tell who should do what when correlated with the patient's interim and final desired outcome states. If case management is isolated to the nursing function, the managed care map may form the basis for the nursing care plan.

RESISTANCE

Any time a new role is created, there is resistance from many quarters. Physicians, in particular, may resist a third party intervening between them and their patients. But if the case manager proves her effectiveness in improving patient outcomes, attitudes soon change.

Nurse resistance may equal or exceed physician resistance when case management is initiated. For example, the head nurse may resent another authority figure, the case manager, on her unit. The head nurse may feel threatened if the case manager has the power to decree, "This isn't working, let's try that." Staff nurses may believe that the authority of the case manager infringes on the autonomy of their practice.

The easiest way to surmount resistance to case management is to institute the system slowly, unit by unit, starting with cases for which trajectories have been carefully mapped. Nothing succeeds like success, and soon units without case management begin to demand it for their patients, too.

DURATION OF SERVICES

The duration of case management service varies in different institutions. In the acute care institution, it often extends from initial hospitalization to discharge. Other organizations may be prepared to case manage from case finding through the end of the illness episode or into a permanent monitoring plan for those with chronic diseases. Often, the extent of case management is related to the reimbursement system and the goals of the organization using case managers. As mentioned earlier, case managers are found in many settings.

MODELS OF CASE MANAGEMENT

There are many successful arrangements for case management. Indeed, any institution must decide what model will work most effectively in its unique setting. A few common designs are presented here.

One popular case management model is unit-based, with a single nurse filling the primary nurse and case manager roles simultaneously. This person is responsible for patient care from admission to discharge (or later), with emphasis on LOS, writing the nursing care plan and the nursing orders, and delegating to care associates on all shifts. This model has the advantage of using assignment patterns closest to those already in effect in many places. In essence, the case manager in this model is not too different from the primary nurse except for the strong focus on outcomes.

Other models separate caregiving and case management. The case management role shifts to a planning/evaluating mode and is less associated with direct caregiving. As with the direct care model, the case manager in this design is responsible for a patient's care and related outcomes throughout the entire episode of illness, no matter who delivers the actual care.

Sometimes, nurse case managers are linked with case-specific attending physicians. Sometimes, the caseload is determined based on geography, keeping a nurse's caseload on one or a limited number of units. Other criteria are possible, of course, ranging from assignment according to nursing specialty to assignment simply based on admissions and discharges. One model is presented in detail just to illustrate the decisions that need to be made in putting a plan in place.

ProACT Plan, Robert Wood Johnson Hospital, New Brunswick, New Jersey

The ProACT plan (Tonges 1989a,b) involves three separate registered nurse roles: the head nurse, the primary nurse, and the clinical care manager (the case manager). Licensed practical nurses (LPNs) and nurses' aides are also used in direct care. This plan called for expansion of clinical and nonclinical support services, employing hosts at the unit level. As the title choice indicates, the host role is envisioned as patient-oriented rather than unit-oriented (like the older ward manager role).

The clinical care manager (case manager) orchestrates the entire hospital stay for a caseload of patients on the same unit, coordinating with physicians, nursing staff, and other professionals to ensure that patient outcomes are achieved in established time frames.

The clinical care manager assesses each patient before admission, provides clinical consultation for primary nurses, and has 24-hour accountability for patients in her caseload. She assesses each patient's progress throughout his hospital stay. Also, she plans for his discharge and for necessary discharge teaching.

Approximately three clinical care managers operate on each unit, with a caseload of 10 to 11 patients each. The salary range for this case manager role falls between that of the head nurse and assistant head nurse. In the ProACT plan, the clinical care manager is accountable to the head nurse of her unit.

The primary nurse in this plan manages the patient's care on a 24-hour basis, participating in direct and indirect care delivery. She assesses her patients each shift, delegating tasks to LPNs and aides. Her caseload of patients changes only as patients are admitted or discharged.

The head nurse in this model has the traditional managerial responsibility, coordinating the work of all the nursing staff, including primary nursing, clinical care managers, and others.

IMPLEMENTING A CASE MANAGEMENT SYSTEM

Many steps are involved in implementing a case management system. The first step is researching alternate systems and setting goals for one's own system. For example, a different design might be selected if the system were planned specifically to achieve budget saving versus a plan focused primarily on improving care.

Whatever the system goals, it is important to determine projected costs from the start. Even when the objectives of the system do not focus on economy, one should have an idea of whether the plan is budget neutral, adds costs, or saves money. Keeping track of system costs also keeps advocates from developing unrealistic systems.

Next, one must identify proper candidates for case management. In some models, every patient is case-managed; in others, only patients with conditions for which case trajectories have been designed. By this time in history, many institutions have protocols for almost all likely patient conditions.

Deciding which conditions/patients need case management requires decisions tailored to the institution's needs and its patient populations. Often, the most common or the most costly cases are the first targeted.

Gaining the acceptance of higher (often corporate) management is a necessity if case management is to be initiated successfully. Corporate management should be kept informed from the outset and as each step of the system is devised. Approval from the top is essential in gaining the cooperation of other groups and individuals who must interface with the case managers and the case management system.

A careful "needs to know" assessment will ensure that no one critical to the system or its success is left in the dark. Any major change in a nursing system involves many other departments. To implement a major change such as case management requires that one cast a wide net and consider carefully all who will be affected. The nurse executive cannot consider the installation of case management as a change merely internal to the nursing division.

Implementing the plan is the next step, usually starting on a trial unit or with one or more patient groups. In any change of this magnitude, there will be problems and glitches. Starting small allows these failures to be corrected on a small scale rather than having a negative effect on the larger system. Even when the test units are working satisfactorily, evaluation should be continuous as the system grows.

CASE MANAGEMENT AND BED UTILIZATION REVIEW

In one respect, the case manager role is the mirror opposite of the old bed utilization role. Whereas the utilization nurse focused on the institutional task of releasing beds in an organization that tended to be patient-oriented, the case manager imposes a patient-oriented design on an organization that tends to be task-oriented.

The utilization review role was often after the fact (i.e., a retrospective evaluation when census data revealed a patient with a long LOS). In contrast, case management occurs during the fact (i.e., it involves ongoing case monitoring and management). Case management is prospective, concurrent, and retrospective, designed to change ongoing care not just to promote the discharge of patients who have been in the system a long time. Utilization review, at least the early versions of it, focused on the bed; case management focuses on the patient.

More modern utilization review professionals may work closely with case managers, their roles designed to complement each other.

EDUCATION FOR CASE MANAGERS

With the growing popularity of the case manager role, nursing schools have been quick to set up master's level programs leading to a degree in case management. An interested prospective student should survey various programs to see what sorts of knowledge are identified as case management requisites. As yet, there is no universally accepted curriculum.

Some schools prefer not to prepare nurses for this role, claiming that case management skills are inherent in any good master's degree program. The danger of a degree that is tightly role-related, of course, is that the degree may become obsolete if the delivery system should change, eliminating that role.

Case managers will be needed as long as restructured practice is the practice design, but no practice pattern lasts forever. When social and political patterns change, care delivery models are likely to change, too. Still, what has been learned in a focus on outcomes management is likely to be incorporated, in some form, in subsequent delivery systems.

SUMMARY

Case management is an outgrowth of many factors, especially the increasing focus on outcomes of care in the light of the continuing need to constrain costs. Outcomes assessment has entered the value system of not only the care delivery system but of the agencies evaluating health care organizations as well. This fact ensures that institutions will be directing attention to outcomes.

Case management is a feedback/control system superimposed on a task-oriented system,

creating management by matrix rather than by hierarchy. The role has the merit of joining together diverse health care providers in a common focus: the patient's outcome.

Case management represents a new and unique opportunity for nursing. Case managers (usually nurses) have become important players in the organization because of their bridging function and their control over system inputs and outputs.

Although the specific forms of case management—and the role design for all involved parties—may change with time, it is unlikely that the focus on patient outcomes will lose its position in the center of the health care system and its values.

REFERENCES

Cohen, E.L., and T.G. Cesta. 1993. *Nursing case management: From concept to evaluation.* St. Louis: C.V. Mosby Co.

Tonges, M.C. 1989a. Redesigning hospital nursing practice: The professionally advanced care team (ProACT) model, Part 1. *Journal of Nursing Administration* 19, no.7:31–38.

Tonges, M.C. 1989b. Redesigning hospital nursing practice: The professionally advanced care team (ProACT) model, Part 2. *Journal of Nursing Administration* 19, no.9:19–22.

SUGGESTED READINGS

Applebaum, R. 1990. *Long-term care case management.* New York: Springer Publishing Co., Inc.

Del Togno-Armanasco, V., et al. 1993. *Collaborative nursing case management.* New York: Springer Publishing Co., Inc.

Enthoven, A. 1988. Managed care of alternative delivery systems. *Journal of Health Politics, Policy and Law* 13, no.2:304–321.

Fralic, M.F. 1992. The nurse case manager: Focus, selection, preparation, and measurement. *Journal of Nursing Administration* 22, no.11:13–14, 46.

Giuliano, K.K., and C.E. Poirier. 1991. Nursing case management: Critical pathways to desirable outcomes. *Nursing Management* 22, no.3:52–55.

Hicks, J., et al. 1992. Nursing challenges in managed care. *Nursing Economics* 10, no.4:265–276.

LeClaire, C.L. 1991. Introducing and accounting for RN case management. *Nursing Management* 22, no.3:44–49.

Lijon, J.C. 1993. Models of nursing care delivery and case management: Classification of terms, *Nursing Economics* 11, no.3:163–169.

Lulavage, A. 1991. RN-LPN teams: Toward unit nursing case management. *Nursing Management* 22, no.3:58–61.

Mahoney, K. 1992. Case management lessons from a public/private partnership to finance long-term care. *Journal of Case Management* 1, no.1: 22–25.

Marschke, P., and M.T. Nolan. 1993. Research related to case management. *Nursing Administration Quarterly* 17, no.3:16–21.

Michaels, C. 1991. A nursing HMO—10 months with Carondelet St. Mary's Hospital-based nurse case management. *Aspen's Advisor for Nurse Executives* 6, no.11:1, 3–4.

Newman, M.A., et al. 1991. Nurse case management: The coming together of theory and practice. *Nursing and Health Care* 12, no.8:404–408.

Pierog, L.J. 1991. Case management: A product line. *Nursing Administration Quarterly* 15, no. 2:16–20.

Possin, B. 1991. A consortium introduces RN case management regionwide. *Nursing Management* 22, no.3:62–64.

Quinn, J. 1993. *Successful case management in long-term care.* New York: Springer Publishing Co., Inc.

Redford, L. 1992. Case management the wave of the future. *Journal of Case Management* 1, no.1:5–8.

Ritter, J., et al. 1992. Redesigned nursing practice: A case management model for critical care. *Nursing Clinics of North America* 27, no.1:119–128.

Rogers, M., et al. 1991. Community-based nursing case management pays off. *Nursing Management* 22, no.3:30–34.

Savarese, M., and C.M. Weber. 1993. Case management for persons who are homeless. *Journal of Case Management* 2, no.1: 3–8.

Tahan, H. 1993. The nurse case manager in acute care settings: Job description and function. *Journal of Nursing Administration* 23, no.10:53–61.

Wilson, A.A. 1993. The cost and quality of patient outcomes: A look at managed competition. *Nursing Administration Quarterly* 17, no. 4:11–16.

Zander, K. 1988. Nursing case management: Strategic management of cost and quality outcomes. *Journal of Nursing Administration* 18, no.5:23–30.

Zander, K. 1990. Differentiating managed care and case management. *Definition* (Newsletter for Center for Nursing Case Management, Inc., South Natick, Massachusetts) 5, no.2:1.

Part IV

Building the Culture and the Values

Underneath the nursing division and the organization lie many shared and unique values systems. A health care organization has many parts and many people—boards, professionals, nonprofessional workers, consumers, and communities. The lifeways of those who work in a health care institution represent diverse ways of thinking, multiple cultures, and different attitudes toward people, illness, and the process of work itself.

In such an environment, it is a challenge to find common ground. Yet, if a shared value system can be developed, an organization has a good foundation on which to build. Sometimes, the only possible goal may be to develop a respect for diverse values and beliefs and the patterns arising out of them.

In a sense, it is artificial to pull out a section of this book labeled values because the underlying values affect everything that happens in an organization—the goals it selects, the methods by which it approaches its goals, the ways it manages problems, and the way it treats its clients and its employees.

Nevertheless, in Part III, we examine some of the basic values issues, not to isolate them but to throw light on their importance. Chapter 14 looks at values-based leadership asking, What can the leader do to make evident his underlying

values? Can a culture be designed to foster certain values over others? Is it better simply to let values emerge? Or can the emergence of desired values be fostered and clarified?

Chapter 15 takes a closer look at ethical issues, specifically those that have an effect on care and care decisions. This chapter also discusses the effect of so-called new age values on nursing care.

Chapter 16 examines staff empowerment. A strong commitment to staff empowerment is a value that characterizes many nursing cultures today. In truth, one could justify placing staff empowerment under many titles in this book. It constitutes a part of how a nursing division is organized—effectively conceived, staff empowerment contributes to productivity—and it certainly relates to goals and outcomes. The notion that staff *should* be empowered is itself a value judgment, but one on which there is much agreement.

Values, then, form an integral part of nursing administration and, like other aspects of the work, are better analyzed and applied than overlooked. Often in a resource-restricted environment, a commitment to values is tested in difficult ways not found in times of more abundant resources. Limited resources call for tough decisions, decisions that do not please everyone.

Add to that the dilemmas raised by ever-increasing technological possibilities for care and the emergent concerns of this society over the quality of human life and we come to appreciate the important role of values in our modern organizations.

14

Values-Based Leadership

All organizations have cultures. Some of these cultures have been practically planned and developed as part of a values-based organizational development plan to create the kind of culture necessary to achieve the strategic mission and vision. Other organizations have cultures that developed without any direction. These cultures evolve over time as influential staff establish the values and key operating principles within the organization.

In some organizations, many little cultures exist side by side without any overriding framework that pulls the separate cultures together. In these situations, turf wars are the inevitable outcome of self-serving cultures that have been allowed to grow independently.

INFLUENCE OF NURSING ON THE VALUES CULTURE

In most of our institutions, the nursing division is so extensive that its characteristics have a major influence on the total organizational culture. When the managerial and caregiving cultures are in conflict, an organization has severe problems. We discuss the more positive case here, the one in which the nurse executive has influence in both directions: downward to the care giving components of the facility and upward to the corporate management staff.

One major factor in developing the culture of the organization is the role modeling that the nurse executive provides. She must be acutely conscious of the messages she sends to the organization. These verbal and nonverbal messages go far in determining the culture of the organization. Just as staff nurses in the units take on the characteristics of the nurse manager, so the organization is likely to take on the characteristics the nurse executive models.

Values drive people and organizations. If the nurse executive's leadership is based on positive values, over time the organization will assimilate these characteristics. If the nurse executive lacks integrity or trust, so will the organization. As the nurse executive actualizes her role, so the organization will actualize similar values and characteristics in building the culture—barring the strong influence of contradictory values from higher powers.

Basic to her success are the values on which the practice of the nurse executive and the resultant culture are based. Highly articulated values with potential to become shared values in the organization form the underpinnings of the nursing program. The mature nurse executive will have carefully thought through the values by which she lives and those by which she practices.

Through a process of values clarification and the eliciting of shared values, the organization can come to a foundation of values around which the organization forms itself. When there is a set of shared values, decisions are easier. In a tricky situation at 2:00 A.M. in the morning, for example, the staff know what to do because they know the foundation on which the practice of the facility is based.

For example, if a shared value is that of integrity, the staff nurse will know that certain information must be shared with a patient to ensure informed consent. Other values, such as always striving for excellence rather than just doing whatever is necessary to just get by, can become the basis on which a program is built. It is important that such values be identified and shared by all.

Staff come from many backgrounds and belief systems. The newly hired staff person will be socialized into the value system of the organization either through a conscious effort of the orientation program or through an informal process on the job. If values can be articulated early and the new staff can share these values, a highly productive team can be developed quickly.

Even within the overall pattern of shared values, subtle differences will evolve. Various units will develop unique value structures. On one unit, for example, the value of a collegial supportive relationship may be fostered whereas it is not so valued on another.

Within a nursing organization, many different kinds of people come together to deliver patient care. Nurses with different personalities tend to gravitate to units that fit their preferences. For example, one can see a basic difference between rehabilitation nurses and cardiovascular/intensive care nurses. They share very different idealized versions of the kind of patient care that is personally satisfying. Compared with each other, they share very unique views of how to provide patient care.

In most institutions, it is possible to contrast the work values between these two units. In rehabilitation units, multiple disciplinary teamwork with much group thinking and planning is usually valued. In high-acuity cardiovascular/intensive care units, often the nursing staff values autonomy and quick response to critical

situations. Neuhauser (1990) described organizations as consisting of many tribes holding separate values and beliefs and even unique languages. Tribal warfare results in a failure to incorporate various factions into the organization under a set of shared values according to Neuhauser.

The challenge for the nurse executive is to express the highly productive synergized culture out of the many different kinds of values and cultures that one finds within a nursing organization. With an overall program for the development of shared values, an overriding umbrella can be put in place that still allows for individual unit cultures. However, the prevailing values, principles, and expectations of the culture become the overarching culture in all the units.

TAKING THE LEADERSHIP

The literature on leadership presumes that the successful leader must impart a sense of integrity. Bennis (1989) identified three parts of integrity: self-knowledge, candor, and maturity. When describing self-knowledge, he noted that the leader never lies to himself, consistently knows his strengths and weaknesses, and deals with these directly. Bennis also noted that part of integrity is trust (i.e., something earned over time as people watch the actions of the leader).

Autry (1991) took the concept a bit further, stating that "Management is not simply a skill or a technique or a profession" (p. 14). Instead, he saw it as a calling and a sacred trust in which the well-being of staff is put in the hands of the executive during the time they are at work. We can take the next step and say that the nurse executive holds a sacred trust for staff and for the patients and families under the staff's care. The trust extends to the community in which she works, a trust from society that resources will be spent wisely and that the profession will be managed effectively under this executive's influence.

Autry pointed out that there are two kinds of managers: those who practice management as a skill and those who approach management as a calling (i.e., a lifetime engagement that enables people to grow personally and contribute to the common good). He made the point that if a person does not care about people, he cannot be effective. The nurse executive who creates a sense of trust by acting with integrity will instill this value as part of the culture.

In the corporatization of health care (i.e., the push to see health care as a business and the rush to show a bottom-line performance), we cannot lose sight of the fact that the effective nurse executive operates within a system of values-based leadership. She exhibits for the organization a positive proactive mode in which people are really cared for and cared about and treated with integrity. When staff can do their work in this kind of culture, they can give this kind of respect to patients.

If people do not feel cared for, they cannot care. In an intensive, caring profession such as nursing, the values of integrity and caring for each other as well as for patients, are highly important. They affect the kind of nursing care outcomes for which the staff strive. By incorporating values such as integrity and caring in the leadership function, the organization will also incorporate these values.

The nurse executive creates a highly cohesive, bonded community held together by a system of shared values and a shared mission and vision. Without values-based leadership, the culture loses its rudder and its main sails and gets buffeted by volatile winds. Developing a culture of shared values creates a feeling of community, a clear sense of direction for all staff. A highly committed and energized staff is developed because they have the shared values around which their community is organized.

IMPLEMENTING A VALUES-BASED PROGRAM

Implementing a values-based program involves discussion and clarification sessions in which a few simple values can be agreed on to be part of the value system. Then, these values must be integrated into the life of the organization through written documents, role modeling, hiring and orientation programs, and continual dialogue. Values statements and credos are examples of written materials that can be used to guide the implementation of a values-based system.

Values statements also appear in the division's philosophy and theory of nursing, as well as in its selection of goals. Yet, no written statement has the same impact as the opportunity for staff members to come together to discuss and analyze values. Values are not so much a cognitive decision as an emergent, an underlying system to which voice may be given when staff are challenged to think about their values, the values of their leaders, and the values of the organization.

SUMMARY

When a system of clearly articulated and shared values is the basis of the practice of the care program, staff will clearly understand expectations and a solid positive culture will be the result. Because of the highly interpersonal nature of nursing care, nurses expect, deserve, and need a high level of professional support and a supportive climate in which to do their work. Poor financial outcomes, low productivity, poor quality of patient care, high absentee rates, and high turnover rates are associated with staff who are in constant turmoil and have low organizational commitment.

When nurses are distracted from their work with patients by flaws in the organizational climate (or because a system of shared values is not in place), quality and productivity suffer. It is important for the nurse executive not only to articulate the values and desired climate but to assess periodically the organization through employee surveys and other assessment tools to make sure that a climate has been constructed that will support the highest level of productivity and job satisfaction on the part of the staff.

REFERENCES

Autry, J. 1991. *Love and profit: The art of caring leadership.* New York: William-Morrow & Co.

Bennis, W. 1989. *On becoming a leader.* Reading, Mass.: Addison-Wesley Publishing.

Neuhauser, P. 1990. *Tribal warfare in organizations.* New York: Harper Business.

SUGGESTED READINGS

Barker, A.M. 1991. An emerging leadership paradigm: Transformational leadership. *Nursing and Health Care* 12, no.4:204–207.

Dickson, G.L. 1993. The unintended consequences of a male professional ideology for the development of nursing education. *Advances in Nursing Science* 15, no.3:67–83.

Evers, J.M., et al. 1989. New directions for nurse managers. *Journal of Continuing Education in Nursing* 20, no.5:200–205.

Gralnick, A. 1988. Cultural aspects of the psychiatric hospital. *Psychiatric Quarterly* 59, no.1:3–9.

Llewellyn-Thomas, H.A., et al. 1989. Measuring perceptions of the exemplary nurse. *Journal of Nursing Education* 28, no.8:336–371.

Sovie, M.D. 1993. Hospital culture—Why create one? *Nursing Economics* 11, no.2:69–75.

Vincent, P., et al. 1993. Are we teaching leadership as a value? *Nursing Management* 24, no.7:65–67.

Ziegenfuss, J.T., Jr. 1991. Organizational barriers to quality improvement in medical and health care organizations. *Quality Assurance and Utilization Review* 6, no.4:115–122.

15

Ethics: Impact on Goals and Practices

Issues of ethics assume prominence when traditional principles fail to give answers to new problems. We live in such a time today, a time of rapid transitions that leave our past moral premises in doubt. Changing technology and changing economics have left behind old ethical and legal answers by raising new and complex questions. At one time, ethical quandaries could be settled by reference to established laws and accepted practices of human conduct. Today's ethical dilemmas often concern situations that have not yet been codified in laws or ritualized in normative conduct. The nurse executive is managing in a complex environment where few answers exist as to what is right to do.

The ethical problems caused by advancing medical technologies are well known to those working in health care facilities. For example, is it good (or right) to use new procedures on the prematurely born infant that may sustain his life at the price of many physical and cognitive limitations? Is this subjecting the infant to experimentation and therefore unethical? Or is it unethical to withhold such experimental techniques when they may save the infant's life at the cost of permanent defects? Technology raises ethical questions that are as new as the technology itself. Should manipulation of genes be allowed to improve human beings? If so, who determines what constitutes improvement?

What about the blurring between business and science as commercial enterprises enter health care? Take, for example, the human genome project seeking to discover the rest of the human genetic code. What will happen subsequent to this investigation, when even more overt intervention is possible into what constitutes being human?

Should life be prolonged when that life lacks the quality desired by the patient? Does the patient have the right to die in such circumstances? Or should his wishes be ignored in favor of the physician's value of prolonging life at any cost? Is assisted suicide acceptable if the patient wants it? When does the practice of medicine become a disservice rather than a service? If the technology *can* maintain life, must life be maintained? These are just a few of the ethical questions raised by the existence of new technologies.

Improved technology raises additional questions concerning distribution of scarce resources. Which baby should get the liver transplant? Who should receive the available kidney? Should distribution of organs depend on ability to pay? On seriousness of the threat of loss of life without the surgery? On the person's ability to bring the media to focus on his case? On the probability of survival postsurgery? On predicated additional years of life? Should the patient who has destroyed the original liver through poor life-style habits be a candidate for a scarce transplant? Who sets the criteria for selection of patients when their numbers outstrip available resources?

The ethical problems surfacing in obstetrics continue to create new challenges. Should the 60-year-old woman who desires it be impregnated by new techniques, even though she may die leaving an immature child to be raised by others? Is it ethical for the mother to lend a womb to a daughter who lacks one? Just as society became relatively comfortable with children created by *in vitro* fertilization, these new challenges arose. What questions will arise next year or even next week?

Just because a technology is possible, should it be developed? Even if the cost is astronomical? Is it fair that the cost of a heart transplant be invested in one person, when a similar expenditure could have helped hundreds if used in preventive health for immunizations? Is this view narrow? Will the expensive technology become cheaper as the techniques develop?

The medical technology and the related cost questions set new dimensions for ethical considerations. Economics assumes more and more importance as technology outstrips our ability to pay for it. The issue of rationing first enacted politically in Oregon has yet to be resolved. What do we do when there simply are not enough organs, enough competent practitioners of a technology to meet the need?

Should medical technology be allowed to place a drain on the society? Is it right not to do all that is possible? Or is it moral to do what is possible when it places cruel demands on the economy and when it robs the nation of fiscal resources that could be devoted to other values? What portion of the gross national product should be spent on health care? Ultimately, the present administration may give a political/administrative answer to that question, but whatever the National Health Plan, not all the ethical issues will be answered.

PHILOSOPHIC POSITIONS ON
ETHICS

To perceive the complexity of morality and the involved issues, a brief review of the philosophy of ethical decision making is necessary. Unfortunately, such a review only adds to the complexity of the situation. The nurse executive who acts from information rather than ignorance, however, is always in a superior position.

Ethics here means the critical study of standards for judging the rightness or wrongness of conduct. Ethics, then, pertains when things are denoted by terms such as *good* or *bad, right* or *wrong, ought* or *duty.* Ethics is the systematic study of morality. There are many conflicting and contradicting positions concerning the meaning of ethics.

The first contradiction concerns whether ethics is real or illusory. Because ethics concerns conduct, it applies only when man has a real choice. If all behavior is seen as the predicted effect of prior vector forces, then ethical choice is as illusory as is free will itself. In a philosophic position of determinism, ethics is merely a label misapplied in a world where everything happens inevitably because of antecedent causes.

Among the positions that accept human choice as a reality, there are many ways to differentiate ethical positions. And some of these nondeterministic philosophies still deny the existence of ethical choice. For example, some philosophies believe that man's acts are basically selfish (i.e., he acts in terms of what he thinks is his own best interest at all times). Although subtle differences can be made between various positions in this category, it is not essential to do so for purposes of this chapter. Terms such as *hedonism, psychological egoism,* or *ethical egoism* may be applied. These philosophies agree that man has free choice but that he always chooses from self-motivated calculations rather than from considerations of rightness or wrongness.

Usually, when one thinks of ethics, one thinks of philosophies that assert that choice exists and can be made on principles of rightness or wrongness. Of these philosophies, two basic types may be found. Teleological philosophies propose that the ethics of an act can be found in the ends achieved by the act. In contrast, deontological positions claim that the rightness or wrongness of an act is found by determining whether the act preserved some given rules or principles.

Teleological philosophies primarily divide into those that determine the rightness or wrongness of an act based on the intention of the actor and those that derive their basis by analysis of the actual consequences of the action. In the first case, a person who performed an act that she perceived would benefit many, would be termed to be acting morally even if her assessment were wrong and many persons were harmed by the act. In contrast, the second position would call the act immoral because of its factual consequences.

Whether the act is judged on the basis of intention or consequences, one can still ask what values mediate the choice. Here, one again finds differences among philosophic positions. Some philosophies call the greatest utility a moral principle (i.e., the good act results in the greatest benefit for the greatest number of persons). Nor are utilitarian positions without their own problems. What can be said, for example, about the act that benefits a few greatly yet harms others minimally? Or contrast an act that does a great benefit for a few with an act that does a minimal good for a greater number. Which is the more ethical act?

Some teleological positions advocate other values than utility. Some judge the act in terms of the number of values that it achieves. Maximizing values becomes the goal in this position. Other positions may be cast in terms of maximizing self-actualization. Many different values may underlie ethical positions, whether they seek to judge an act by the intention of the actor or the consequences of the act.

Deontological positions stem from different origins. Here, the rules or principles that determine the morality of an act arise from many different sources. Chief among these espoused sources are the self (one's *conscience*), *God* (whatever god is espoused by the given system), or *law* as the societal source of moral principles.

Again, there is no easy answer, for two gods may direct their disciples toward different acts. And two consciences may lead their possessors to opposite conclusions. Even the meaning of *conscience* changes in various philosophies. In one, it means an instinctive sentiment that automatically tells one what is moral. In another

system, the conscience may be a learned process, based on the norms of the society that instills the conscience. In others, conscience may be based on a rational principle.

Kant's categorical imperative is an example of the latter sort. Kant said that everyone should judge his act based on its universal applicability. Hence the would-be suicide must ask, What if all persons killed themselves? Because this would lead to the end of humanity, the would-be suicide is led to see (rationally) that the considered act is immoral.

The reader must appreciate that many philosophic niceties have been sacrificed in the preceding discussion. But it should make the point that many persons act in ways that they consider to be moral and that these acts may stem from radically different belief systems. Further, these acts (and the decisions underlying them) may be in conflict even though each person believes his choice to be the right one. This should explain why ethics by committee is not always successful. Consensus is not always possible even among well-intentioned persons.

ETHICAL ISSUES FOR THE NURSE

Nurses are not able to escape dealing with ethical issues. Of course, some issues will be settled by the society at large, but even here, the nurse has a special civic duty to participate in the deliberations. Other decisions will fall to the nurse because of her role as custodian of the patient. Indeed, such decisions already are part of her practice. When, for example, the physician determines to prolong the life of a suffering patient, the nurse is the one who confronts the effects of that decision as she spends time with that patient and the family.

The nurse is the one who must cope when the patient and the family disagree on extreme measures. The nurse may be faced with choosing between patient and family preferences if the question of whether or not to resuscitate arises.

The nurse executive has a special obligation to the staff in such a complex situation. Structures must be devised that allow for ethical decision making of the highest quality. The rights of the staff must be protected so that no one feels her own moral integrity has been compromised.

Zablow's (1984) study of staff nurses showed that they were not particularly introspective concerning ethical questions. Indeed, they seldom debated over which course of behavior was moral. Instead, the question was whether they had the courage to assert the positions that they believed to be the moral ones. Often, this situation arose when what the nurse believed to be the right thing to do conflicted with the action ordered by the physician.

Unfortunately, large numbers of nurses in the Zablow study sacrificed their own adjudged position to the wishes of another. Usually, that other was the physician but at times it was the institution (or one of its representatives). In most cases, the staff nurse yielded to another person who was perceived as more powerful, as holding more authority.

It may be that nurses lacked the courage of their convictions because those convictions were not well conceived. It is more likely that the nurses thought that they did not have the power to assert their positions over those perceived as having more status. The nurse executive needs to be sensitive to the perceptions of her staff in this regard. She must do all she can to see that nurses are not placed in positions in which they believe their integrity is compromised.

Jameton (1984) described three types of ethical problems faced by nurses. Moral uncertainty is experienced when the nurse is unsure what moral principles or values apply. Moral uncertainty includes those cases in which the nurse is not sure what the moral problem is. Jameton's second classification is the moral dilemma. In this case, two or more moral principles apply but lead to inconsistent courses of action when applied. The third type of ethical problem is termed *moral distress*. Here, one knows the right thing to do, but institutional constraints make it nearly impossible to do so. Jameton's third problem, moral distress, closely resembles Zablow's findings.

One of the most difficult chronic ethical problems that staff nurses face is the deception or attempted deception of patients by physicians

and families. Although many physicians have changed this practice, families have been slower to change. Often, the deception involves masking the incipient death of the patient. The nurse may be requested to maintain the deception whether or not she agrees with this decision.

The moral problem that lying to a patient may create for a nurse is heightened because she is the frequent target of the patient's testing. When, for example, the patient does not believe what he is told about his health status, the nurse is doubly a victim—of her own doubt concerning the wisdom of deception and of the demand that she affirm a lie even when the patient evidences his doubt.

Fortunately, the tide of deception in medical practice started to change after the President's Commission for the Study of Ethical Problems in Medicine and Biomedical and Behavioral Research (1982) recommended that such deceptive practices be discontinued in most patient–physician relationships.

MANAGEMENT OF ETHICAL PROBLEMS

Given the complexity of ethical issues in today's health care institution, what should the nurse executive do? She must look simultaneously at ethical implications of nursing practice and of institutional policies and strategies. She also needs to keep current on legal precedents that may have an effect on ethical decision making in the institution.

The *Code for Nurses* produced by the American Nurses Association (1985) serves as a general guideline, presenting broad ethical principles generally accepted in this country, as well as offering brief explanations for each principle. Unfortunately, the principles are too broad to suggest specific actions to be taken. Take, for example, the item, "The nurse assumes responsibility and accountability for individual nursing judgments and actions." Few would argue with the principle, but it serves little purpose in solving an issue of accountability.

For the subordinate staff, the nurse executive can set up structures that prevent the staff nurse from being caught in the middle between her own convictions and the orders of others with more power in the institution. There should be a channel by which nurses can refuse to participate in treatments or in patient management strategies when to do so presents them with valid moral crises. The structure should be devised so that a nurse can refuse participation for personal ethical reasons without being faced with threat or coercion. Certainly, the nurse should not face psychological (or other) penalties for enacting her own personal code.

The nurse executive also may elect to provide inservice education to make nurses more able to make effective discriminations in cases of ethical decision making. One of Zablow's case studies was instructive on this point. A nurse was extremely upset when a liver available for transplant went to another patient rather than hers. The nurse clearly had assumed an advocacy position for her patient but failed to understand that the mere fact that he was *her* patient was not sufficient rationale for the hard choice that had to be made.

As new laws are enacted to cover new problems, the nurse executive must keep informed. Both changes in the law and in case decisions setting new precedents are important. When major changes occur, the nurse executive will need to review divisional and institutional policy for conformance with the new dictate. Obviously, some institutions may elect to have ethical positions that uphold differing ethical positions. For example, many Catholic institutions refuse to perform abortions. Such an ethical position should be made clear to clients. The patient who wants an abortion should be told that this institution does not perform abortions but that others do so.

An institution can take its own position on such issues. The fact that abortion is legal does not mean that every institution must perform abortions. Obviously, to refrain from performing a legal service is quite different from performing an illegal act. At present, the nation is embroiled in legal debate concerning the many right-to-life groups that protest vehemently and sometimes violently at women's clinics. The issue here is to what lengths one can go to impress one's own position on others.

Because institutional finance is a driving force in decision making, the nurse executive is faced with many ethical dilemmas. What happens, for example, when the institution limits its treatment of charity cases to stay solvent? Here is an ethical problem with no simple answer. Indeed, most ethical problems involve not a right versus a wrong but two conflicting goods. Obviously, it is good to treat charity patients who cannot pay for needed services. But it also is good to stay economically solvent and keep one's doors open. Few ethical choices are easy; few are entirely satisfactory. But it is important that the nurse executive know her own position and her institution's position so that she will be able to supply leadership in interpreting such difficult issues to her staff.

Because of the complexity of extant ethical issues, most institutions appoint an ethics committee to handle unique ethical patient problems and to judge the ethics of research proposals. Although such committees may confront difficulties, they provide a forum in which ethical problems can be scrutinized. They also allow for shared decision making under difficult conditions. Because such committees should represent the best in thinking concerning ethical problems, some institutions provide an ethicist to guide committee deliberation. The nurse executive will want to make sure that nursing has representation on the ethics committee. After all, the nurses live most closely with the ethical dilemmas.

The nurse executive has a special obligation to the staff to be concerned about preventing the moral distress that Jameton discussed. Frontline staff are frequently confronted with ethical disparities between their value system and that of patients and their families, physicians, or even hospital administrators.

The stress of constant, intense interactions with patients can itself become burdensome to the staff. Albrecht (1990) defined the term *emotional labor* as a way to conceptualize this tremendous hardship. As customer relations become more important, an extra burden is placed on frontline staff, not only to be therapeutic but to operate in a way that will bring the greatest level of patient and family satisfaction.

Sometimes, this consumer focus brings patient ethics in conflict with nurse ethics, creating moral distress. Many nurses leave nursing and bedside care because they have no support systems to help them work through the moral and ethical dilemmas that they face on the front line. The nurse executive must be sensitive to the nurse who feels moral distress because of family/patient/physician disagreements.

Staff on the front line need to feel the presence of a continuous support system to handle these issues. When nurses feel moral distress, they become detached and disengaged. A nurse who raises issues and questions cannot be cast as a troublemaker.

The effect of moral distress on the quality of care and issues such as turnover is seldom discussed, yet nurses who feel detached and disengaged cannot provide quality care. Nursing satisfaction is a strong measure of nurse retention. It is important that the nurse executive know how nurses perceive the institution's support for ethical issues and moral dilemmas.

The visible and sustained presence of the nurse executive around issues of ethics communicates concern to the staff members. Brown-bag lunches with staff allow for discussion of ethical issues. Roundtable discussions on individual units are another mechanism. Members of the ethics committee are often eager to be available to the nursing staff for open forum discussions. Monthly meetings of a facilitywide ethics roundtable is another structure in which issues having to do with ethics can be examined. By critiquing issues with peers, clarification can be sought and support provided.

ETHICS FROM THE PATIENT'S PERSPECTIVE

Not all ethics problems relate to staff. The nurse executive also must be the patient's advocate in relation to moral issues. This involves patient care systems and information systems of all kinds. There are many questions that must be addressed to the nursing management systems:

1. What systems are devised to see that patients can make informed consent?

2. What systems are devised to keep patient records confidential? (This question becomes more complex in an era when interfacing computer systems complicate the confidentiality issue.)
3. What cross-subsidization exists in the billing systems, and who is penalized by the system?
4. Does the reimbursement system encourage a two- or even three-tier system of health care? If so, is that an ethical issue?
5. What issues of access arise in patient admissions? Are groups of persons systematically disenfranchised from health care in a given community?
6. What surrogate is appointed for the patient who cannot make his own decisions? Is there a system to see that such a surrogate is appointed?

IMPLICATIONS OF THE NEW SPIRITUALITY

Some new and rather unique problems in health care ethics arise under so-called new age beliefs. One of the underlying beliefs of many of these philosophies is that each of us creates his own world. A simplistic application of this belief may cause a person to blame the patient for his own illness. The blamer may be the nurse, the family, or even the patient himself.

Such a simplistic interpretation of some new age philosophies creates a new layer of judgment where once there was none. Look, for example, at the following description of nursing theory by Watson and consider how a thoughtless reader might interpret illness:

A troubled soul can lead to illness, and illness can produce disease. Specific experiences, for example, developmental conflicts, inner suffering, guilt, self-blame, despair, loss, and grief, and general and specific stress can lead to illness and result in disease. Unknowns can also lead to illness; the unknown can only be known by experience and may require inner searching to find. Disease processes can also result from genetic, constitutional vulnerabilities and manifest themselves when disharmony is present. (Watson 1988, p. 48)

If disease is disharmony, the patient is at fault and need only create harmony to solve his illness—so might the conclusion be drawn by someone applying little depth to understanding the philosophy. Coming to grips with accountability for illness used to be a problem related to patients with obvious life-style illnesses such as alcoholism and drug abuse. Now, one often finds the same judgmental attitudes expressed toward cancer patients and others with conditions once judged to be entirely external to the patient's thoughts and actions.

When all or part of one's staff hold beliefs such as those expressed in Watson's theory of nursing, there is a need to explore what such beliefs mean as they relate to the giving and receiving of care and concern. Whether nurses deal with their own attitudes and those of patients or families, blame-placing is not productive of the harmony Watson hoped to invoke.

Introspection into causes of illness is a part of many new age philosophies, but if the belief that one participates in his own illness is held, that is not equivalent to placing blame. Nor can the new age nurse assume that imposing her value system on a patient holding alternate belief systems is any less offensive than is the missionary zeal of some proselytizing religious sects.

When her beliefs are not a part of the patient's philosophy, the staff member has no right to impose her philosophy and its ethical implications on the patient.

SUMMARY

Any philosophy of patient care is influenced by certain ethical tenets. It is important that a nurse executive has a sense of moral direction. In an age when many decisions are made on economic criteria, it is important to remember that health care facilities exist to deliver health care. A nurse executive should be able to identify the values that underlie nursing and institutional practices and decisions.

Because ethical problems assume prominence in an era undergoing great change, it is important that education and support be offered around these issues for both staff and patients.

REFERENCES

Albrecht, K. 1990. *A service within: Solving the middle management leadership crisis.* Homewood, Ill.: Dow-Jones-Irwin.

American Nurses Association. 1985. *Code for nurses with interpretive statements.* Kansas City, Mo.: American Nurses Association.

Jameton, A. 1984. *Nursing practice: The ethical issues.* Englewood Cliffs, N.J.: Prentice Hall.

President's Commission for the Study of Ethical Problems in Medicine and Biomedical and Behavioral Research. 1982. *Making health care decisions: Vol. 1.* Washington, D.C.: U.S. Government Printing Office.

Watson, J. 1988. *Nursing: Human science and human care: A theory of nursing.* New York: National League for Nursing.

Zablow, R.J. 1984. *Preparing students for the moral dimension of professional nursing practice: A protocol for nurse educators.* Unpublished dissertation, Teachers College, Columbia University.

SUGGESTED READINGS

American Nurses Association, Center for Human Rights Taskforce. 1993. *Compendium of position statements on the nurse's role in end-of-life decisions.* Washington, D.C.

Beck, L., et al. 1993. Use of the code of ethics for accountability in discharge planning. *Nursing Forum* 28, no.3:5–12.

Blancett, S.S., and P.A. Sullivan. 1993. Ethics survey results. *Journal of Nursing Administration* 23, no.3:9–13.

Bushy, A., and J.R. Rauh. 1991. Implementing an ethics committee in rural institutions. *Journal of Nursing Administration* 21, no.22:18–25.

Cannon, P. 1988. The professional ethics and practice committee: A step toward the achievement of excellence. *Nursing Administration Quarterly* 12, no.4:53–56.

Corley, M.C., and D. Raines. 1993. An ethical practice environment as a caring environment. *Nursing Administration Quarterly* 17, no.2:68–74.

Cunningham, N., and S. Hutchinson. 1990. Myths in health care ethics. *Image* 22, no.4:235–238.

Curtin, L.L. 1993. Keepers of the keys: Economics, ethics, and nursing administration. *Nursing Administration Quarterly* 17, no.4:1–10.

Davis, A.J. 1982. Helping your staff address ethical dilemmas. *Journal of Nursing Administration* 12, no.2:9–13.

Edwards, B.J., and A.M. Haddad. 1988. Establishing a nursing bioethics committee. *Journal of Nursing Administration* 18, no.3:30–33.

Fenton, M. 1988. Moral distress in clinical practice: Implications for the nurse administrator. *Canadian Journal of Nursing Administration* 1, no.3:8–11.

Haddad, A.M. 1992. Ethical problems in home healthcare. *Journal of Nursing Administration* 22, no.3:46–51.

Holly, C.M., and M. Lyons. 1992. Ethical practice in acute care nursing: Are we there yet? *The Journal of the New York State Nurses Association* 23, no.4:4–7.

Institute of Medicine. 1983. *Nursing and nursing education: Public policies and private actions.* Washington, D.C.: National Academy Press.

Jacques, R. 1993. Untheorized dimensions of caring work: Caring as a structural practice and caring as a way of seeing. *Nursing Administration Quarterly* 17, no.2:11–17.

Kerfoot, K.M. 1992. Preventing moral distress: Our ethical obligation. *Aspen's Advisor for Nurse Executives* 7, no.5:1, 3–5.

Long, L., and P. Prophit, Sr. 1981. *Understanding/responding: A communication manual for nurses.* Monterey, Calif.: Catholic University Press of America.

Luguire, R., and S. Houston. 1992. Ethical concerns regarding cardiac retransplantation. *Nursing Economics* 10, no.6:413–417.

McDaniel, C., and G.A. Wolf. 1992. Transformational leadership in nursing service: A test of theory. *Journal of Nursing Administration* 22, no.2:6–65.

Menzel, P.T. 1983. *Medical costs, moral choices: A philosophy of health care economics in America.* New Haven, Conn.: Yale University Press.

Milner, S. 1993. An ethical nursing practice model. *Journal of Nursing Administration* 23, no.3:22–25.

Morath, J.M., and M. Manthey. 1993. An environment for care and service leadership: The nurse administrator's impact. *Nursing Administration Quarterly* 17, no.2:68–74.

Nyberg, J. 1989. The element of caring in nursing administration. *Nursing Administration Quarterly* 13, no.3:9–16.

Nyberg, J. 1993. Teaching caring to the nurse administrator. *Journal of Nursing Administration* 23, no.1:11–17.

Oleson, M. 1990. Subjectively perceived quality of life. *Image* 22, no.3:187–190.

Palmer, R.H. 1991. *Striving for quality in health care: An inquiry into policy and practice.* Ann Arbor, Mich.: Health Administration Press.

Parker, R.S. 1990. Measuring nurses' moral judgments. *Image* 22, no.4:213–218.

Reverby, S.M. 1987. *Ordered to care: The dilemma of American nursing, 1850–1945.* New York: Cambridge University Press.

Rodney, P. 1989. Towards ethical decision-making in nursing practice. *Canadian Journal of Nursing Administration* 2, no.2:11–14.

Schwarz, J.K. 1993. Surrogate decision-making and ethics committees: The new role of the New York State nurse. *The Journal of the New York State Nurses Association* 24, no.2:4–8.

Somers, J.B. 1993. The struggle for the soul of health insurance. *Journal of Health Politics, Policy and Law* 18, no.2:287–317.

Stevens, P.E. 1992. Who gets care? Access to health care as an arena for nursing action. *Scholarly Inquiry for Nursing Practice* 6, no.3:185–200.

Sullivan, P.A., and T. Brown. 1991. Common-sense ethics in administrative decision making. Part I. *Journal of Nursing Administration* 21, no.10:21–23.

Sullivan, P.A., and T. Brown. 1991. Common-sense ethics in administrative decision making. Part II. *Journal of Nursing Administration* 21, no.11:57–61.

Weeks, L.C. 1987. Ethics committees. *Journal of Nursing Administration* 17, no.10:31, 35.

White, G. 1993. *Ethical dilemmas in contemporary nursing practice.* Washington D.C.: American Nurses Association.

Woolery, L.K. 1990. Professional standards and ethical dilemmas in nursing information systems. *Journal of Nursing Administration* 20, no.10:5–53.

Yeo, M., ed. 1991. *Concepts and cases in nursing ethics.* Petersborough, Ontario, Canada: Broadview Press Ltd.

16

Empowering Staff in Today's Care Environment

Nursing, like other fields, passes through phases in which certain concepts are popular and then, in turn, are replaced with newer notions. Today's idea of empowerment replaces yesterday's notion of power. This is not to say that nursing no longer seeks power; it simply seeks to extend the notion of power through the method of empowerment.

Empowerment is often contrasted with power in terms of its expansion or contraction. Power contracts; it is the authority that one takes to oneself as opposed to others. Usually, power is seen as power *over* others. Empowerment, in contrast, expands; it is authority purposefully shared with others.

An important notion in empowerment is that the total quantum of power is not diminished when power is shared. Effectively used, empowerment in a nursing division increases the total amount of nursing's influence in the organization rather than each participant receiving a small quantum from some defined and limited amount.

Power, then, is *convergent,* centered in a single person or small group, whereas empowerment is *divergent,* distributed, spread over many people. Although power and empowerment are separate notions, they need not be separate in practice. An effective nurse executive who shares power with his staff (empowerment) may concurrently and for that reason increase the power of his own role.

HISTORICAL PERSPECTIVE

One of nursing's historical vulnerabilities has been the lack of empowerment of nurse professionals. It is easy to see why this happened: Others operating on a perception of power rather than empowerment worked to keep nursing from exerting influence.

Of course, this was not true in every setting in every era. The history of public health nursing is full of instances of great nurse empowerment: The creation of the Frontier Nursing Service in the Kentucky mountains, the establishment of the Henry Street Settlement, indeed the entire era of building the Visiting Nurse Association illustrate times and places in which nursing was empowered.

Of course, one might observe that nursing has effectively empowered itself in places that did not beckon to competition, situations that did not offer great financial enticement to others. This is not to make light of the fact that in each of these cases nurses saw a problem, knew what could be done about it, and responded with great strength and determination.

Whatever the era, nurses like anyone else fulfill their mission better when they are empowered to work to their full capacity. It is not surprising that better nursing, better health care, and more role satisfaction occur in such circumstances.

Most nurse executives, then, attempt to spread power among their nurses, not only increasing the total amount of influence within the nursing division but also increasing the satisfaction that nurses derive from their roles.

SOURCES OF EMPOWERMENT

How does empowerment come about? There are at least four common sources of its enhancement: expanded expertise, new legal powers, new roles, and changed self-perceptions. The nurse executive has more ability to manipulate some of these variables than others, but each deserves attention.

Expanded Expertise

Expertise is always power: more skills, more power. This is true for the individual and for the group. For decades, nurses have complained that they were prevented from practicing at the peak of their expertise, but that is not today's situation. The economic environment is changing; as we noted in Chapter 12, it has become cost-effective to get the most mileage out of a nurse's ability. Today, restructured practice aims to fully use each nurse's skills and knowledge level. Nurses are seen as scarce resources, knowledgeable workers who cannot be spared to do lower-level tasks.

Within nursing, enhanced experience and advanced preparation are the best routes to increased empowerment. As the nurse's knowledge and skills increase, so does her acceptance by and respect from others in health care.

Benner's (1984) research tells us of the difference made by increased expertise. Using the Dreyfus Model of Skill Acquisition (Dreyfus and Dreyfus, no date), Benner constructed a model of nursing research designed to explore clinical excellence. The Dreyfus model describes five separate levels of skill acquisition, and Benner, accordingly, differentiated nursing practice into these five levels: (1) novice, (2) advanced beginner, (3) competent performer, (4) proficient performer, and (5) expert.

Briefly, the levels can be characterized in the following way. The novice learns context-free rules to guide his action. He gains few subtleties in understanding; he simply applies the objectifiable rules. The advanced beginner starts to appreciate some "aspects of the situation" that require prior experience for recognition. The advanced beginner still needs help in setting priorities and sorting out what is important from what is not. He is only beginning to recognize recurrent meaningful patterns. The competent performer (a level reached after 2 to 3 years of practice) begins to see his actions in terms of long-range goals and plans. He lacks speed and flexibility but has a feeling of mastery and the ability to cope with many contingencies. The proficient performer sees situations as wholes rather than being concerned with isolated aspects. He recognizes when the expected picture fails to materialize and no longer relies on rules or analytic principles. Instead, he has an intuitive grasp of each situation and zeroes in on problems and solutions without wasting time considering alternatives. For these nurses, the knowledge imbedded in practice starts to become visible. At the expert level, the thought processes become intuitive, as if the expert had escaped the rules entirely. The growth is toward seeing and responding to the situation as a whole.

The Dreyfus educational model allowed Benner to segregate and rank anecdotes about excellent practice among nurses. Benner found the need for a rigidly controlled practice system was greatest for the novice or advanced beginner but that such high control actually impaired the work of the expert nurse. In essence, the nurse is empowered, freed for creative and effective response, by his developing expertise.

If Benner described the experience factor as one element of expertise, then master's and doctoral education serve as hallmarks of formalized advanced knowledge. Yet, the history of nursing reminds us that knowledge alone may be insufficient if others have the power to control what a nurse may and may not do with his knowledge. This consideration leads to the next source of empowerment.

New Legal Powers

As a profession, nursing has failed to agree on goals and strategies for seeking new legal status to empower the average nurse. Most commonly, the disagreements have centered on the beginning credentials/educational criteria for nurses and/or the difference between professional and technical nursing.

This failure reflects our inability as a profession to create adequate vehicles for resolving internal disputes. Ironically, as long as nurses are busy disagreeing with each other, they are not a threat to anyone else's power. Sadly, any answer to these internecine wars would have been better than the two-decade debate that continues today.

Despite the internal struggle over nurse licensure, nurses have made great strides in legalizing various outlying nurse roles, particularly those of nurse practitioners. This has not occurred without challenge. Midwives, for example, were long challenged by physicians as practicing beyond their nursing licenses. Not surprisingly, these challenges grew when midwives began to deviate from their pattern of delivering the poor and uninsured (i.e., when they began cultivating a middle- and upper-class clientele who wanted birthing to be a more positive experience).

Other nurse practitioners (not midwives) also have been sued for practicing medicine without licenses. Again, this happened when their roles emerged as threats to physician power, namely, when they were perceived (not inaccurately) as in competition for the paying customer.

Despite these suits and struggles, the practitioner movement has achieved legal empowerment (although differing slightly from state to state), and nurses in these roles usually feel empowered to practice at the peak of their preparation.

As nurse practitioner roles became integrated into the health care system, the fear they evoked in others was mitigated, and now nurse practitioners generally are accepted. The nurse practitioner is empowered legally because he may act independently of physician orders—or within various cooperative relationships in which, to all intent and purposes, the nurse is free to use his skills and knowledge. Nurses can be rightfully proud of their successes in providing nurse practitioners with legal empowerment.

Further, by hiring nurse practitioners, the nurse executive can take advantage of the cost-containment focus of the era. When a nursing division can provide advanced services at lower costs than other providers, the whole division is empowered.

New Roles

New roles represent another path to empowerment. In the case of the nurse practitioner, the new legal status and the new role go hand in hand. Indeed, the greatest movement in nursing at present has been the conversion of master's level clinical specialist programs to combined clinical specialist–practitioner programs. These programs combine the nursing orientation with the primary care skills, preparing the graduate for practitioner licensure.

The growth of these programs has been supported by several changes. First, insurance companies recognize that reimbursement costs are lessened by allowing nurses to practice at the top of their preparation instead of demanding that higher-paid physicians be used. Nursing did a fine job of making its research into nurse practitioner effectiveness known in the right places (see, e.g., Brooten et al. 1986), but cost savings was the final selling point.

The development of nurse practitioner roles was slowed by the objections of some nurse leaders who thought that practitioner tasks simply were not nursing and that the practitioners would be co-opted by medicine. Some leaders said the movement was a ploy to lead nurses away from nursing into medicine. By now, one seldom hears this sort of resistance. Nor do the nurse practitioners evidence this perspective.

The nursing identity of nurse practitioners not only remains intact but characterizes their approach to the primary care of patients. Unlike physicians who might be more drawn to the esoteric unusual case, the nurse practitioner is at home considering how Mr. Jones with intermittent claudication can get his groceries the five blocks from the closest market.

Nurse practitioner roles mark a great new empowerment in our profession, one that blends at least three criteria for empowerment: expanded expertise, a new legal status, and new role development.

But we do not have to go to the nurse practitioners to find empowered new nursing roles. Another new nursing role empowered, not by legal fiat but by its placement in the care delivery structure, is the case manager role that has emerged with the coming of restructured practice. (Restructured practice and case management are discussed in Chapters 12 and 13, respectively.)

In a restructured care delivery system, the chief function of the case manager is an *integrator role*—bringing together the tasks that have been differentiated across the systems in nursing and in other departments. Because the case manager focuses on each patient's trajectory of recovery, he keeps the task-oriented system controlled by a patient orientation, namely, by looking at individual patient outcomes.

Both the nurse practitioner and the nurse case manager are empowered because of the ways their roles fit into today's care systems. But this does not mean all nursing roles must be changed to empower nurses. This brings us to the last and most important way in which empowerment is achieved.

New Self-Perceptions

Often the power a nurse exercises is more affected by his self-perception than by any legal or role delineation. Indeed, changing the perceptions of his staff may be the most important way in which a nurse executive can enhance empowerment in his division. One hears lots of criticism from noted observers of nursing concerning the way the practices of the field disempower nurses' self-perceptions.

For example, sociologist Hans Mauksch (personal communication, circa 1985) said that nursing and medicine handle their knowledge in very different ways. Paraphrased here, he said that medicine gives its student knowledge in a context that says, "Here's another piece of information to make you more powerful." But nursing hands knowledge to its student as a burden. "Here's something else you must learn. Never forget it or you may kill someone." These contextual assumptions are not said aloud, of course, yet they color subsequent behaviors and self-perceptions.

Historian Susan Reverby (1987) looked at nursing sympathetically and found plenty of justification for such attitudes, but that does not change the self-perception of a nurse who sees her knowledge as a burden. Reverby saw the causes as external to the profession, noting society's unwillingness to value caring.

Nurse historian JoAnne Ashley (1977) looked closer to home and blamed nursing's low status and lack of power on the paternalism of hospital administrators and the sexism of physicians, again seeking an external cause.

But the matter of fact is that wherever the source lies, nursing has a long history of fostering a handmaiden image, playing doctor–nurse games, and yes, of being the silent member when joining physicians on grand rounds. These are the expectations that can be changed by an effective nurse executive. Nurses, like other human beings, tend to live up to one's expectations for them. When a nurse executive expects and demands enhanced self-perception, behaviors change and nurses become empowered.

The greatest danger occurs when nurses accept the limitations put on them by others. When the limitations are not accepted, to a great degree they disappear. Empowerment related to self-perception is a matter of accepting one's own ideas or the ideas of one's leader over those imposed by others who would create limitations. Self-empowerment is a combination of feeling empowered and acting empowered.

Nor is empowerment strictly based on a relationship of nurses with other professionals; it also involves how nurses see and treat each other. A nurse who wants to be empowered must respect the empowerment of other nurses. This means that the nurse executive must build an environment that fosters mutual respect among the nursing staff. It is ironic when nurses are inconsiderate of other nurses, inappropriate in a profession so quick to express empathy for patients.

To empower all nurses, each nurse must learn to have faith in his peer professionals and to accept them as trustworthy, responsible, and capable. Such a value and respect for others must be instilled at the top by the nurse executive.

Granted, there are tactics that help change self-perceptions—teaching nurses assertiveness comes to mind. But setting the tone and role playing the values is an important executive function. Manipulating performance expectations is equally important. A change toward empowerment means that the executive must develop systems to support those nurses who exercise their professional autonomy.

The behaviors of empowerment have been identified by many researchers. In nursing, Gorman and Clark (1986) can be credited with early work on the concept. Although they called their variable *power,* today we would call it *empowerment.* The study was an early attempt at empowering nurses, to get staff nurses to assume more power over themselves and their professional performance. In their work, Gorman and Clark identified four major variables that still apply today:

1. Analytic nursing—they taught nurse subjects to apply the same problem-solving skills to understanding their organization as they applied to understanding their patients' conditions. Obviously, to really understand a situation is the first step in changing it. The study group identified cases in which they were able and not able to achieve their objectives. In analytic nursing, the staff nurses learned not to assume that the organization could not change and not to assume that what is must be accepted as unchangeable.

2. Change activities were the next set of behaviors identified in the study. Project leaders taught the nurse subjects how to remove barriers through planned group activities (i.e., how to become change agents). Nurses in the study group selected projects to be implemented in their own hospitals, getting practice in the change process applied in real organizations. The subjects were amazed to discover their own successes when change was thoughtfully planned.

3. Collegiality was the next aspect of empowerment. The project leaders taught the subjects to respect, consult, and collaborate with nurse peers, counteracting the tendency (present even today in nursing) to view seeking help as a sign of failure. In contrast, of course, physicians readily call on other physicians as consultants. Nurses in the study had to learn this behavior.

4. Sponsorship, identified as the role played by nursing administration, was the last variable in the Gorman and Clark study. Administration of the participating hospitals had to enable staff to achieve goals and to advance in the organization. This applied not merely to general policies but to one-on-one relationships. Mentoring and fostering career advancement of nurses with talent was an essential component. Administration needed to be committed to fostering change efforts initiated by nursing groups. And they had to be approachable by nursing staff.

In the Gorman and Clark study, the variables manipulated were both new skills and enhanced self-concepts. Then, as now, when nurses increase their expectations of themselves, they have a remarkable ability to live up to their own expectations.

ORGANIZATIONAL MODELS FOR EMPOWERMENT

Empowerment can take place under any organizational design, yet there are certain forms that encourage empowerment by their very arrangements. Decentralized nursing models do this because of a commitment to send authority and responsibility as far down the chain of command as possible.

Restructured practice and other forms of management that use a matrix structure also provide for shared and distributed authority and power. When power is shared in any organizational design, empowerment is fostered.

The newer shared governance models make an even greater commitment to empowerment, not only providing for professional autonomy but demanding it. In these models (discussed in Chapter 9), a council of professional nurses is the final court of judgment for professional practice issues. The governance form is gaining favor throughout the United States.

Although it has yet to materialize on a grand scale, nursing has attempted to take responsibility for the gatekeeper function in organized care delivery. At present, many nurses control the exit gate, namely, monitoring patient discharge from a system. Such roles range from bed utilization review in hospitals to making reimbursement decisions in insurance companies to various roles in case management and patient discharge.

Nurses also propose that they take charge of the gate-opening roles, one element of the National League for Nursing proposal for a National Health Care Plan (Hawken 1990). Indeed, there is no reason why nurses cannot be good agents to screen patients and deploy them to appropriate providers. Many already serve that function in emergency department care.

Although it makes sense that nurses fill such a gate-opening position, it is also clear that gatekeepers (on either side of the gate) hold very powerful positions, empowering not only the role holder but the entire profession that supplies the gatekeepers.

SUMMARY

Empowerment, then, is distributed over many people; it is divergent while power is convergent, limited to a few. The roles of both leaders and followers are important in an empowerment model. Traditionally, power has been associated with the highest executive. Empowerment, in contrast, filters down through the whole organization.

An important discovery of our era is that these two principles, power and empowerment, are not incompatible. Indeed, they work hand-in-glove. By encouraging empowerment (distributive), the nurse executive may also increase the (convergent) powers of his own office. An empowered staff creates a powerful leader in a win-win situation for all.

REFERENCES

Ashley, J. 1977. *Hospitals, paternalism and the role of the nurse.* New York: Teachers College Press.

Benner, P. 1984. *From novice to expert: Excellence and power in clinical nursing practice.* Menlo Park, Calif.: Addison-Wesley Publishing Co., Inc.

Brooten, D., et al. 1986. A randomized clinical trial of early hospital discharge and home follow-up of very-low-birth-weight infants. *New England Journal of Medicine* 315, no.15: 934–939.

Dreyfus, S.E., and H.L. Dreyfus. No date. *A five-stage model of the mental activities involved in directed skill acquisition.* Unpublished report, United States Air Force Office of Scientific Research (Contract F49620-79-C-0063), University of California at Berkeley.

Gorman, S., and N. Clark. 1986. Power and effective nursing practice: A report on the findings of the Nursing Knowledge Project. *Nursing Outlook* 34, no.3:129–134.

Hawken, P.L. 1990. NLN's national health strategy: A plan for reform. In *Public Policy Bulletin.* New York: National League for Nursing (NLN).

Reverby, S.M. 1987. *Ordered to care: The dilemma of American nursing, 1850–1945.* New York: Cambridge University Press.

SUGGESTED READINGS

Bullough, B. 1992. Alternative models for specialty nursing practice. *Nursing and Health Care* 13, no.5:254–259.

Calkin, J.D. 1984. A model for advanced nursing practice. *Journal of Nursing Administration* 14, no.1:24–30.

Chandler, G.E. 1992. The source and process of empowerment. *Nursing Administration Quarterly* 16, no.3:65–71.

Clifford, P.G. 1992. The myth of empowerment. *Nursing Administration Quarterly* 16, no.3:1–5.

Connelly, L.M., et al. 1993. A place to be yourself: Empowerment from the client's perspective. *Image* 25, no.4: 297–303.

Cronin, C.J., and J. Maklebust, J. 1989. Case-managed care: Capitalizing on the CNS. *Nursing Management* 20, no.3:38–43.

Curtin, L. 1990. Designing new roles: Nursing in the '90s and beyond. *Nursing Management* 21, no.12:7–9.

Gawlinski, A., and L.S. Kern, eds. 1994. *The clinical nurse specialist role in critical care.* Philadelphia: W.B. Saunders, for the American Association of Critical-Care Nurses.

Gunden, E., and S. Crissman. 1992. Leadership skills for empowerment. *Nursing Administration Quarterly* 16, no.3:6–10.

Hambric, A.B., and J.A. Spross, eds. 1989. *The clinical nurse specialist in theory and practice,* 2nd ed. Philadelphia: W.B. Saunders.

Johnson, L. 1992. Interactive planning: A model for staff empowerment. *Nursing Administration Quarterly* 16, no.3:47–57.

Mason, D.J., et al. 1991. Toward a feminist model for the political empowerment of nurses. *Image* 23, no.2:72–77.

McGraw, J.P. 1992. The road to empowerment. *Nursing Administration Quarterly* 16, no.3:16–19.

Morath, J.M. 1988. The clinical nursing specialist: Evaluation issues. *Nursing Management* 19, no.3:72–80.

Price, M.J., et al. 1992. Developing national guidelines of nurse practitioner education: An overview of the product and the process. *Nursing Education* 31, no.1:10–15.

Snyder, M. 1990. Specialization in nursing: Logic or chaos. In *The nursing profession: Turning points,* ed. N. Chaska, 107–112. St. Louis: C.V. Mosby Co.

Styles, M.M. 1989. *On specialization in nursing: Toward a new empowerment.* Kansas City, Mo.: American Nurses Foundation.

Styles, M.M. 1990. Clinical nurse specialists and the future of nursing. In *The clinical nurse specialist,* eds. P.S.A. Sparacino et al., 279–284. East Norwalk, Conn.: Appleton & Lange.

Tierney, M.J., et al. 1990. Cost accountability and clinical nurse specialist evaluation. *Nursing Management* 21, no.5:26–31.

Zerwekh, J.V. 1992. The practice of empowerment and coercion by expert public health nurses. *Image* 24, no.2:101–105.

Part V
Managing Productivity

One of the most important functions of the nurse executive's office is the management of productivity. In an era of scarce resources, it goes without saying that productivity is critical. With fewer resources, each must be used to its full potential. Resources come in many forms, most importantly, people, the focus of Part V.

This section then looks at how people are used in the conversion of goals into efficient activities. Chapter 17 looks at the comprehensive divisional goals and reviews the process of converting them to human activities and functions. Chapter 18 looks at the production of administrative policies that facilitate that process, and Chapter 19 looks at the pragmatic deploying of personnel. Chapter 20 takes the other side of that task, looking at the work-impinging characteristics of patients and how they may be manipulated to produce productivity. However it is framed, productivity deals with getting the work done in the most efficient manner at the least cost in use of resources.

17

Concretizing Goal Statements: Functions and Standards

To identify the mission and objectives of a nursing organization is not the end of the administrative task. The executive must then determine how the goals are to be achieved. Two mechanisms come into play: (1) determining what activities must be performed to achieve the goals (i.e., deriving functions and activity plans), and (2) setting expectations as to how well those activities must be performed (i.e., determining standards). It is here that ideas are translated into action, when notions become—or fail to become—reality.

In this chapter, three different types of functions are presented: nursing divisional functions, job functions, and the functions of the nurse executive. These functions are derived primarily from the mission and objectives for the division, the set of job constellations for workers, and the executive role, respectively.

FUNCTIONS OF THE DIVISION

The functions of a nursing division represent the critical juncture at which goals are translated into acts. These comprise the constellation of key activities perceived as necessary and sufficient for the achievement of the divisional goals (usually elaborated as a mission and subsequent set of divisional objectives). Objectives are assumed to achieve the divisional mission if they themselves are achieved. In essence, the functions of the division represent the ongoing work that provides for day-to-day operations, often while executives are more concerned with strategic contingencies.

When additional strategic goals are added to the mix, they also require action plans. Although strategic plans may be more dynamic, for that very reason they require a definitive set of actions to be taken. A strategy requires implementing tactics.

The first step in organizing a nursing division is to ask what actions must be taken to achieve each objective (mission-related or strategic). When a single objective is considered alone, the requisite actions designed for its accomplishment are identified in what is commonly called an *activity plan*. An activity plan is detailed; it tells who will do what, when, where, and how. This level of detail is possible because the activity plan addresses a single objective.

When several objectives are considered together, the actions required to achieve them jointly are usually called *functions*. Functions are broad-based key activities that, if taken together and successfully completed, ensure attainment of a group of objectives.

The functions that achieve the divisional objectives usually do not match objectives one for one. For example, a single function may accomplish three objectives. Conversely, another objective may require a number of functions for its achievement. For example, the objective "to provide adequate and able nursing staff for competent care delivery" might be partially achieved by each of the following four functions:

1. Develop job descriptions for each level of personnel within the division.
2. Establish criteria and procedures for hiring, evaluating, promoting, and dismissing personnel.
3. Maintain an effective staffing plan that considers patient acuity needs.
4. Hire nursing division personnel as needed to fill the staffing plan.

One usually considers divisional objectives and functions as a constellation rather than individually, asking: Is this group of functions necessary and sufficient for the achievement of the objectives? Do these functions identify the key activities of the division?

Strategic plans more often are handled by separate action plans for each major effort. The difference is that most strategic plans are more targeted, less likely to be spread over organizationwide activities.

Activity plans must consider not only actions directly involved in reaching objectives but also those that are prerequisites or supportive. Drucker (1974), for example, identified four kinds of functions: result-producing activities, support activities, hygiene and housekeeping activities, and activities of top management. All these activities may be necessary to achieve a given objective.

STANDARDS

Although *functions* along with action plans (or strategies and accompanying tactics) tell what is to be done, they do not give a mechanism by which to measure the performance. Standards provide this necessity. Standards are operationalized, allowing the user to rate the actual performance of an activity.

An additional term, *criterion*, sometimes is used interchangeably with *standard*. Other times, a standard may be broken into several criteria, all or a portion of which must be achieved to achieve the standard.

DISTRIBUTION OF FUNCTIONS

Like divisional objectives, divisional functions represent an early phase of *differentiation* in the nursing organization. Indeed, divisional specialization begins when specific functions are assigned to different organizational units. Functions must be viewed together as a whole. Only in this way can the *integration* of the nursing division be achieved. The organization of a nursing division is designed through finer and finer discriminations but always with a view from the whole. It is the function of top management to integrate and orchestrate that view from the whole.

Divisional functions and their coordinated objectives are distributed downward through the organizing frameworks, the departments, units, and committees. Indeed, the organizing frameworks themselves may be determined by the way in which functions are separated or combined. Thus, one might create a staff education department if most staff education functions are kept together. If, however, staff education functions are dispersed, there might be no need for a single education department, and each nursing unit might be responsible for its own unique staff education program. In other instances, the nurse executive might treat her organizing framework of departments, units, and committees as givens, determining which functions she wishes to distribute in each of these given organization entities.

Functions are distributed through several organizational structures. First, they are distributed by departments (main subclassifications of the nursing division) and by nursing units (usually subclassifications of the nursing department). Some functions, in contrast, are distributed within the committee structure of the division. Within those departments, units, and committees, functions are further delegated through various job descriptions and role expectations. Specific activities also are delegated through the assignment system.

The rules for derivation of divisional functions may be summarized as follows:

1. Identify the constellation of key activities necessary for achievement of divisional objectives.
2. Add functions required to *support* the activities identified as achieving the objectives. In a nursing division, such activities as continuing education and research might be considered supportive to a divisional objective of patient care.
3. Include essential hygiene and housekeeping activities required to maintain the division (e.g., recordkeeping, employee health services, or secretarial services).
4. Add the key activities of nursing top management that have not been addressed under objective-achieving activities. These might include such activities as organizing the division or developing management staff.
5. Check to see if the selected functions are compatible with one another as a constellation of coordinated activities; revise as necessary.
6. Ensure that key functions are necessary and sufficient for achievement of divisional objectives.
7. Ensure that functions can be achieved within the division, given its departments, units, and committee structure; revise either structures or functions accordingly.

The same set of rules will serve for departmental and unit functions as well. All organization subunits need to specify their particular functions, those unique to the subunit and those in which they participate jointly with other subdivisions. Just as one objective might be distributed over several functions, so a single function may be distributed over several departments or units. Conversely, a given function might be assigned to a single department or unit if it requires specialization for its enactment.

Not all functions of a nursing division reach downward. The division will also participate in institutionwide functions as well as in corporate-level functions. Taken together with strategic planning, it is evident that the organization is a web of mutually facilitative functions directed toward a unique set of goals and missions.

JOB FUNCTIONS

Divisional functions (key activities) ultimately are differentiated into the specific tasks and responsibilities of which they are comprised. These discrete tasks and responsibilities are then sorted into relevant job constellations, codified in job descriptions. It may be easier to codify jobs at lower levels in the organization than for those at higher offices. For example, the functions of a chief nurse executive may undergo many changes over time as the organization shifts to meet changing environmental presses.

When designing those relatively stable roles, each constellation of functions should conjoin items of equivalent complexity, and the assortment of tasks and responsibilities in a single job should be of a compatible nature. Each job classification should represent a reasonable work pattern for a qualified individual.

Obviously, the number of workers required for each job classification will depend on quantitative calculations: How many times do the job activities need to be repeated? The constellation of jobs clumped together in any one role is changing rapidly in the delivery of nursing care. Restructured practice has caused nurse executives to examine tasks anew, asking what tasks can be performed by workers with what level of preparation. Few institutions have exactly the same number and design of positions as existed a decade ago.

Considered as a whole, the job classifications of a nursing division should provide for completion of all tasks implied by the divisional functions. Job classifications are the final step of differentiation in organizing a nursing division and ultimately stem from the divisional functions. However, just as functions interplay with organizational departmentalization, so specific job tasks interplay with organizational policies. Policies may make the completion of tasks easier or more difficult.

In a world without constraints or traditions, the nurse executive would determine her job classifications simply by logic and her sense of fit. Even today, the nurse executive is free to create many job classifications of her own choosing, but she is limited in the skilled professions by state licensing laws that restrict certain functions to certain classes of workers. Legislation places some constraints on how job functions are bundled together. Even with legal dictates, today's job descriptions and their functions are likely to differ significantly from institution to institution.

The historical move to create institutional licensure was an attempt to do away with all constraints on job classification. Indeed, the topic has arisen again in relation to restructured practice. As long as certain licensed groups of workers retain rights and privileges regarding performance of certain tasks, the nurse executive will have limitations on how she can bundle tasks and responsibilities. Some see this limitation as a small price to pay (in managerial flexibility) for the benefits gained by maintaining discrete professional and occupational groups within nursing.

Today, many nurse executives are experimenting with different job mixes to promote optimal effectiveness and economy. One sees two contrasting approaches. In the more common design, the nurse executive returns to a mix with an increased proportion of lower-level caregivers (e.g., an increase in nurse aides or licensed practical nurses). The objective of this approach is primarily one of economy, and it is accompanied by attempts to assign all tasks to appropriate levels of employees.

An opposite approach tries to increase professional staffing. In some instances, all-registered nurses (RN) staffing is achieved. The argument offered for this tactic is that the RN is the best all-purpose employee. Not only can she do all tasks, but she can do so without spending time in coordination, direction, and teaching of lower-level personnel. This can be an important factor in situations in which lower-level workers have poor motivation or have negotiated contracts that delimit what the workers may do.

The move toward all-professional staffing has lost momentum in many parts of the nation as RN salaries have risen. The salary increments, although perhaps overdue, have had the effect of limiting the number of professional staff who can be hired on inelastic budgets.

Yet, the answer for one institution may not be the answer for another. The variables concerning patients, staff, and circumstances all must be taken into account in determining a staffing strategy. In all cases, the nurse executive should *have* a strategy.

General principles in creating job classifications include the following:

1. The job classifications of a division should arise primarily from the necessary work to be performed, not merely from tradition and legal constraints.
2. Job classifications should clearly differentiate the expectations for different levels of workers, and the salary structure should reflect both required skills and job responsibilities. Although not all assigned tasks can be included in any job description, those described should indicate level and nature of expected performance.
3. Job classifications should be added, removed, or revised if the work of the division significantly changes. For example, some institutions with a high level of medical technology find fewer and fewer tasks for the unskilled or semiskilled worker. This might necessitate eliminating some traditional lower-level jobs or substituting new classes of technicians.
4. In addition to considering each job classification singly, there may be a need for radical redistribution of all divisional tasks into new job classifications at some time in the history of a given institution. Some job enrichment programs focus on creating more meaningful collections of tasks within each given job.
5. In some institutions, job classifications are coordinated and classified institution-wide, according to the level of difficulty and responsibility. In this case, the nurse executive must see that her job classifica-

tions are appropriately placed and coordinated with other institutional job classifications according to their required skills and responsibilities. Retrospective job analysis often is used in making such judgments or in revising obsolete job classifications.

Sometimes jobs are reorganized in an attempt to get around constraints built into union-administration labor contracts. In some states where head nurses are found in many unions, the tactic of reorganizing the head nurse job has been used to pull managers out of the union. The nurse executive has the authority to make real changes in jobs, but they must not be simply cosmetic changes masquerading under a new role title.

When job descriptions are significantly changed, it is common practice to allow those holding present jobs to apply for the new positions. If these persons fail to qualify, however, they need not be selected. A nurse executive can be challenged in making a job change if her only change is one of qualifications. Suppose, for example, that a nurse executive decides to create a new qualification for head nurses (e.g., that they hold master's degrees). To make such a change, she must substantiate that the new qualification is essential to the head nurse job today.

Often, when a change involves primarily a shift in qualifications rather than in job responsibilities, it can be enacted by grandfathering in those already holding the job but lacking the new qualification. Newly hired persons, thereafter, can be held to the new requirement.

Job Descriptions

Constellations of job functions are documented in job descriptions, but these contain many other elements in addition to tasks and responsibilities. An adequate job description contains at least the following elements:

1. a specific job title
2. a job number or coding that indicates the level and classification of this job in rela-

tion to other jobs in the division or institution
3. reporting relationships (to whom one is responsible and for whom one is accountable)
4. summary description of the position, its key functions, and major responsibilities
5. substantive detailed list of responsibilities and/or tasks
6. real and potential hazards of the position: environmental, psychological, physiological, chemical, biologic
7. qualifications for holding the position, usually educational and experiential; some institutions also identify requisite personal characteristics if they can be clearly associated with success in the job

Some cautions are in order in writing job descriptions. First, a job description should tell what is specific to a given position. A job description should not contain a majority of functions that are assistive in nature: "assists head nurse to . . .," "assists head nurse in developing . . .," "assists head nurse in managing. . . ." A job description of this sort does not give clear criteria for determining performance of the incumbent.

Second, as the position responsibility increases, the job description will be less programmed; as the responsibility decreases, the job description will be more programmed. For example, the job description for the nurse executive may describe many responsibilities but few specific tasks. This is because the nurse executive has the freedom to select those mechanisms by which to achieve the job responsibilities. The nurses' aide job description, in contrast, should list fewer responsibilities, and the way in which those responsibilities are to be carried out should be specified as tasks: "takes temperature, pulse, respirations (TPRs) as assigned" (as task) rather than "evaluates patient's physiologic status" (a responsibility).

Even in constructing a job description for a position of limited responsibility, the nurse executive must be careful to allow leeway for unspecified tasks at the same level of skill and responsibility. The list of tasks can be headed "characteristic tasks" to indicate the incompleteness. Another device is the inclusion in the list of an element that reads "other tasks as assigned." It is impossible to imagine and include all possible job eventualities in the job description.

FUNCTIONS OF THE NURSE EXECUTIVE

The executive function is at least a two-way position, with corporate responsibilities (institutional management) upward and responsibility for nursing practice downward. One cannot neglect either aspect.

Divisional

The executive function includes those specific tasks and responsibilities for nursing that can be achieved only with a view of the whole division. Only the nurse executive or those few managers whom she allows to share her perspective are capable of performing the executive function. The executive function includes several critical functions: providing vision, setting goals, solving problems, bridging, negating, and unifying. These are intellectual activities, and her decisions in respect to them affect her entire division and the entire organization.

In providing vision, the executive blends two images: the desired status of nursing as a profession and the desired quality of practice for the given nursing organization. This is the aspect of vision, requiring today a broad comprehension of the environment as well.

Her vision directly affects the major goal-setting activities of the division. Yet, the vision itself is more than the specific goals selected; it is the ethos of nursing and nursing care that permeates the organization. The nurse executive bears the burden of setting the tone of the division.

This is the ultimate, if subtle, meaning of leadership in nursing administration. The nurse executive who directs a division without vision, albeit with efficiency, fails in the greatest obligation and the greatest opportunity.

Nor can this vision simply be equated with the goals set. Compare two nurse executives with a similar vision of nursing as a developing scientific, independent profession. One nurse executive might exemplify this vision by establishing an active nursing research department; the other, instead, might foster inquiry-based practice among her staff nurses. The vision is broader than any specific goal exemplifying it, although it directs what goals will be selected.

Similarly, the vision of the nurse executive will have an impact on executive problem solving. To a great extent, the executive's vision determines what problems are recognized, how they are cast, and what sorts of solutions are sought. Problem solving, here, refers to major problems whose resolution will affect the entire nursing division. Such problems typically are nonroutine, unique, and nonrepetitive.

In addition to providing vision, goal setting, and problem solving, the nurse executive plays a bridging role. Bridging takes at least three forms. First, the executive bridges among the various departments and components of her division. This bridging is represented in the well-known linchpin function; the executive simply makes the organizational components fit together and function as a single machine.

The second form of bridging is between the conceptual and the actual. Here, the nurse executive bridges the gap from the world of idea, represented in the plans and planning documents, to the world of actual performance. This bridging includes interpreting the environment and what it means in terms of the nursing division. In this bridging, the ideas take on reality by affecting nursing practices.

The third form of bridging is a temporal one from the present into the future. Present acts are created with future desired states in mind. Development of human resources for future organizational needs is a part of this bridging. Trend setting and working toward enactment of planned changes are part of the picture.

Another significant executive function, that of negating, is often overlooked. Yet, it is critical that the dysfunctional, the impairing, be weeded out. Negating (or nest cleaning) is required if the nursing division is not to be weighed down with burdens of obsolete policies and practices. Nest cleaning should be used like sunset laws (wherein an agency is not renewed unless it can substantiate its productivity and utility). In this case, the nurse executive needs to eliminate dysfunctional policies, practices, and procedures that have accumulated over time within the nursing division.

Corporate Function (Institutional)

The nurse executive is or should be a major corporate or institutional officer. In this capacity, she participates in corporate or institutionwide planning and decision making. In today's environment, the corporate responsibility of the chief nurse officer is greater than in the past. In an era of shrinking resources, her input is essential.

As a corporate officer, the nurse executive will be involved in decisions and planning that extend corporationwide, often concerning nonnursing matters as well. In the capacity of corporate officer, the nurse executive will need to study the institution norms for executive behavior. She may well find that a different set of rules pertain from those practiced in the nursing division.

For example, a norm of cooperation may be replaced by a norm of competition among corporate officers. I think, for example, of a trusting nurse officer who was inveigled into sponsoring a program that her peer corporate officers knew would displease the president. This nurse shot herself in the foot by not understanding the corporate environment.

Another nurse executive, when given an opportunity to speak to the board of trustees, relayed her division's problems, failing to perceive that the president had a prevailing practice of only giving the trustees the good news. No two corporations will have the same set of unspoken rules of operations, but all will have them. The nurse executive needs to learn them quickly, never making assumptions in advance.

In both roles (corporate and divisional), the nurse executive must communicate from one constituency to the other. She conveys nursing needs, achievements, and problems to other or-

ganizational executives without putting these narrow concerns above the corporate perspective. Similarly, when decisions are made for the good of the total organization, she communicates and interprets these to the nursing constituency.

Sometimes, the chief nurse executive is the only nurse who participates in corporate top management. In larger corporations, there may be two or more layers of nurse executives who participate in executive management: the corporate nurse executive and nurse executives at different institutions within the corporation.

PERSPECTIVES ON CONCRETIZING GOAL STATEMENTS

This chapter has taken the position that the concretizing of goal statements is a rational act of matching resources with goals. Several assumptions underlying this position are open to debate. First, the position assumes that one always knows the tasks that need to be performed to achieve one's objectives. Although it may be true that one can determine a set of activities likely to achieve any given objective, it is not necessarily true that one instinctively happens on the best set of functions, the best set of activities.

One cannot be dogmatic in making the linkages between goals and the activities that achieve them. For any given set of goals, there may be alternate ways in which they could be achieved. And as the environment is subject to sudden, unanticipated changes, the most effective activity patterns may change overnight. The job of the nurse executive is not simply to achieve goals but to do it in ways that meet additional criteria: efficiency, vision, and perhaps even flair.

A danger of a highly rational, planning model such as proposed here is that it requires environmental stability. If one is to plan ahead for a given time period, there must be enough stability for those plans to be enacted accordingly. Whether this can be achieved in today's rapidly shifting environments is questionable. Rapid shifts in plans and activities may be essential.

Indeed, institutions will fail if they cannot make rapid adjustments to the changing environment. The planning sequence offered in this chapter, then, may be too static. It may be, however, that a rational stable planning model can be combined with a more rapid, adjusting model. One is reminded of Mintzberg's (1973) early differentiation of strategies into planning, adaptive, and entrepreneurial. One probably needs a combination of all three to thrive (or survive) today. This chapter has focused on the rational element rather than the adaptive or entrepreneurial models needed to complement it.

SUMMARY

The functions in the nursing division represent the enactment of purpose and objectives. Functions are the key activities that achieve the various goals of the division; divisional and job functions are two major types formalized in the operating documents of a nursing division. The functions of the nurse executive combine the divisional focus with a corporate focus, roles that must be enacted simultaneously.

REFERENCES

Drucker, P.F. 1974. *Management: Tasks, responsibilities, practices*. New York: Harper & Row.

Mintzberg, H. 1973. Strategy-making in three modes. *California Management Review* 16, no.2:44–53.

SUGGESTED READINGS

American Nurses Association. 1977. *Standards of rehabilitation nursing practice*. Washington, D.C.: ANA.

American Nurses Association. 1980. *A statement on the scope of medical-surgical nursing practice*. Washington, D.C.: ANA.

American Nurses Association. 1981. *Standards of cardiovascular nursing practice*. Washington, D.C.: ANA.

American Nurses Association. 1981. *Standards of perioperative nursing practice*. Washington, D.C.: ANA.

American Nurses Association. 1985. *The scope of practice of the primary health care nurse practitioner*. Washington, D.C.: ANA.

American Nurses Association. 1985. *Standards of child and adolescent psychiatric and mental health nursing practice*. Washington, D.C.: ANA.

American Nurses Association. 1986. *The role of the clinical nurse specialist*. Washington D.C.: ANA.

American Nurses Association. 1987. *The scope of nursing practice*. Washington, D.C.: ANA.

American Nurses Association. 1987. *Standards of addictions nursing practice with selected diagnoses and criteria*. Washington, D.C.: ANA.

American Nurses Association. 1987. *Standards of oncology nursing practice*. Washington, D.C.: ANA.

American Nurses Association. 1990. *Standards of psychiatric consultation-liaison nursing practice*. Washington, D.C.: ANA.

American Nurses Association. 1991. *Standards of clinical nursing practice*. Washington, D.C.: ANA.

American Nurses Association. 1993. *The scope of cardiac rehabilitation nursing practice*. Washington, D.C.: ANA.

Butler, R. 1991. *Designing organizations: A decision-making perspective*. New York: Routledge.

Curtin, L. 1990. Designing new roles: Nursing in the '90s and beyond. *Nursing Management* 21, no.12:7–9.

Duncan, W.J. 1989. *Great ideas in management*. San Francisco: Jossey-Bass Publishers.

Grohar-Murray, M.E., and H.R. DiCroce 1992. *Leadership and management in nursing*. Norwalk, Conn.: Appleton & Lange.

Poulin, M.A. 1991. The nurse executive role: A structural and functional analysis. *Issues in nursing administration: Selected readings,* ed. M.J. Ward and S.A. Price, 199–205, St. Louis, Mo.: Mosby-Year Books, Inc.

Simms, L.M., et al. 1991. Nurse executives: Functions and priorities. In *Issues in nursing administration: Selected readings,* ed. M.J. Ward and S.A. Price, 206–214. St. Louis, Mo.: Mosby-Year Book, Inc.

Swansburg, R.C. 1990. Committees. In *Management and leadership for nurse managers,* ed. R.C. Swansburg, 298–322. Boston: Jones and Bartlett Publishers.

18

Policies, Procedures, and Practices

Policies, procedures, and practices provide guidelines for how action plans and functions will be enacted in an organization. They constrain and direct specific events; they are the rules that together determine the nursing systems of the division. These systems should be revised periodically for efficiency, safety, and effectiveness.

POLICIES AND PROCEDURES

A policy is a guideline that has been formalized by administrative authority and directs action to some purpose. A policy system is the total constellation of events and rules related to that policy. The three major components in a comprehensive policy system are (1) a purpose, (2) a policy rule, and (3) a written directive on actions to follow in implementing the rule (i.e., a procedure).

A procedure also is a formalized guideline but a secondary one; it details the means to be used to achieve the ends specified in the purpose and delineated further in the policy. A procedure may or may not allow discretion in application of a policy statement. A procedure specifies the way in which a policy is to be implemented if the mode of implementation is restricted. Many but not all policy statements are accompanied by procedures.

Policies and procedures contrast with practices in that practices are the actual habitual behaviors of organization personnel. Policies and procedures are prescribed, but practice, prescribed or not, is what actually happens.

Policy Systems

The components of a policy system are demonstrated in the following illustration. Suppose an institution has a policy that no new employee will be granted vacation time for the first year of employment. Such a policy rule requires a written directive on actions to be followed, for the policy itself is still open to multiple interpretations. For example, is the end of the eleventh month or the end of the twelfth month considered as completion of a year's employment? Does the policy refer to all vacation time or only to vacation time with pay? Does this policy mean that the new employee earns no vacation time at all during the first year or simply that he must take the earned vacation during the second year?

Clearly, this policy needs a procedure if diverse managers are to apply it consistently. Typically, both policies and procedures (together or separately) are recorded in a policy book and are referred to as policies. The common use of the term *policy* for both policy statements and procedures is misleading. Yet, nurses tend to reserve the term *procedure* for those interventions done to or with patients.

The purpose of a policy is as important as the procedures it requires for implementation. Simply by examining a policy statement one cannot always determine the purpose for which it was derived.

There is no way to derive the other two components from any one given component of a policy system. For any given purpose, as an illustration, many different policy statements could be derived. For example, even an apparently simple purpose of establishing racial equality in hiring practices could lead to several contradictory policies such as (1) hiring on a quota system designed to reflect local population percentages, (2) hiring on a system that gives certain compensatory advantages to minority candidates, or (3) evaluation of candidates' qualifications without reference to race.

Nor is one able to deduce the purpose from the policy. For example, if a company has a policy of evaluating candidates without reference to race, there is no assurance that the purpose is one of racial equality. The purpose may be simply to get the candidate with the best qualifications for each job, or it may be one of having policies that qualify the institution for desired federal funds.

For any given policy statement, any number of different procedures might be devised. And many procedures have effects far different from that intended.

Unanticipated Outcomes

Unanticipated results, beneficial or detrimental, may occur when a procedure is put into place. Not every outcome can be anticipated. Other negative effects occur when a policy stays on the books long after the purpose it served has disappeared. One sees instances of this problem every day. Take, for example, staff members assigned to 10:45 A.M. lunches, a practice started when an old cafeteria could not handle the full employee load over regular lunch hours.

If the purpose of the excessively early lunches is lost, the practice may continue even though a new and efficient cafeteria has long since replaced the old one. If no one remembers why the 10:45 A.M. lunches were begun in the first place, then it is difficult to calculate the effects of a proposed change in the time schedule. Hence, a detrimental effect may occur when the original purpose is covert, unknown, or forgotten.

The reason even courageous administrators fear to change a policy once it has been established is that no one can anticipate all the possible effects of a proposed change. One effect that *can* be anticipated is that someone will object to every proposed change, even in the case of a clearly bad policy. For example, some workers will fight for maintenance of the 10:45 A.M. lunch hour.

If all a person knows about a policy is that it cured some problems of the past—and it must have when it was created—it is not surprising that the nurse administrator hesitates to change it, possibly reinstituting old difficulties.

Given the inherent risk in any change, two rules for drafting and implementing policies are evident: (1) Test any new directive on a small population (one unit) before applying it throughout the institution, and (2) identify the purpose in the policy statement.

In general, policies may be seen as facilitative or inhibitive. They should exist for situations in which those facing the need for action are not equipped to make the needed judgments, but they should not be devised in situations in which they hamstring autonomous, professional judgment.

Policies also provide conformity from unit to unit when the choices are too broad and when different decisions made by various subordinate managers might appear to give certain employees unfair advantages over others.

FORMULATING NURSING POLICY

Nursing policies are no longer set in isolation. Indeed, it is difficult to find any nursing policy that does not have an effect on other arenas within the institution. Further, policies made throughout the organization have an impact on nursing. Policy formulation is a complex function requiring consideration of potential impact on various groups.

Content of Policies

When formulating nursing policy, one must ask several questions: How does nursing policy relate to other institutional policy statements? What content should be included in a manual? How specific should policy statements and procedures be? What are the mechanics of creating a usable policy manual? What content belongs in nursing policy statements?

Nursing policy must coordinate with other administrative policy. Policy established at higher organizational levels should not be contradicted by nursing policy, but nursing policy need not be limited to areas covered under these general policies.

One arena in which problems commonly occur is the interaction between personnel and nursing divisions. As a condition of hire, for example, a personnel division may have a policy that all employees of a particular job classification receive 4 weeks of vacation yearly. Unless he cares to challenge the policy at a higher organizational level, the nurse executive is bound by this commitment.

However, the personnel division has no right to direct the nurse executive in operational application of the policy. The nurse executive has the right to make further restrictions on when and under what conditions that vacation time is given, as long as it is, in fact, given. The method of implementing administrative policies remains the operational prerogative of the nurse executive.

A special instance in policy formulation is that of the coordinated policy, an agreement between two or more divisions or departments as to some aspect of their relationship with each other. Nursing and Medical Records, for example, may have agreed on a routine for the handling of readmission charts.

Validation of coordinated policy requires consent and signature of both division heads on the published directive. Nursing manuals may be planned to integrate or to separate such coordinated policies and institutionwide policies.

Selection of content is an important factor in formulating any policy manual. When should a policy statement be made? A policy should be established when its creation solves a problem that recurrently affects the work of the division.

Another perspective goes further, namely, deriving policy to describe the total scope of the division's autonomous responsibility, not just the problem areas. Sometimes, it is difficult to identify all relevant areas for autonomous policy formulation. When one decides to capture the full scope of responsibility, two measures can be used to identify content gaps in policy.

One system asks new employees to log carefully those questions for which there is no policy statement and for which they have to rely on word-of-mouth information. Another measure is to categorize the policy manual into a comprehensive topical arrangement. Each topic can then be studied for omissions.

Two types of policy require different formulations. Policy meant to give facilitating information requires detailed procedures. For example, if the nurse needs to find out the policy for renting a piece of equipment not available in the home institution, she needs to know precise facts. Such a document will be heavy on procedure and light on policy. Similarly, if she needs to know nursing's responsibility (as opposed to the laboratory's) for an unusual test, she needs exact information.

The second type of policy provides a basis for administrative problem solving. These policies need procedures that establish boundaries, reference points, and guidelines without limiting the nurse manager's ability to use judgment. If a policy of this sort is too exacting, a nurse manager may be forced to make a less than desirable decision. For example, a nurse executive might find himself unable to finance the needed education of a coronary care nurse if a tuition policy is written with only college credit courses in mind. Policies meant to guide management decisions should leave room for unanticipated qualifications and conditions.

Levels of Policy Participation

The nursing division represents the largest unit within most health care institutions in terms of number of employees and budget. Also, it is a 24-hour, sustained operation—always functional—whereas many other services only require part-time (e.g., nine-to-five) operations. Nursing, as the custodian of the patient, is affected by policies made throughout the organization.

Because of its critical organization function, nursing cannot afford to be insular. The chief nurse executive must be involved in policy determination at the institutional level. His perspective and special knowledge must color organizational decision making.

As the complexity of the health care organization increases (e.g., through horizontal and vertical intraorganizational expansion) and as external controls increase (e.g., through multifarious payment systems), it is essential that nursing take an organizational perspective.

The nurse executive needs to participate in strategic policy setting in the institution, and he also needs to convey the institutional perspective to his subordinates. In an era when financial retrenchment prevails, the nursing division often cannot avoid retrenchment/conservation activities. If staff do not understand the organizational perspective, the nurse executive may be seen as failing to hold the line on the nursing division's needs. He may become a scapegoat for circumstances beyond his control if he is not able to explain policy changes with credibility.

POLICY FORMAT AND PROCEDURES

Another major question concerns the process by which policy decisions are communicated within the institution and within the nursing division. Some institutions have a central clearinghouse where policies are codified and checked for compatibility with other extant policies. In such a situation, nursing policies may be integrated along with other institutional policies. It is important, in such cases, that the clearinghouse function be understood as one of processing; it is not a step in which policy decisions are reconsidered or changed by another party.

In other instances, the nurse executive may produce a separate manual containing only nursing division policies (a supplement to the institutionwide policy publication). Other nurse executives may elect to combine nursing policies with selected institutional policies that have major impacts on the nursing division. To a great degree, these decisions will be influenced by the sheer number of policies, and that, in turn, is influenced by the size of the institution/corporation.

This section sets forth some simple guidelines for establishing a nursing policy manual. The chief criteria for policy format selection are simplicity and utility. If the policies are complex and difficult to follow, the manual will not be used. There is no one ideal format for policies, but a few principles can be given:

1. If possible, the title of every policy should use the most common terminology (for easy location).
2. A brief description of the policy should be set out at the top of the document so that the reader can rapidly tell if it contains the desired information (without having to read the entire procedure).
3. Objectives (purposes) for the policy should be stated. This facilitates periodic manual review. If the policy no longer meets the original objectives, it will be apparent.
4. A code system should be used to enable the reader to find related policy and procedural statements.
5. All policies should be authenticated by date, by the nurse executive's signature, and by his title.

Pagination of policies is a potential problem area. Some manuals are constructed with policies placed in alphabetic order by title, with page numbers assigned in sequence. This causes two problems: (1) If one cannot guess the correct title of the desired policy, there is no way to locate it except by reading the entire index until the particular policy comes up; and (2) every new policy that is added to the manual, if placed in alphabetic order, requires new pagination for the rest of the manual.

It is easier to locate material and to add new policies if the content of the manual is divided into mutually exclusive sections or subsections, each of which has its own pagination. Then, the reader need consult only a small area of the index to find a relevant policy. Cross-indexing facilitates policy location also.

In those institutions that now have their policy books on-line in a computer system, the search procedure is simplified. However, that is not yet the norm.

Common variations are found in policy format. Some institutions intermix institutional and nursing policies in a single manual. The advantage is that the employee need only deal with one manual, but it may be so extensive as to make it difficult to locate specific policies, not to mention physically cumbersome.

Some institutions separate policies and procedures into two manuals. (The nursing procedure book is one instance of this practice.) The advantage is that the policy book usually is terse and easy to use, but one must seek out cross-indexed procedures frequently.

Also, the mechanics of creating and maintaining a nursing policy manual are complex. The manual should be constructed so that policies can be readily removed or added to appropriate sections of the book. A simple loose-leaf system fits this criterion. Along with the simplest design, the most complex, namely, computerization of the policies, also provides for swift and efficient updating. In addition to a system for replacing obsolete policies, a plan should be evolved for periodic review and updating of the contents of the manual.

It is important that outdated copies of revised policies be thoroughly destroyed (except for a historical copy in nursing division files). Nothing is more frustrating than to follow what appears to be the most recent policy, only to find out that it was superseded but not replaced in the manual. Furthermore, staff members should be instructed to disregard undated and unsigned (unauthorized) policies; such pieces of paper only confuse an already complex system. Finally, a policy manual is only as useful as it is accessible; up-to-date copies should be available to all nursing staff.

PROCEDURES

In some instances, it may be difficult to determine where the policy leaves off and procedure begins. Generally, two types of procedures are found within the nursing division: those addressed to managerial aspects and those specific to clinical nursing methods. The first type usually is included with the related policy directives in a policy book or manual. The second type (clinical nursing directions) usually is contained within a manual traditionally called a *procedure book.*

There are both substance and form issues to consider in producing a clinical procedure book. Many of the criteria stated for a policy book also apply here. The manual should be simple to read and use; titles should use the most common terms for easy access. Outdated copies should be destroyed except for historical records. Where applicable, citations should be given to related managerial policies and procedures. Appropriate clinical references should also be included for the staff member who wishes further information concerning the procedure.

Clinical procedures should indicate whether they are suggested methods or required ones. Most procedures are of the former kind, but for legal purposes, some methods may need to be followed without exception. These differences should be made clear in the manual.

It is critical that one's clinical procedures are up to date. An expert in the related clinical knowledge should determine the content for each procedure. Then, content may be put into standard format by a person assigned to this task. Clinical procedures should be checked for accuracy by a small group of additional experts.

Some institutions buy procedure books available on the market. There is nothing wrong with using prepared books, provided that they are checked for compatibility with a given institution's equipment, practices, and policies. Each institution need not reinvent the wheel.

PRACTICES

Practices may or may not implement policies. Yet, policies and practices should not conflict.

Indeed, court or arbitration cases are likely to hold employees to the common practice, not to the published policy, when the two differ. The nurse executive needs to examine any practice carefully before countermanding it. Some practices grow up as compensation for poor work policies and systems.

All new policies need to be widely displayed, particularly if they have wide impact on present practice. In a contested case, the nurse executive may have to prove that the employee not only had the opportunity to become familiar with a new policy but that the conditions were created so that he *necessarily* was made familiar with it.

SUMMARY

Policies, procedures, and practices define the more stable events of the nursing division. Together, they comprise the rule structures of the organization. Policies serve several purposes; they (1) provide information, (2) guide decision making, (3) substitute for some decision making, (4) define and limit roles with relation to decision making, (5) create standard operating procedures among organizational units, (6) solve recurrent problems, (7) eliminate likely areas for conflict, and (8) make choices among equally attractive alternatives. Procedures detail the way in which policies are to be carried out if a specific means is to be preferred. Practices include all behaviors, arising by habit or tradition or those created by policy decisions and problem-solving behavior.

SUGGESTED READINGS

Jones-Schenk, J., and P. Hartley. 1993. Organizing for communication and integration. *Journal of Nursing Administration* 23, no.10:30–33.

Lee, J.B., and L.R. Eriksen. 1990. The effects of a policy change on three types of absence. *Journal of Nursing Administration* 20, no.7–8:37–40.

Smeltzer, C.H., and P.D. Vrba. 1991. Standard compliance: The process and art of preparation. *Journal of Nursing Administration* 21, no.4:45–54.

Swansburg, R.C. 1990. Nursing service policies and procedures. In *Management and leadership for nurse managers.* ed. R.C. Swansburg, 212–225. Boston: Jones and Bartlett Publishers.

Van-Koot, B., and P. Laverty. 1992. A research foundation for policies and procedures. *Canadian Nurse* 88, no.1:39–41.

Warner, D.C. 1991. Nursing and public policy. *Journal of Nursing Administration* 21, no.5:52–57.

Williams, M.T. 1988. Policies and procedures for scheduling student nurses. *Journal of Nursing Administration* 18, no.9:32–37.

19

Assigning, Staffing, and Scheduling

The conversion of objectives into functions represents the first translation of goals into actions. The subsequent distribution of functions through departments, units, committees, and job descriptions is the next step in organization of those actions. A further distribution and differentiation of actions is done through assigning, staffing, and scheduling of personnel. Here, the quantification of divisional actions occurs.

In the prior decisions concerning departmentalization, committee structure, and job descriptions, work was distributed by type; but in assigning, staffing, and scheduling, work is allocated by specific tasks (or responsibilities) and concrete amounts of work to be performed by concrete numbers of workers. This chapter looks at assigning, staffing, and scheduling as they pertain to patient care units.

In most cases, the nurse executive will have specialists do the actual assigning, staffing, and scheduling of personnel. Most institutions now use computerized systems, at least for staffing and scheduling. And most have a senior nurse manager who is skilled in designing and applying these programs. In a few institutions, head nurses still produce all these final determinations.

Whoever does the actual work, it is important that the nurse executive understand the principles on which these systems work as well as how they interface. If the nurse executive lacks this basic understanding, she may find herself at the mercy of a computer programmer or system operator with a commitment to the wrong system. Computerized or not, a system is only as good as the data and decision rules designed into it.

The nurse executive must understand that there is no such thing as a variable that cannot be factored into a system. The best way to judge the effectiveness of one's systems is to assess the satisfaction of staff and the degree to which "coverage" meets patient needs. Of course, these two items may not always correspond. A contented staff may be receiving more weekends off than can be justified by patient needs, for example.

Because assigning, staffing, and scheduling affect every staff member, they can be the source of major discontent if the systems do not work. They can also affect patient care and budgets. The nurse executive, who oversees the systems at least to the extent of determining the principles driving the systems, must be capable of judging when the systems meet or fail to meet their objectives.

Definitions

Assigning refers to the manner in which the total work of the nursing unit is divided up among personnel. Assigning plans cover the clock as do staffing and scheduling plans. Assigning places accountability for patients and tasks.

Staffing refers to the plan for how many nursing personnel, of what classifications, will be needed for each unit on each shift. Generally, the staffing plan is a prototype, a standard. Each unit where patient care is delivered has a basic plan.

Scheduling is the ongoing filling (or approximating) of that staffing pattern by designating individual personnel to work specific hours and days. Scheduling, therefore, represents the enactment of the staffing plan adjusted for intervening variables.

Assigning and staffing decisions interact in the same manner as do decisions about functions and departmentalization. Two patterns are seen: (1) departmentalization designed to optimize delivery on a specific group of functions or (2) a conjoined group of functions selected to be compatible with already extant departments. Usually, decisions concerning functions and departmentalization are derived by considering both aspects simultaneously. A similar situation occurs with assigning and staffing.

If the planned or actual number and mix of personnel (staffing) is relatively fixed, it places constraints on the selection of an assignment system. For example, a staff with minimal or less prepared personnel may dictate a compensatory functional or restructured assignment system. In the opposite case, suppose there is a commitment to a primary nursing assignment system, and the resources to afford it are available. Then, the staffing can be planned to allow for the assignment model.

Ideally, an assignment system should be selected first, based on a decision concerning what best serves the patient care goals of the division. Next, a staffing pattern would be devised to fit the demands of that assignment system, and finally, a schedule would be devised to implement the staffing plan. Seldom, however, does the ideal situation exist. For example, if the community has a surfeit of professional nurses and few licensed practical nurses (LPNs) or nurses' aides, the staffing may require a modification of the assignment system. Similarly, if

the institution has limited financial resources for salaries, staffing may need to be shifted toward greater use of nonprofessional personnel, thereby affecting assignment decisions. Typically, the staffing pattern and the assignment system are mutually determined.

ASSIGNMENT SYSTEMS

Assignment systems have an interesting evolution in nursing. Each new system is greeted as if it were the answer to all the problems of nursing care delivery. Indeed, each new assignment system can be seen to cure the major deficiency of the preceding system. Each system, in its turn, brings forth its own set of problems and deficiencies. See Chapter 12 for an analysis of this process.

Even today, one still sees evidence of three historical assignment systems: functional, team, and primary nursing. Commonly, a restructured practice adding a case manager function may be superimposed on any one of these basic designs. At least four criteria are important for evaluating each assignment method: (1) administrative efficiency, (2) patient needs satisfaction (effectiveness), (3) staff needs satisfaction (happiness quotient), and (4) economy (insurance/societal satisfaction).

Functional Assignment

In theory, the functional assignment system is the most administratively efficient method because it divides labor according to specific tasks. Each employee has a clearly defined set of tasks, different from the assignments of others. There is little likelihood of confusion over who will do what. Minimal time is spent coordinating activities among staff members. Further, each member can become highly skilled if he does the same task repetitively.

A functional system underlies many elements of restructured practice, especially if nursing technicians and mixed-skill teams are used. Nurses find the functional method most efficient during pressing personnel shortages. A functional assignment is designed to take advantage of different skill levels among workers. Economy may be realized here by always assigning tasks to the lowest possible level of personnel who may legally perform the function.

Sometimes today, a functional assignment is combined with a team approach in various amalgams of the two work designs.

Team Assignment

The team method of assignment evolved as an attempt to increase patient and staff satisfaction even at the cost of administrative efficiency. The sources for potential loss of efficiency include the fact that each staff member is curtailed to the care of a limited group of patients and that increased time is spent in coordinating delegated work. Because individual assignments are less regularized than under the functional method, more time is spent by head nurses and team leaders in checking up on workers. Further, the delegation of work to team members may be performed by a team leader with minimal managerial experience, further decreasing efficiency.

Not all experts agree that the team system is less efficient than the functional method in actual practice. Many believe that the closer interaction among the staff members provides an esprit de corps that compensates for time expended in delegation and coordination. Most advocates of the team system, however, rest their support on the increased satisfaction of patient and staff needs.

Theoretically, the patient's needs are better met by the team system because he is cared for by a limited number of personnel who know him better. Increased effectiveness in care, so it is reasoned, results not only from identification and resolution of patient needs but from the opportunity for more therapeutic, closer patient–nurse relationships.

These gains in effectiveness, however, may be somewhat offset by the increased likelihood of errors. Workers doing multiple different tasks are more likely to make mistakes than are workers repeating the same tasks over and over. In almost all cases, the team assignment system is associated with patient-based rather than task-based division of work. Each staff member is likely to be doing many different tasks for a limited number of patients rather than a single task for a large number of patients.

Theoretically, each staff member should feel greater satisfaction in team than in functional assignments due to increased guidance from a team leader and better matching of worker skills to patient needs. Also, by working with fewer patients, the team member has a clear sense of his own contribution to patient outcomes.

From a fiscal perspective, team assignment is probably the most expensive mode of delivering patient care. Limiting use of staff to one team requires more staffing. When team members and leaders are frequently changed, the original advantage of a nurse knowing intimately a few patients is lost.

Primary Nursing Assignment

In primary care, each patient is assigned to one nurse for his total hospitalization. She is responsible for planning and organizing his care. The focus in primary care is on who *plans* the care more than on who delivers it. The registered nurse (RN) may be assisted in the care of her patients by other staff members assigned through various systems. Interestingly, this is the first assignment system that can subsume other assignment systems within it. This is because of the predominance of planning over doing; it is a system that gives predominance to the cognitive acts of nursing.

In primary nursing, each primary nurse has a certain number of patients, and she is responsible for all nursing care planning for these patients. Usually this care planning is seen as a 24-hour responsibility. The primary nurse may be called at irregular hours for important changes in her patient's nursing needs. In some restructured care systems, the primary nurse may also be responsible for case management functions.

Administrative efficiency is lost by limiting each nurse's knowledge and mobility to the care of only a few patients. The system permits, however, mobile use of other staff members—important if there is a downward shift in personnel mix.

However, it is possible that the primary nurse will generate more nursing orders than would appear in any other assignment system. Efficiency gained through clarity of orders and mobility of lower-level personnel may be lost through the increased work generation. Clearly, efficiency may be traded for increased care effectiveness in this system. The amount of work generated may be limited by use of case management tools that set clear expectations concerning the "amount" of work anticipated for any given patient.

One source of gain in efficiency in primary nursing care is the elimination of many positions in the chain of communication. The physician and other health workers are encouraged to deal directly with the primary nurse; less time is spent in passing on orders. Improved effectiveness also is due to decreasing care errors that occur with multiple relaying of orders.

Effectiveness is usually improved by the primary care mode, and the system scores well on the criterion of patient needs satisfaction because each patient has his private nurse planner. The method ensures that at least one staff member has a vested interest in his case, and his problems are more likely to be identified and resolved under this system.

Primary care is an attempt to increase the professionalism of nursing by establishing accountability for individually designed and administered nursing care. Theoretically, primary care should increase the RN's satisfaction with her career because she has clear products: patient outcomes that are the direct result of her own work and decisions. This form of assignment allows the nurse to operate at the peak of her professional capacity. The system is not overly concerned with the satisfaction of staff members other than the primary nurse, although they may benefit from her clear nursing orders and guidance.

In real situations, staff and patient needs satisfaction is greatly dependent on the preparation of the nurse for a primary care role. A nurse who does not feel secure in nursing care planning will feel threatened by primary care assignments. Also, the patient whose primary nurse is not capable is much worse off than the patient under team or functional nursing who is exposed to many nurses, any one of whom might plan for his needs.

Economically, there is little agreement as to the cost of primary nursing versus team or functional. Conflicting positions have been offered in both the popular literature and in nursing studies. Primary nursing has been touted as more expensive, equal in cost, and less expensive by different sources.

Restructured Practice

Restructured practice combines elements from these traditional formats for staff assignment in various ways. Moreover, a new role of the case manager is filtered into the mix in many cases. Chapter 13 reviews various assignment systems that impose this new role on the structure.

Comparison of Head Nurse Role under Various Methods

The role of the head nurse varies within the major assignment systems. In functional care, the head nurse is a manager in the strict sense; only she has the overall view of the whole unit. Only she is responsible for seeing that all the pieces of work are delegated, completed, and coordinated. Because many different nurses are likely to see each patient under the functional system, the head nurse is fairly sure that any gross defects or omissions in care will come to someone's attention.

Under the team system, the head nurse delegates many of her day-to-day management duties to team leaders. This allows her more time for long-term planning for patient care and staff education needs. This ideal may not be realized, however, if she must spend extensive time evaluating and educating team leaders to the skills of management.

In a primary care system, the head nurse becomes even more of a teacher and evaluator. As the care systems limit the patient's contacts to fewer professional nurses, the head nurse must assume the role of clinical care evaluator. It is vital that the head nurse evaluate the care planning of each nurse. In this system, the nurse's mistake or error of judgment is not likely to be corrected unless the head nurse finds it.

In the evolution from functional, through team, to primary nursing systems of assignment, the head nurse role evolves from that of an organizer and manager of tasks to an evaluator of clinical care and a teacher of nurses. These role variations demand distinctly different abilities. Hence, an excellent head nurse under one assignment system may be a poor head nurse under another.

In many ways, the head nurse role under restructured practice resembles that under functional nursing. The head nurse is the person who orchestrates the performance of all tasks by various personnel. The role often is enacted in a matrix where she must work alongside a case manager in designing effective systems of care.

Further, she is no longer protected from corporate goals, and often her management decisions must include consideration of corporate initiatives for fiscal management. In essence, the head nurse role in restructured practice has become a corporate role, requiring exquisite managerial skills.

STAFFING

Staffing and assignment systems interact to deliver on the goals and functions of the nursing division. When any of these elements are changed, the impact on the others must be reviewed. Some assignment systems tend to use more or less staff than others; other variables in the environment affect the relationship between staffing and assigning.

For example, the assignment system that is efficient in use of manpower in a large complex medical center using high technology for seri-

ously ill patients may be inefficient in a skilled nursing facility with few critically ill patients and a lower level of technology. Patient acuity and the level of technological therapy used are critical factors that must be considered in any decision concerning staffing. The following section reviews staffing as if it were a separate entity; the reader is cautioned to remember its interaction with the other components of the total nursing system.

Staffing has two main components: (1) a *staffing pattern* indicating how many persons of what job classification should be on duty per each unit, per shift, per day, and (2) the *staffing plan*, a scheme mathematically derived to indicate how many people of what job classifications must be hired to deliver on the staffing pattern. These two components each present a different set of problems for the nurse executive.

Staffing Pattern

A staffing pattern for a single patient care unit is given in Figure 19–1. A final staffing pattern is the cumulative design; it incorporates counts for all units of the nursing division.

A staffing pattern is a relatively permanent document, built on several assumptions:

1. that each given unit will continue to admit the same type of patients (similar acuity) in the same numbers for the total period in which the staffing pattern is in effect
2. that patient needs can be "averaged out" per unit on a daily basis and can be converted into the number of required nurs-

3 WEST	Days	Evenings	Nights
	1 HN		
	4 RN	2 RN	1 RN
	2 LPN	1 LPN	
	2 NA	2 NA	2 NA
	9	5	3

Note: HN, head nurse; LPN, licensed practical nurse; NA, nurse assistant; RN, registered nurse.

Figure 19–1 Staffing Pattern for a Single Patient Care Unit

ing hours (as reflected in the determined staffing)
3. that the converted number of nursing hours will remain relatively constant from day to day

If these assumptions fail to hold up, then the *constancy* of the staffing pattern is called into question. The working assumptions (and the efficacy of the staffing pattern) can be overturned by any change that causes a deviation in the estimated nursing hours per patient day, for example, alterations in

1. patient acuity levels
2. actual patient days
3. nursing or medical technologies (when those changes cause a difference in nursing time required)
4. assignment systems
5. nursing care goals
6. interface with other departments and divisions (when those altered interfaces cause more or less "work" for the nursing unit)
7. physical plant or equipment
8. nursing delivery or management systems

When trends in these variables can be forecast, staffing patterns can be adjusted accordingly. The staffing pattern of a nursing division usually is reviewed at least yearly for modifications required by changes in patient numbers, care trends, or contextual variables.

Determining the Staffing Pattern

The staffing pattern is a quantitative statement of patient care delivery. It reveals how many hours per day per shift per unit will be worked by each level of personnel. This critical conversion to a finite number of hours of work as compared with patient needs can be derived in two distinct ways.

1. Patient acuity/classification systems focus on patient needs: Patients are sorted in various categories, related to acuity and number of nursing hours required per patient in that category per shift.

2. Task-quantifying systems focus on nursing acts: Common nursing tasks are related directly or indirectly (through various patient care units [PCUs]) to a time-per-task measure. This measure may be derived through past experience or time and motion studies. These systems are also called task analysis methodologies.

These conversion systems may be primitive or complex, accurate or inaccurate, or correctly or incorrectly applied. The more sophisticated systems of both sorts break down final hours to be worked according to the level of nursing personnel required to give the care. Some sophisticated systems combine a patient classification mechanism with a task quantification system. Task analysis systems have undergone a resurgence with the notion of restructuring. Both types of systems are discussed in Chapter 20.

One system of determining the staffing pattern is presented here, although it oversimplifies a complex process:

• Develop a system of identifying and codifying individual patient needs. (This usually involves use of a patient acuity/ classification system.)

   1. Sum all patient needs per unit per shift for a per-day tally.

   2. Differentiate needs as to complexity and summarize by complexity level.

   3. Cumulate need tallies for a long enough period to derive a needs norm per unit per shift per day.

• Develop a system of relating patient needs to number of patients on that unit for the day (the census norms to quantitative care delivery data). Thus, one might calculate norms. This requires that one

   1. Determine the quality and quantity of nursing care that will be given in response to patient needs.

   2. Apply a nursing task quantification system.

   3. Include relating complexity of needs to level of personnel.

- Develop a mechanism for relating care delivery data to job descriptions of care deliverers. (Either job descriptions may be constructed to fit care delivery data or care delivery data may be compared with extant job categories to determine number of employees of each job category necessary to deliver the required quantitative sum of care hours.)

  1. Remember to include indirect nursing time if the quantification system used did not do so.
  2. Remember to correct norms if there is a goal of improving quality of care delivered. (It is true that nurses can work smarter in the same amount of time, but most upgrading also involves increased expenditure of nursing time. It is not reasonable to expect more and more for no increased cost in time involvement.)

Staffing that takes into account patient needs and/or specific nursing tasks to be performed is an advancement over old systems based on (1) number of beds per unit or, slightly improved, (2) average census per unit. These old norms ignored the fact that even if census were stable, one group of 30 patients might need far more care than another group of 30 patients.

This fluctuation of amount of care needed (even among equal numbers of patients) was long reflected in a common quantitative measure of nursing care, the nursing-hours-per-patient-day (NHPD) unit. This measure is calculated by adding together all nursing personnel on a unit for 24 hours, multiplying them (singly or together) by the number of hours worked, and dividing this figure by the number of patients on that unit for the day (the census data). Thus, one might calculate:

January 5, 1995:

20 personnel × 8 hours each (over 3 shifts) for 40 patients = 4.0 NHPD

One of the first alterations in staffing patterns based on the NHPD was the intensive care unit staffing. Here, it was possible to group all patients requiring excessive hours of nursing care, determine the NHPD norms of this unit as compared with average nursing care units, and charge patients higher fees for more nursing hours.

Today, ironically, as patients on all inpatient units grow more acute, some units are finding it less essential to make a daily adjustment according to level of acuity or required nursing care hours. This occurs simply because the consistent high-intensity care needs show less variance than was once the case.

The NHPD is a norm that may be useful to the nurse executive. For example, she may compare typical NHPD figures for like units among different hospitals. Such data reach most nurse executives whose organizations participate in nationwide data collection through the American Hospital Association. Past data from her own organization also will be useful in providing normative values.

The use of the NHPD unit in reaching staffing decisions is limited, however. First, it is normative rather than prescriptive (i.e., it tells how many hours of care [roughly] *are* being delivered, not how many hours *ought to be* delivered in relation to patient needs). Further, those hours incorporate all nursing staff hours, both those used in giving care and those used in administrative and other activities.

The NHPD calculation also fails to differentiate among employees with different levels of skill training and education. Finally, the NHPD index combines three shifts without any mechanism for differentiation, despite the fact that the work loads may differ significantly on those shifts.

There was a time when most staffing patterns were based on the NHPD (or census, or number of patient beds). Once a staffing number was determined for a whole day, then the nurse executive distributed that number over three shifts based on either her intuitive or her investigated notion of the proportion of care that was needed on each shift. Again, another set of norms arose—those of percentages of staff per shift. One common pattern was that of days, 45 percent of the staff; evenings, 35 percent; and nights, 20 percent. Alternate patterns also were given and supported.

Obviously, such a percentage distribution is interesting but useless in any given case because the tasks assigned per shift vary from institution to institution as do patient needs per shift. Present staffing systems, relying on data concerning patient needs during a shift or nursing tasks during a shift, make the shift, not the day, the unit for consideration in staffing decisions. In this way, one avoids unnecessary extrapolation concerning how the shifts compare in work load.

It is important to consider the NHPD index and its historical impact on nursing administration. First, it has the advantage of being a figure that is easily calculated and that allows for comparison among institutions. Indeed, many unsophisticated nurse executives found themselves prisoners of this index. Hospital administrators who failed to understand professional nursing did—and some still do—see the NHPD as a norm applicable to any institution. The administrator with such limited understanding was not above using this figure as a measure for the achievement of the nurse executive in administering her division.

Indisputably, this norm became a burden in situations in which contextual or patient variables significantly increased the nursing care tasks. Further, the calculation of this norm became more problematic. As numbers of workers on a nursing unit increased in types, calculations were made differently by different nurse executives. One nurse executive might include secretarial personnel if those employees were personnel of the nursing division. Another nurse executive might not count secretarial personnel if they reported to another division. It is not surprising that some nurse executives manipulated the NHPD counts to their statistical advantage.

What is important is that the nurse executive recognize the limitations of this calculation and that she be able to explain her NHPD data in the light of the nature of that calculation.

Both the patient classification system and the task quantification system are attempts to create indices that overcome the poverty of the NHPD index. Both of these systems ultimately aim to relate patient needs (or nurse tasks) to staffing. NHPD only relates time-put-in to staffing, reflecting neither patient needs nor nursing tasks.

Variables Affecting Staffing Pattern Determinations

As indicated throughout this discussion, many variables may affect staffing determinations. These include

- nursing organization factors
  1. patient care objectives
  2. determined levels of patient care
  3. nursing division/department/unit functions
  4. assignment systems
  5. services to staff (e.g., inservice hours allowed)
- patient factors
  1. variety of patient conditions
  2. acuity
  3. length of stay
  4. patient numbers
  5. age groups
  6. general health status and health goals
  7. care expectations
  8. fluctuations in numbers, acuity, variety, etc.
- staff factors
  1. job descriptions of the division/organization
  2. educational level of staff
  3. experiential level of staff
  4. work ethic of groups of staff members
  5. expectations of staff from the organization
- health care organization factors
  1. financial resources available
  2. personnel policies, especially regarding work time
  3. support services within the organization
  4. number and nature of interfaces within the total institution
  5. number of beds per unit or module
  6. architecture and functional space layouts
- extraorganizational factors
  1. staff mix available in the community
  2. staff number available
  3. coordinating patterns with community health agencies

There are too many variables to allow one to derive a single simple formula for staffing. Staffing judgments often are a mixture of scientific (or logical) derivations plus pragmatic knowledge of what works in a given situation.

Problems Related to Staffing Patterns

Several problems that make staffing decisions difficult are briefly reviewed here: (1) staffing mix, (2) use of supplementary staff, (3) peaks and valleys in the work load, (4) planned alterations in levels of care, and (5) effects of prospective payment.

Staffing Mix

The nurse executive must determine how many RNs, LPNs, nursing assistants, or other workers are to man each nursing unit. This includes determining how many RNs of what categories are to be used (when a nursing ladder or other plan differentiates among RNs).

Decisions concerning mix will be dictated partially by the supply of skilled personnel available in the community (or who can be attracted to the community). Also, the types of patients to be cared for will influence such decisions. More seriously ill patients and patients requiring highly technical care will require higher levels of professional staffing. Efficiency in use of personnel and quality in care are the basic criteria for determining mix.

Often, mix is determined by a task quantification system. Here, each task is assigned to a given level of worker, and by a cumulative count of tasks per level, one can establish a ratio of staff mix. This method may be deceptive if it is applied without thought. First, many systems that time tasks only time activities performed in direct contact with a patient. Hence, they may allow no time for professional planning and just plain thinking.

Such a system tends to recommend a staff mix at a lower level than actually required. Further, such a system may overlook that a low-level task in any given instance may need to be performed by a higher-level worker than normal because of other intervening patient-related factors. Just because taking temperatures is assigned to an aide level, one cannot assume that every temperature should be taken by an aide. Nevertheless, in a cost-conscious society, it is certainly reasonable to aim for a situation in which most employees are working, at most times, at their highest capacity.

Some nurse executives believe that the use of tasks to estimate levels of staff personnel is not the way to attain maximum efficiency. Nurse executives favoring professional staffing give the following argument: When staff is heavy with lower-level personnel, there is an increased need for supervising, directing, and follow-up.

This need for management alters the role of the professionals; their time is used in management, not in patient care. By staffing with higher-level personnel, whose role concepts and education prepare them for self-direction, one produces more and higher-quality patient care with a smaller total number of personnel. Elimination of the heavy amount of supervising, directing, and follow-up enables fewer personnel to deliver more advanced nursing care. A decrease in the number of staff is compensated for in the quality of care provided.

Other factors support this argument in favor of increased professional staffing. One is the increasing complexity of nursing technology, decreasing the need for employees with little education and few skills.

At one time, the argument was enhanced by the comparatively high salaries for nursing assistants (often unionized). These salaries once were so high as to allow for replacement of the aide by a more highly skilled worker, with little extra investment. Indeed, a decade or more ago, Aiken (1984) concluded that the RN was the best all-around general health care worker when viewed from perspectives of cost and capabilities. With the extensive increments that many nurses have received in the intervening decade, the argument no longer applies.

Still, we have two opposing theories of cost containment in staffing. One advocates aiming for as low a staff level as permitted, given the normative tasks to be performed in the nursing division. The other theory aims, in contrast, to staff at the highest level possible. Probably both arguments have substantial merit, and the right strategy for one institution might be the wrong strategy for another institution—one with a different case mix or with different impacting environmental contingencies.

It also is possible that both these opposing strategies would be effective in the same situation. And both strategies might be better than a strategy that fell somewhere along a continuum between these two extremes. It is important to realize that there are no eternal truths in such practical decisions. The right choice in strategy is the one that proves effective in reaching one's goals in a given situation.

At present, the pendulum may have swung too far in the direction of relying on lower-level workers. By that, it is meant that reports of ill-prepared lower-level workers are on the rise. Nursing's major organizations have been so disturbed that they are presently campaigning to increase the use of RNs. It is always difficult to know where self-interest (many nurses are presently unemployed as this book is being written) and professional accountability meet. It seems, however, that the danger is not restructured practice itself (and its use of lower-level employees) but abuse of the system with ill-prepared lower-level workers or unjustified cuts of needed professionals.

Also, the mixes of personnel for patient care, mixes of nursing and non-nursing personnel on the unit, must be considered. Use of supplemental non-nursing staff is another factor in determining a staff mix. Hosts, unit managers, or secretaries are common to most health institutions; these workers take over various unit activities, freeing the professionals for actual nursing care.

This division of nursing and non-nursing functions on the unit probably has solved more problems than it has created, but the division has brought with it a set of difficulties in coordination. Such difficulties can be forestalled by accurate understanding of and preparation against potential conflict situations.

Two sorts of problems occur with the various non-nursing workers: logistic problems and power struggles. Logistic difficulties occur, for example, when secretaries, hosts, or unit management staff give less than peak performances.

When support staff manage the unit's supplies (always depending on the actual job descriptions), their function can be compared with the supply lines that serve an army. The soldier on the battlefield gives little thought to such supportive service until the ammunition fails to arrive; then, suddenly, the supply services have a direct and critical effect on his ability to fight.

The nurse is in a similar position. Stocking of sterile supplies, for example, is not really important to her until she cannot obtain materials to do a dressing. When this occurs, one no longer can say that stocking of supplies is not a critical function in nursing care.

When hosts or unit management services are perceived clearly as *means* to the *ends* of nursing care, the division of functions is effective and everyone works toward the same goals. A problem arises, however, when a unit manager develops a sense of his job as an end in itself. This can happen easily, and the person who takes extreme pride in his work may be more susceptible to this fault than is the less conscientious worker.

Compared with the world of the nurse, the world of the traditional unit manager is orderly, routinized, and relatively stable. He deals with inanimate objects that stay where he puts them (except for interference by nurses); he has supplies that are used up at regular rates (except when nurses unpredictably use too much of an item at one time); and he has supply charges that can be processed through clearly defined standard operating procedures (except when the nurse forgets to write down which patient used the supply).

Clearly, from the perspective of the unit manager, the biggest obstacle to his work is the professional nurse. This obstacle is particularly frustrating if the manager sees his job as an end in itself. The unit manager has a job with a high degree of task routinization and a low level of technology; the nurse, however, has a job with great variation in tasks and a high level of technology. The nurse cannot develop routinized behavior when patient needs, priorities, and surrounding events cannot be predicted with certainty.

When the unit manager sees his job as one of helping the nurse to cope with this irregular environment, the relationship between nurse and manager can be effective; such a manager can take pride in his ability to assist professional staff in meeting exigencies. Unit managers are most likely to develop this attitude when they are responsible to the head nurse.

When a unit manager is a coequal with the head nurse, then means (support systems) have been equated in value with ends (nursing care). A manager in such a system may try to substantiate the equality of his position by adapting the environment to the needs of his own job of low technology and routinized tasks. This presents the problem of two bosses demanding that the same environment conform to the needs of diverse work perspectives.

A relatively simple solution to these potential problems is to make the unit manager directly responsible to the head nurse. In this way, better nursing care will remain the objective of the support systems.

In many newer job configurations, hosts or unit managers have additional direct responsibilities for patients. These may include such tasks as greeting patients on their arrival to the unit, serving a customer relations function, and performing various service amenities for patients. Such direct patient relations may sensitize these non-nursing personnel to the human relations aspect of caring for patients.

Appropriate staffing decisions concerning the numbers of secretaries, hosts, or unit managers to be hired can be made by assessment of the kind and number of non-nursing tasks completed on each nursing unit. In restructuring, constructing a non-nursing role is intrinsic to designing the whole system.

The secretary-host-unit manager issue also illustrates a situation in which nursing staffing may be constrained by the organization of personnel in other divisions. For example, if other divisions house the unit managers, secretaries, or hosts, the nurse executive may find herself in a position of trying to divest other institutional power sources of positions to expand positions in her own division or of trying to change the nature of those non-nursing roles.

Although such moves may be called for on the basis of current patient care needs and system restructuring, her intervention may be perceived as a power move and meet resistance. Negotiation across divisional lines where other positions interface with and affect nursing positions is a delicate matter, certainly one requiring much backup data and cool, logical argument.

Use of Supplementary Staff

The staffing pattern may or may not allow for use of supplementary staffing. The justification for these additional staff is that the regular staffing pattern is based on the average, the normal situation, and that situation simply does not always exist.

Emergency staffing and float staffing function on different principles. The emergency staffing pattern describes the redistribution of nursing personnel for an emergency situation. Some fortunate hospitals have extra personnel in the community who can be called in for an emergency situation, but that circumstance is rare. Typically, an emergency staffing pattern rearranges regular staffing for management of the crisis situation. Such an emergency staffing pattern often is devised along with a disaster plan. These documents may be simple or complex; there may be one staffing pattern or alternates designed to meet the contingencies of specific types of disasters. The emergency staffing pattern typically reduces patient care unit staff to the lowest level at which patient safety is assured, freeing staff members for duties elsewhere during the emergency situation.

The float staff pattern consists of a design for regular employees who are not assigned to specific patient care units but who are regular workers, either full-time or part-time. The float staffing is planned to compensate for two variables: increases in patient needs, and absences among the unit-assigned staff members due to illness or other contingencies.

The organization that is unable to maintain a float staff has to have a larger unit-assigned staff. Float staffing, however, enables an institution to "cover for" those units on which the work load is temporarily heavier than the norm.

By using a single staff for this purpose (the float staff), there is less need to move unit-assigned personnel to balance work load. Movement of unit-assigned personnel is less desirable than use of float staff (see the scheduling section).

The float staff size and composition are determined by data on the institution's total work load variance from the norm for the units. In some instances, to preserve flexibility of staff, the normal unit staffing pattern will be set to cover the *low normal* work load. Then, there is heavy reliance on the float staff.

Most institutions, however, staff for the norm, recognizing that on days when work load is below that norm there will be some waste of staff time. Few institutions are able to adjust staffing for periods of decreased activities. The rare institution that has a monopoly on hiring of health personnel due to absence of other employing agencies in the area may be able to send employees home when the work load is light. In most instances, this is not possible, and the nurse executive does well to have a constructive plan for the use of personnel when such a condition exists. Self-teaching inservice projects are used at such times, and other productive use of employee time can be devised with a little thought.

Use of a float staff is a partial solution to increased activity needs, but it brings its own set of problems; the first is that of finding the right persons for it. An ideal float staff has full-time workers who like the challenge of working with different types of patients in different settings. The problem is the scarcity of nurses who enjoy this challenge. The vast majority of workers prefer the stability of working with a known group of patients and staff.

Many institutions man a float staff with either part-timers or new personnel waiting for permanent unit positions to become available. Unfortunately, part-timers and new personnel are the workers least likely to succeed in meeting the changing demands of float positions. The institution that desires a good float staff needs to evolve a reward system that recognizes the difficulty of float work.

Another supplementary staffing pattern is on-call staffing. Typically used in operating room and other specialty units, this pattern determines how many people of what sort need to be on-call at any given time. Usually, on-call staffing is filled with regular employees who receive some remuneration for being on-call whether or not they are called. Such employees often receive further remuneration when they are, in fact, called. In a system of decentralized scheduling, an on-call system may not exist formally; yet, the head nurse may be familiar with the life styles of her employees, knowing who can be reached and where for emergencies. Such a decentralized scheduling system also uses peer pressure to ensure expected work attendance.

Peaks and Valleys in the Work Load

Peaks and valleys in the nursing work load occur on several levels: (1) daily differences in what may be performed, (2) irregular peaks and valleys on various days or months, and (3) seasonal yearly peaks and valleys.

Daily peaks and valleys are caused by the natural flow of events on a patient care unit. Hence, there may be times when staff are literally unable to proceed with their work because of intervening events. The aim of the unit must be to even out those events insofar as is possible. Otherwise, one needs a larger staff if all the work must be achieved in shorter work periods.

Some unit events are within the control of the nursing division. For example, if a head nurse demands that all patients receive morning treatments between 9:00 A.M. and 11:00 A.M., she is creating her own peak activity period. Examination of the nursing system routines enables staff to even out many peaks and valleys in the work load.

Other events are perceived as outside the control of the nursing division, although that may not necessarily be the case. For example, some nursing divisions have been successful in getting physician staff to stagger their rounds; other nursing divisions have managed to stagger or rearrange visiting hours to fit care needs. In any case, the aim is to establish a constant work flow as this allows for optimal work achievement by minimal nursing staff.

In instances when it is not possible to remove a major peak or valley, the nurse executive should plan for it. Unnecessary events should be eliminated from peak work time periods, and supplementary work or education activities may be planned for the valleys. For example, if patient mealtimes cannot be staggered given the dietary department's limitations, then the nursing staff on a unit with many dependent patients would be freed of other tasks at this time to see to feeding needs.

Peaks and valleys also occur in units in which patient occupancy rates vary considerably. This condition is more likely to exist in small specialty units, with units short of staff one day and overstaffed the next. Because they are specialty units, it is difficult to cover shortages with nurses from other areas. More often, however, the problem of such a unit is overstaffing. For example, one must have a nurse stationed in Labor and Delivery whether or not any patients are immediately in the unit; similarly, the Emergency Department must be ready at hand. In these instances, it is a challenge to make the unit cost-effective.

One common solution not in the realm of staffing is that of combining services when several hospitals serve a single community. For example, if three hospitals are located in the same small town, they might agree to move all pediatric facilities to one, emergency department functions to another, and obstetric facilities to the third. By having each specialty cater to a larger total population, the waste in staff coverage can be better controlled.

When unpredictable patient occupancy rates occur in nonspecialty units, the problem can be partly cured by float staffing for staff shortages or variable staffing for both staff shortages and oversupply of staff. (Variable staffing is discussed later in this chapter.)

In some instances, the variance in occupancy rate is a seasonal factor and can be predicted ahead even when it cannot be controlled. For example, a ski town with lodges and tourism expects skiing accidents in the winter. In cases of predictable variances, the nurse executive may have two or more staffing patterns for a single year. In some situations in which tourism is responsible for the increase in patient admissions, the tourist population may increase the nursing population available for hire to fill the heavier staffing needs.

When nursing moves toward specialization and when variance occurs in the specialty units, it may be difficult to find the staff who can cover such units. One possibility is to encourage nursing staff members to develop two, rather than one, special areas of knowledge and expertise.

Planned Alterations in Levels of Care

As nursing moves toward cutting the cost of nursing services, it is logical that nursing divisions begin to relate costs to the level of nursing care received. Certainly, no institution will tolerate a level of care that qualifies as unsafe. Yet, it is feasible that levels will be developed and that the consumer will elect the care level he desires (directly or indirectly through a choice of insurance coverage that specifies a level of care).

Often today, luxury units have different staffing patterns from their identical sister units on economy models. Indeed, there might even be a swing unit that is staffed for A-level care at one time, B-level care at another, depending on the choices of the particular patient body of the moment. Although number of staff is not directly correlated with quality of care, it is reasonable to assume that the higher-level care will require more staff and a higher ratio of professional staffing.

Some nurses may reject the idea of staffing for the level of nursing care. Indeed, they assert that every patient deserves top-quality nursing care. In the absence of the resources to deliver it, however, the demand for universal highest-quality care merely produces disillusionment.

Ultimately, nursing can advance as a profession only when the client sees what he is getting for his investment. Nursing must be prepared to tell the client realistically what services he will receive for what fees. Once nursing has specified different levels of care, it must be prepared to deliver on what is promised. Obviously, in differential levels of care, the diverse staffing patterns would be tied closely to corresponding plans for care.

Some for-profit health care chains already market their level of health care versus that of competitors. For example, one chain offers new parents a postdelivery dinner of lobster and champagne. Of course, such luxury amenities do not describe the quality of nursing care delivered.

Often nursing faces real moral dilemmas in which prospective payment has led some institutions to reject certain patients on financially determined criteria. Here, the two-tier level, unfortunately, means one level of care and one level of noncare. Nationwide attempts to hold the line on health care costs will produce such disjunctures in the health care system as answers are sought in the shifting health care industry and in the national debate on health policy.

There is another subtle sense in which two-tier nursing care exists in many institutions. This occurs when different levels of care delivery occur in routine operations. For example, the weekend service is inferior in some places because of large numbers of days off extended to personnel. Unfortunately, patients have little say about this depletion of services. Certainly, they receive no compensatory adjustment in the fees they pay for nursing services.

Effects of Prospective Payment

The preceding discussion assumes that the staffing decisions are based primarily on some defined or intuited notion of the nursing care that patients need to receive. In many institutions, the systems of reimbursement may curtail resources returned to the nursing division. Because nursing is labor-intensive, such curtailing usually means a loss of staff. When staff (resources) are arbitrarily cut or limited, reviewing the basis for staffing is essential.

When this situation exists, the nurse executive must be clear about setting a baseline for nursing services. She must know when service reaches a dangerous level. She must have clear criteria that enable her to know when a unit must be closed for the safety of its patients, present or future. These criteria should be available before the fact, not after a dangerous situation makes itself felt.

Such a situation (i.e., one in which nursing resources are highly limited) calls for extensive examination of nursing policies, practices, and procedures. Productivity becomes essential; each employee must be used to the maximum. Quality alone is no longer enough; quantity of work also assumes major importance. Streamlining is the essence of management, and all methods of care delivery must be scrutinized with this in mind.

Such a situation puts nursing in competition with other components in the health care institution for limited resources. Nurse executives need to recognize this shift from a cooperative to a competitive model of management. The nurse executive who cannot defend her need for resources will surely lose them.

In a labor-intensive operation, staffing is the first item affected by a cut in institutional resources. And staffing decisions may, more and more, need to be made in the light of clear, hard data. Some form of variable staffing (discussed next) may carry the day in most institutions.

Variable Staffing

Variable staffing is an alternate to the permanent staffing pattern. This method does not make assumptions about care units and their patients. In variable staffing, the pattern is determined daily, based on present input data from patients on each unit. This eliminates the problems that arise when staffing is based on stagnant predictions of patient needs. In variable staffing, the number of workers on any patient care unit may change daily.

Variable staffing usually relies on a patient acuity system that is able to convert patient care needs to hours of nursing care needed to deliver on those needs. Today, most acuity systems reflect the real hours of care given to patients rather than the hours of care actually needed. Nevertheless, whatever the base of the acuity system, it enables one to make judgments as to the relative need for staff from one unit to the next. With such weighted needs for staff, one can adjust staff numbers per unit accordingly.

In some institutions, the total number of staff to be distributed was originally determined by adding together all staff used in a staffing plan conceived by a different method (perhaps an estimate of unit norms). In some places, the available staff is simply a matter of how many workers the organization can afford or attract in a competitive market. In other places, staff total numbers are themselves a derivation of cumulative hours normed out from a system that uses the acuity counts over time.

In most places, variable staffing quotients are produced by computer, although manual calculations are possible. The sophistication of the system varies, depending on the institution's resources. Some systems can give an estimate of levels of workers; others only derive a total number of care hours needed per unit. In all cases, equity in distribution of staff depends on the accuracy of the data concerning patient acuity that is fed into the system.

Variable staffing combines two elements discussed separately in this chapter: staffing and scheduling. Work hours are scheduled, but unit placement is not planned ahead; staffing is planned only as a number of personnel for the whole institution.

Variable staffing is a mathematical solution to the problems of staffing in an uncertain world, but it is not necessarily a solution to the human relations aspect of the staffing problem. Many staff members do not like to participate in a system that treats them as interchangeable cogs. Many prefer the constancy of working on a single unit, with a single patient population. Most variable staffing plans allow for a base staff per unit, so that transfer of personnel is minimized. When this tactic is not followed, there is additional wastage of time if staff must learn new units and new groups of patients too frequently.

Some variable staffing plans do not consider the institution as a whole but distribute available staff over subunits of two or three companion floors. In this plan, the employee is assured that he must learn only these related units. This may be a good compromise between hard data (acuity hour needs) and human data (a need for stability in one's work environment). In other institutions, the variable is much like the older notion of a float staff. In all cases, the issue is how to balance two needs: patient quantity of work to be performed and staff need for stability in a work environment.

Staffing Plan

Recall that staffing has two components, the staffing pattern, which decides how many staff of what sort are needed on each unit per shift per day, and the staffing plan, the determination of how many people must be hired to deliver on that staffing pattern.

Suppose one were to calculate a staffing plan, in other words, how many persons needed to be hired to fill a single RN position on a day shift on a given patient care unit. One might make calculations of the following sort:

1. Each RN works a determinable number of days per year.
2. By dividing days worked per nurse by the number of days in a year, one derives the number of staff required to fill one positional slot for the year (i.e., on a full-time basis).

Figure 19–2 illustrates such a calculation, using the number of days of vacation, sick time, holidays, and inservice days that are the norm in the hypothetical hospital.

Notice that the mathematical calculation shown in Figure 19–2 is just the beginning of the estimate, not the finish. Several obstacles and problems remain to be solved. First, no one worker would realistically agree to work 65 percent of a full-time job. And if someone did, the payroll and personnel offices would be irate at the necessary calculations.

Even if one found another worker to fill the 65 percent, the work of this employee would complement (and complete) the work of the full-time worker (so the job is filled 100 percent of the time) *only if* the two were never on duty on the same day. Note, however, that the calculation included sick time, an entity that specifically cannot be planned ahead. Further, there is no guarantee that these two employees will use exactly the correct, normed-out percentage of sick days.

Note also that the formula is incomplete in that the 65 percent employee would not actually get the exact prorated number of sick days allowable, vacation days, and so on, as the full-time

Staffing for One RN Slot on 3 West for a Year (364 days)

I. Deduct days not worked, for total work days for an individual full-time employee	364	days (calculated at an "even" 52 weeks)
	−104	days off (two days off per week × 52 weeks)
	260	days remaining
	− 10	paid holidays
	250	days remaining
	− 5	sick days (the institutional norm)
	245	days remaining
	− 5	paid inservice days (institutional norm)
	240	days remaining
	− 20	days paid vacation
	220	days remaining = total work days
II. Divide year by number of days worked by a full-time worker, to get number of full-time workers needed to fill the position	$\dfrac{364.00}{220}$ = 1.65 RN workers to fill one job

Figure 19–2 Calculation of Staff Required to Fill a Single Full-Time Position

employee. Once again, the formula proves only to give an estimate of number of employees.

Such calculations allow one to consider the work of a larger group of nurses together. Suppose, for example, that a given unit was staffed with three RNs on days, for a total of 1,092 work days in a 52-week period (364 days × 3 positions). Here, five RNs would appear to be able to fill three positions (220 work days each × 5 RNs = 1,100 days, or slightly more than that required). Notice, however, that a single personnel policy such as every other weekend off makes this coverage impossible. Furthermore, the plan would require vacations spread out evenly through the year.

The staffing plan, accordingly, is calculated on a basis of mathematical design plus modification required by policies of the institution and by interfacing with the scheduling office (whose policies also may have an effect on what days what workers may be used). At its best, the staffing plan delivers an approximation of the staffing pattern. Approximation may be brought closer with more flexibility and shifting of staff from unit to unit, but there are prices to be paid for this approach in terms of human relations and possibly quality of care.

Nor can one come up with a norm for the staffing plan (e.g., 1.65 employees per position). This figure would diverge in an institution with a different number of holidays, days for vaca-

tion, or a different norm for sick time used. When different categories of workers are entitled to different lengths of vacation, calculations must be performed separately for each class of worker.

Calculating a Staffing Plan from Care Hours

In the previous illustration, the staffing pattern was a given, and the staffing plan was calculated to fill that pattern. It also is possible, when an institution has a good mechanism for estimating patient care hours, to move in the opposite direction—to go from patient care hours per unit per shift, to total number of nursing hours required per year, to number of staff required to deliver those hours (staffing plan), to number of positions required to deliver that staff (staffing pattern).

Suppose, for example, that the institution represented in Figure 19–2 used a system of PCUs that converts to nursing care hours. With appropriate historical data, it would be possible to calculate backward to see what sort of staffing pattern would apply.

The main administrative objective in the staffing plan, however devised, is one of even distribution of staff. Every event or policy that mitigates against equal distribution of staff makes the staffing plan more difficult to calculate, removing it farther from the mathematical model that serves as its base.

For example, if unionized staff gain every other weekend off, this will throw off staffing calculations because 50 percent of staff will be off at the same time. This prevents any three-for-one (or five-for-three) sort of arrangement among staff hours. Hence, an every-other-weekend-off policy is costly even when a competitive environment calls for it. A nurse executive who agrees to an every-other-weekend-off policy is left with two equally unattractive alternatives: (1) She can use deficient staffing every weekend, allowing the quality of care to drop, or (2) she can search for supplementary weekend staff for coverage. The latter is not ideal as a personnel system, but at least it enables the nurse executive to build a rational staffing plan to deliver on a staffing pattern. The first solution, differential levels of care, will meet with disapproval from accrediting agencies.

Another staffing plan dilemma is whether to rotate employees among shifts. Ideally, each shift should be handled separately, but the ideal may not be possible if there are few nurses in a community who voluntarily work the evening or night shifts. Obviously, shift work breaks most of the rules nurses teach others concerning circadian cycles, but this is a reason outside the domain of the staffing plan. When workers rotate shifts, it is not possible to derive a staffing plan separate from the scheduling plan. It also makes it difficult to use the shift as the basis for various work load calculations.

SCHEDULING

Scheduling is the final step in the assigning-staffing-scheduling system, the step whereby workers are assigned specific days and specific hours of work. The schedule approximates the staffing pattern using the resources (people) designated by the staffing plan. The chief goal is balance (i.e., distribution of workers evenly throughout the given scheduling period).

Difficult as it is to determine staffing patterns, filling these patterns can be a greater problem. First off, the 7-day week was created to con-

found managers. At least, this is true in a society in which 5-day work weeks predominate. Suppose that one wished to fill two RN positions on one unit for one shift for 1 year. Using our earlier case, it is necessary to hire 1.65 nurses for one position or 3.30 for two positions. Given that nurses are unlikely to apply for 30 percent positions, the closest approximation for these two positions will be three RNs full time.

When one tries to fit the three nurses into an average week, however, problems arise. (An average week here is taken to be one in which no holidays, vacations, or sick time occurs.) In this arrangement, the following pattern shown in Figure 19–3 emerges.

The pattern reveals the problem that 1 day per week the unit is overstaffed. There are, however, solutions to this problem. Now and then, one credits one staff member's time on the overlap day to inservice education. When this is done, overlapping on several units is made to coincide as to day to be able to collect a large enough group of workers eligible for a planned inservice program.

Few if any institutions can afford to offer the nurse an inservice day once every 3 weeks, however, although the actual total of inservice days is greatly reduced once vacations, holidays, and other interruption days are added to the schedule.

Another solution is to use the overstaffing to solve internal variations in work load. In this procedure, one ensures that overstaffed days do not coincide from unit to unit, so the extra RN can be transferred to the unit with the heaviest patient activity.

A third solution to the problem of overstaffing is to find a nurse who is interested in working a 4-day week. This ideal solution, however,

X = days worked in the week							
RN A	X	X	X	X	X		
RN B			X	X	X	X	X
RN C	X	X	X			X	X

Figure 19–3 Three Nurses Filling Two Staffing Positions

may be difficult to arrange. Yet another solution to the overstaffing problem is to balance the excess staff scheduling against a deficient staff scheduling pattern. Suppose, for example, that on the same unit four LPNs were filling three positions. Here, a deficiency pattern arises, as shown in Figure 19–4.

With four workers for three positions, one deficiency occurs per week. Thus, a floor that had the good fortune to have a staffing pattern requiring two RNs and three LPNs per day could minimize losses by seeing that the day with the extra RN coincided with the day deficient by one LPN.

Notice that this sample schedule fit was attained by having complete freedom for placement of days off. In this pattern, the RN would have every third weekend off, and the LPN would have only one weekend out of every four. This small sample of interplay between staffing and scheduling may give the reader an appreciation of the complexities involved in the process. It should be adequate to demonstrate that hours could be spent in trying to figure out work hours. When the scheduling process is compounded with holidays, vacations, and personal requests, the job becomes mammoth.

Scheduling Formats

Several basic types of scheduling ease the complexity of the process, including block scheduling, cyclical scheduling, and computer scheduling. Each of these represents an improvement on the preceding form, but examples of all three still are in effect today.

In block scheduling, the work schedule for a unit is planned in a block of weeks. The term *block* originally was applied to this scheduling because days to be worked often were blocked together, forming patterns such as that illustrated in Figure 19–5.

Block scheduling often is done for 4 to 8 weeks at a time. It can be calculated without great difficulty and has flexibility in that the next block of time need not necessarily follow the pattern of the preceding block.

Cyclical scheduling is an improvement on block scheduling in that it has repetitive work patterns assigned to personnel. Because each employee has a permanent pattern, he can calculate even months in advance when he will be on duty. A cyclical schedule has a repeated pattern of interweaving schedules.

These interlinking parts are a permanent plan, a fixed cycle of, usually, 4 to 6 weeks. The employee may have a different schedule for each of the weeks contained in the cycle, but the pattern repeats without change. Some assignment slots within a cycle may be perceived by employees as more desirable than others. Typically, the choice of assignment slots is handled on a seniority basis. Figure 19–6 illustrates a cyclical schedule.

Several things should be noted in this cycle. First, the employee schedules have been meshed so that (1) there are never less than two RNs on duty, (2) there are never more than two persons (RNs and LPNs considered together) off on the same day, and (3) there is never a day without at least one LPN on duty. These are the factors that dominated the interlinkages of these employee schedules.

X = days worked in the week

Worker A	X	X	X	X	X		
Worker B			X	X	X	X	X
Worker C	X	X			X	X	X
Worker D	X	X	X	X			X

Figure 19–4 Four Nurses Filling Three Staffing Positions

X = days worked in the week

Week	RN	M	T	W	Th	F	Sa	Su
I	A			X	X	X	X	X
	B	X	X			X	X	X
	C	X	X	X	X			X
II	A	X	X			X	X	X
	B	X	X	X	X			X
	C			X	X	X	X	X

Figure 19–5 Three Nurses Filling Three Staffing Positions

✗ = *days worked in the week*

Staff	Week I							Week II							Week III							Week IV						
	S	M	T	W	T	F	S	S	M	T	W	T	F	S	S	M	T	W	T	F	S	S	M	T	W	T	F	S
RN 1	✗		✗	✗	✗		✗	✗	✗	✗			✗	✗	✗	✗	✗		✗	✗			✗	✗	✗	✗	✗	
RN 2		✗	✗		✗	✗	✗	✗	✗		✗	✗	✗			✗	✗	✗		✗	✗	✗	✗		✗	✗	✗	
RN 3	✗	✗		✗	✗	✗			✗	✗	✗	✗		✗	✗	✗		✗	✗			✗	✗	✗	✗			✗
RN 4	✗		✗	✗		✗	✗	✗		✗	✗	✗	✗			✗	✗	✗	✗	✗	✗	✗	✗	✗			✗	✗
LPN 1		✗	✗	✗	✗	✗			✗	✗	✗		✗	✗	✗		✗	✗	✗	✗	✗		✗	✗		✗	✗	
LPN 2	✗	✗	✗		✗			✗	✗	✗			✗		✗	✗	✗		✗	✗			✗	✗	✗	✗		✗

Figure 19–6 Cyclical Staffing Pattern

Also, the cycles consider the individual employees insofar as each employee has at least one full weekend off per 4-week cycle. Beyond this general principle, it is obvious that some cycles would be preferred over others. For example, RN 2 actually has two weekends per period (as one cycle joins the next with Saturday and Sunday off). Also, this schedule never has the nurse working more than 5 consecutive days. In contrast, RN 4 usually has split days off, and she has one period in which she works 8 days in a row. (The only appealing component in this schedule is the 3-day weekend between weeks II and III.) A nurse new to the unit would probably be given the fourth rotation pattern. She would probably bid for a change of schedule if another RN were to leave the unit.

Even though some cycles are less than perfect, nevertheless the employee can plan ahead because the pattern (in this case a 4-week pattern) keeps repeating. Moreover, a schedule need only be developed once per staffing pattern. Because it repeats without change, the only schedules that need attention are those in which exceptions occur, as in a week containing a holiday.

Computerized scheduling enables the user to devise a plan that considers more variables than would be possible for hand calculations. For example, one might design a computer program for scheduling with the following dictates:

- patterns that must be maintained
  1. Miss G goes to school every Friday; she must have that day off.
  2. Mrs. T's religion will not allow her to work on Saturdays; she must have that day off.
- first-priority options when possible
  1. Mr. F must hire a babysitter if he works Tuesday or Wednesday; he would prefer to have these as his days off.
  2. Give every employee one weekend off per 4-week period if possible.
  3. Where possible, give an employee 2 days off together instead of split.
- secondary priorities (to be followed if they do not interfere with priority options above)
  1. Preferably, do not have an employee work more than 6 days in a row.
  2. Schedule holiday time off within 10 days of the occurrence of the holiday.

These variables are only a sample of the constraints that may be incorporated into a computer program for scheduling. Most computer programs can combine general directives applicable to all staff with other variables applicable only to individual staff members. Also, a good program can handle those rules that must be applied in addition to rules that are assigned different priorities.

There are instances when staff complain that the computer is less successful than a human scheduler. Usually, this reflects not so much a computer deficiency as a failure to update the program or make it comprehensive. A computer will consider only those elements that are programmed into its circuits. A poor computer scheduling system indicates a poor program.

Centralized versus Decentralized Scheduling

There are many arguments concerning whether centralized or decentralized scheduling is most satisfactory. In centralized scheduling, all work hours for the entire nursing division are planned in a central office by a single scheduler or a staff of schedulers. Decentralized schedules are planned at the unit level, usually by the head nurse. Either of these systems may use block, cyclical, or computer techniques of scheduling.

Arguments offered in favor of decentralized scheduling by the head nurse include the fact that the head nurse knows her staff intimately; she is in a better position to meet their individual scheduling needs. And, because she knows her patients' needs, she can respond to them in her scheduling with a sensitivity that someone in a central office cannot have. Further, when there are differences concerning desired work days, the head nurse can get staff members together for negotiation and problem resolution. Decentralized scheduling places responsibility right where it belongs—at the functional level. The head nurse is the one who will have to live with the schedule; she should have the right to make it.

Counterarguments identify the problems in decentralized scheduling. First, the staff may try to manipulate the head nurse. They may ask for special favors, and she may be afraid not to grant them, especially if the relationship between the head nurse and the staff members is one of close friendship. Staff members may try to get the head nurse to put their needs above the needs of the patients. This problem would not occur if scheduling were performed by an impartial central scheduler.

Another argument against decentralized scheduling is the massive amount of time that it takes, especially if block scheduling still is used. The head nurse puts a significant amount of her time every month or every 6 weeks into an essentially mechanical task. Furthermore, there is likely to be more reworking of the schedule because workers are likely to ask for more schedule modifications from a head nurse than from a central scheduler.

Finally, decentralized scheduling never takes into account the whole division. Hence, it might happen that many floors accidentally select the same night for their shortest coverage. This lack of central planning would make it difficult to pull staff members to meet acute staffing needs.

Arguments for central scheduling contain the following lines of reasoning. First, central scheduling is performed without personal bias; there will be few claims of discrimination. Central scheduling is likely to use advanced techniques and those formats that allow for a long-term projection of hours. This ultimately is more favorable to the employee than weekly or monthly negotiation with the head nurse. Also, the scheduler, who does this as a full-time job or as a major responsibility, will become skilled in coping with the intricacies of scheduling. Better to have one expert than 20 amateur head nurse schedulers.

Not only does central scheduling save professional nursing time (a nonnurse can easily learn the necessary nursing implications for scheduling), but it allows for coordination over the entire division. Also, the scheduler will be in an ideal position to judge how to fill gaps if it becomes necessary to pull personnel because of staff illnesses or changes in patient work load.

Further, a central scheduler is likely to develop efficient systems to deal with personal requests for exceptions or schedule alterations. When this person deals with all the requests of the division, he will probably become less vulnerable to unreasonable or repeated requests. Such a person is likely to build a routine and efficient system for handling such requests.

This same notion can be considered a point against central staffing. The lack of personal relations with staff may make the scheduler insensitive to pressing needs for schedule alterations. If the central scheduler is not skilled in interpersonal relationships, the schedules are likely to become a focus for employee discontent.

When centralized scheduling uses a cyclical pattern, the argument can be made that the system takes little or no account of patient work load. When work load deviations are the rule, perhaps centralized cyclical scheduling is the worst form. However, most new computerized scheduling programs are both centralized and able to consider fluctuations in the patient load. (However, if patient work load changes rapidly, from day to day, then no system that schedules work units ahead will suffice without modifications on a daily basis.)

Goals of Scheduling

Regardless of who does the scheduling or what format is used, the goals for scheduling are universal and can be summarized as follows:

1. achievement of divisional, departmental, and unit objectives, especially those related to patient care
2. accurate match of unit needs with staff abilities and numbers
3. maximum use of manpower
4. equity of treatment to all employees (or equal treatment for all members within a similar job classification)
5. optimization on use of professional expertise
6. satisfaction of personnel (both as to hours worked and as to perceived sense of scheduling equity)
7. maintenance of flexibility to meet care needs while still giving employees maximum ability to know work hours ahead
8. consideration of unique needs of staff as well as patients

Scheduling Problems

Of the many problems that arise in scheduling, only a few major ones are addressed here: (1) management of full-time versus part-time employees, (2) use of supplementary personnel,

(3) creation of policies that control abuse of sick time, (4) use of patient acuity or task quantification in scheduling, (5) legal and administrative constraints on scheduling, and (6) irregular-hour scheduling practices.

Full-Time versus Part-Time Employees

Most institutions combine full-time and part-time workers in a nursing division. When this is the case, it is very important that the nurse executive develop a benefits package for each of these roles that seems equitable to those within the role and to the employees in the alternate time pattern. Some directors, in an attempt to fill position vacancies, offer disproportionate benefits to part-timers. This may draw part-time staff, but full-timers may feel inequitably treated. Equity may involve pay or benefits in compensation for preferential hours. Full-timers may be more understanding of some favoritism in hours extended to a part-timer if they know that they have some recompensing factor, such as vacation prorated at a higher level, a higher pay scale, or some other benefit that compensates and equalizes the situation.

Today, a nurse executive may have several benefit packages attached to different work designs. Some may be packages for full-time employees; others may be packages for part-timers. There may be different packages assigned to differing work conditions within these groups. For example, a full-time package that guarantees all weekends off may have a reduced number of vacation days or a reduced salary base. As long as the nurse executive has the freedom to balance scheduling advantages and disadvantages with system rewards (monies and benefits), there is no reason why she cannot increase her flexibility in use of potential staff. What matters is that her plans are built in a manner that seeks to be equitable to all employees.

Supplementary Personnel and Their Use

Part-time personnel may be seen as supplementary; often, they are regular employees in that they work every week just as the full-timers do. Several other groups of supplementary staff are used at times in various institutions: float personnel, pulled or transferred staff, agency personnel, and emergency staff.

Float staff are persons who routinely are assigned to the most needy unit. (Often, the float staff will be excused from rotating to specialized units, although this is not always the case.) Sometime part-timers are given only float positions; in this case, the terms *float* and *part-time* are interchangeable. Other institutions place newcomers on float until a regular position on a unit becomes available. As mentioned earlier, float work requires more adjustment and more judgment than a stable unit job, so new people may be the least well prepared for this task.

When float staff are not available, most institutions balance the work load by pulling, or transferring, staff members from units that are overstaffed in relation to the patient work load. This policy maintains managerial flexibility, a necessity in coping with unforeseen emergency situations. However, if used as a routine procedure, pulling creates many difficulties. A worker often is resentful when he is pulled from his regular assignment. In being pulled, he faces all the difficulties of the float nurse—having to learn about new patients, new systems, new expectations.

Sometimes, injury is added to insult when the same worker always is pulled. Some supervisors make the error of always sending the worker who can best adjust to a new environment and is most versatile and smartest. It is obvious that the staff member is being punished for excellence in performance—not a practice designed to endear the supervisor to the pulled staff member.

Further, the pulled member may find that he is resented on the new unit and is treated poorly. In addition to the feeling that he is an interloper, he may be met with hostility or indifference from the very staff that he was sent to relieve: "Find the supplies yourself, I'm too busy to orient you." "Didn't they teach you anything on 8 North?" Worse, the pulled staff member may find that he is assigned some of the more difficult patients on the unit. Ironically, the time when a unit is the least prepared to orient and assist a new member is when the unit is overworked. It is not surprising that the pulled staff

member may meet with less than desirable staff attitudes.

Several things can be done to mitigate this situation. First, staff should not be transferred unless the need for extra staff is acute. In most cases, the overworked unit will be better off if it can alter its work load, perhaps by omitting some of the other amenities of care. Other institutions get around the stranger-in-our-midst syndrome by creating sister units in which all members of each staff are systematically oriented to another unit. In this case, pulling is done only from one unit to the sister unit. The manager gives up some flexibility but enhances the likelihood that a transferred member will actually be useful on the new floor.

Agency personnel usually are the least satisfactory supplementary staff. An agency nurse is one who is hired from a nurse employment agency to work as a staff nurse on a given unit for 1 or more sequential days, evenings, or nights. Some agency nurses are kept for months, which gives them time to adjust to the institution and their environment, but others may only work 1 or 2 days. Because an agency nurse is more costly to the health care institution, she will be replaced with its own staff as soon as possible.

The major problem with agency nurses is their unfamiliarity with the institution, its policies, and its practices. This is being remedied by strict rules by both accrediting agencies and agencies supplying nurses. New requirements ensure that a nurse is oriented to an institution before she can work there even temporarily. In this way, all agency personnel can be oriented to a limited number of hospitals, increasing the quality control for the potential employer.

In this era of corporate health care, institutions in the same parent company often form their own internal agency. Other mechanisms allow such chains to optimize on use of personnel. For example, institutions in the same community may actually shift personnel from one corporate location to another. Others offer employees the opportunity to shift from one geographic location to another without losing position, tenure, or benefits. Economies of scale certainly favor the health care chains; their personnel usage is limited only by the corporation's creativity.

Some institutions are fortunate enough to have another source of supplementary personnel: a group of nonworking nurses who will fill in for emergencies, heavy vacation times, or other periods when staff is short. This group, however, fluctuates—declining in tough economic times, when such nurses themselves seek full-time jobs; increasing when economic times improve. Another source of supplemental staff is the unemployed or underemployed nurse.

With the staffing restraint practiced under prospective payment, many areas of the nation have a growing body of nurses unable to find permanent work. Obviously, this group represents a major problem for nursing as a profession, but a convenience for institutions requiring supplementary staff.

When no supplementary staff are available in emergencies, the institution may extend its own personnel with double-shifting and overtime. This poses several problems, including the fact that it is extremely expensive and pushes staff members beyond normal physiologic and psychological limits, decreasing their efficiency and safety.

When supplementary staff are not available, it becomes critical to average out the work load from unit to unit. If staff cannot be brought in or transferred, then another source of control is patient admissions. When patients rather than staff are considered the mobile factor, then control is established in the admissions office. A patient acuity system or a task quantification system will enable the nursing division to compare work load among units, and patients may be placed accordingly. Such a system requires that there be several units to which each patient potentially may be assigned. Also, the admitting nurse or whoever makes such decisions must have enough admission medical information to estimate future patient care needs.

Creating Policies That Discourage Abuse of Sick Time

Abuse of sick time is another factor that can ruin a well-planned schedule. Some employees perceive sick time as time that is owed to them. They take sick days whether or not they are ill. Such practices can be curtailed by good personnel policies concerning chronic absences. Also, a policy that builds in rewards for failure to use sick time will discourage abuse. Some institutions give back a proportion of unused sick days as extra days off. Other institutions allow sick time to accumulate without loss for long periods.

Use of Patient Acuity or Task Quantification in Scheduling

Work load estimates from patient acuity or task quantification systems often are used to make daily alterations in the schedule. As discussed earlier, some workers object to this routine movement of staff according to unit needs. In other cases, work load data are not used routinely to move staff but only when work load deviation is excessive. One problem with regulation by work load is that nurses soon learn to manipulate the system by overweighting unit work load assessments. If the work load data are to play a significant part in staff scheduling, then one must work at developing a system in which nurses cannot or do not manipulate the data unfairly. Use of these systems is detailed in Chapter 20.

Legal and Administrative Constraints on Scheduling

In devising schedules for nursing staff, the nurse executive and the scheduler(s) need to be aware of laws concerning work time. The Fair Labor Standards Act is a federal law concerning the use of workers, and most states have work laws that must be followed. Such laws usually address issues such as

1. minimum number of hours that a worker must have off between shifts
2. maximum number of days that may be worked without a day off
3. maximum number of hours within a single shift

Because work laws vary widely from state to state, it is important that the nurse executive review those pertaining to her own state.

The nurse executive also will need to see that personnel policies of her own institution are followed. It is particularly important that no employee labor contracts be negotiated and agreed to until she has reviewed proposals for their impact on her staffing and scheduling.

Irregular-Hour Scheduling Practices

Periodically, 10-hour, 12-hour, or other irregular-length shifts come into popularity. One advantage of such a shift is that it often gives the employee 3 rather than 2 days off at a time. For some employees, this is a great advantage. For others, the extra time off is little compensation for the fatigue generated by the longer shift. The 10-hour shift has the disadvantage of not fitting evenly into a 24-hour day, which usually is resolved by having employees work staggered shifts or by compensating with some partial-shift workers. When overlaps do occur on 10-hour shifts, overlaps usually are planned for the peak work hours, but these plans often are costly because they end up increasing the number of required personnel.

Although irregular shifts are popular when they are initiated, the novelty is likely to wear off. The nurse executive should not jump into a major shift-time revision without much thought and testing. It is true that some units and some particular staffs manage better with such schedules. Because these schedules seldom correspond with those of most staff members' mates or children, the nurse executive should not be led into massive shift-time revisions on the basis of enthusiasm of one or two units of staff members who prefer the irregular hours.

The present trend is away from irregular staffing because, on the whole, it costs the institution more money. Many institutions are presently negotiating away from these hours, even if their staff would prefer to maintain them.

SUMMARY

Assigning, staffing, and scheduling of employees are the ways in which the goals of the nursing division are converted into concrete acts. In these steps, goals are changed from qualitative formulations into quantitative plans. Assigning, staffing, and scheduling cannot be performed in isolation from the goals of the nursing division. Moreover, because they interact on each other, they must be planned together. No plan is perfect, but each institution must consider its own diverse contextual variables.

REFERENCES

Aiken, L.H. 1984. The nurse labor market. *Journal of Nursing Administration* 14, no.1:20.

SUGGESTED READINGS

Abdoo, Y.M. 1985. Staffing and Scheduling. In *The professional practice of nursing administration*, ed. L.M. Simms, et al., 264–280. New York: John Wiley & Sons, Inc.

Cockerill, R., et al. 1993. Measuring nursing workload for case costing. *Nursing Economics* 11, no.6:342–349.

Marquis, B.L., and C.J. Huston. 1992. *Leadership roles and management functions in nursing*. Philadelphia: J.B. Lippincott Co.

Metcalf, M.L. 1982. The 12-hour weekend plan—Does the nursing staff really like it? *Journal of Nursing Administration* 12, no.10:16–19.

Prescott, P.A. 1991. Forecasting requirements of health care personnel. *Nursing Economics* 9, no.1:18–24.

Prescott, P.A. 1991. Nursing intensity: Needed today for more than staffing. *Nursing Economics* 9, no.6:409–414.

Robertson, S., and M.K. Pabst. 1992. Staffing and scheduling. In *Nursing administration: A micro/macro approach for effective nurse executives*, ed. P.J. Decker and E.J. Sullivan, 505–528. Norwalk, Conn.: Appleton & Lange.

Shamian, J., et al. 1992. Nursing resource requirements and support services. *Nursing Economics* 10, no.2:110–115.

20

Staff and Patient Classifications

Assigning, staffing, and scheduling, as discussed in the previous chapter, are not only interdependent systems but systems that interact with the nursing division's methods of classifying staff and patients. Staff classification includes determining jobs and concretizing them in job descriptions as well as establishing clinical progression ladders. So-called clinical ladders may be constructed for bedside registered nurse staff only or for various types and levels of nursing personnel.

Patient classifications are done through sorting patients according to conditions or nursing needs as well as through acuity systems. Patients initially are classified by a decision resulting in their placement on one unit versus another, a pediatric unit versus an adult unit, say, or a medical unit versus a surgical unit. Designation of certain geographic areas as units for placement of certain types of patients is a critical but often unexamined structure for the nursing division. Patients are also classified according to such factors as level of acuity and amount and level of care required. These classification systems are used normatively to establish both long-term staffing patterns and short-term alterations in scheduling.

Staff and patient classification systems are the focus of this chapter.

NURSING STAFF CLASSIFICATION SYSTEMS

Three classification concepts for nursing staff are reviewed here: the clinical ladder, the administrative ladder, and the job responsibility scattergram. Specifics of creating a job description, another classification tool for staff, are discussed in Chapter 17. The systems discussed here are related to the RN, although principles would be identical for classification of other employees.

Clinical Ladder

The clinical ladder allows status and rewards to be conferred on the excellent bedside nurse, promoting retention of excellence at the bedside. It offers another mode of nurse advancement besides the administrative route. In a clinical ladder, nurses are ranked or rated from a beginning competency through diverse levels of clinical practice. Some systems have as few as three levels; others have five to seven; a few have even more levels. In some systems, different job titles are associated with the different levels—a good reinforcement because the job title serves as a status symbol; in other systems a number or letter grade follows a common title (Clinical Nurse II, Staff Nurse C). In all the effective systems, salary is related to classification. Indeed, it would be virtually useless to establish a clinical ladder as an alternate status route if it lacked monetary rewards.

Although the system has the potential of keeping the excellent bedside nurse at the bedside, there are several potential problems with the clinical ladder concept. First, it is built on the assumption that there is room within the nursing practice of the institution for all the expertise that a nurse is capable of using. Certainly, it is always true that a nurse may practice smarter within the same time period, but if an institution is short-staffed to the point of barely having time for nurses to finish standing treatment and medication orders, one may question how much advanced practice really is possible.

Of course, one could argue that a clinical ladder is even more needed in such an environment. In any case, the nurse executive must determine the value of a clinical ladder in her particular environment.

Some institutions, particularly in a period of tight budgeting, have dropped the notion that the nursing division can have all the clinical expertise obtainable. Units may be given quotas concerning how many staff at what clinical ladder levels they may employ. For example, 6 North might be judged to merit no more than two Clinical Nurse IV positions. If those positions were already filled, a Clinical Nurse III on 6 North might have to apply to another unit were she seeking advancement in rank.

Such controls on numbers of nurses within each rank may be necessary if an institution is to control its budget tightly. The open-ended system, in which any nurse may be hired and then periodically ranked based on ability, creates a great unknown in manpower budgeting.

Another potential problem with the clinical ladder is the difficulty of creating a fair evaluation system. Nursing performance may be theoretically on different levels, but to establish and describe those levels and to tell where each nurse fits in relation to those levels is a monumental task.

A third problem is that of deciding what the clinical ladder measures. Typically, the clinical ladder rewards both performance and education. The nurse executive who only wants to pay for services delivered will keep her ladder free of credentialism or consider credentials as qualifying one for testing, not as meeting test requirements. For example, suppose that the Clinical Nurse V position calls for advanced research. The nurse executive will argue that she wants to see the nurse demonstrate that behavior, not merely that she have the credential of a master's or doctoral degree.

However, the nurse executive who uses her clinical ladder as a means to promote and reward advanced education might refuse to promote a nurse to Clinical Nurse V without a master's degree, thereby using the clinical ladder as a mechanism to urge nurses back to school. Although an education factor may be built into a clinical ladder as a prerequisite, the ladder will be a poor one if placement on the scale is automatically related to education, with little consideration of performance. In this case, the nurse executive may pay for services not delivered.

Gradations of financial compensation for clinical rank also present another problem. Although one wants to give status and rewards to excellent clinical nurses, it is a fact that the administrative nurse has greater responsibilities—for staff and for larger patient populations. Hence, it is difficult to justify a system in which one may make more money for less responsibility, no matter how well performed.

One can and should, however, be selective in the use of funds budgeted for clinical care. There is no reason why performance level cannot be a major factor built into the salary scale. Too many present systems are skewed to reward the least experienced, beginning nurse. Salary compression with good beginning salaries yet minimal advancement rewards is a common deficit in nursing.

Methodologically, creation of a clinical ladder involves several steps. First, job descriptions for each level of the ladder must be developed in concrete and highly operational terms. Typically, several major categories of nursing performance are defined and addressed on each job description to allow comparisons from one level to another. Often, systems use some formulation of the steps of the nursing process to serve this function. For example, every job description might address the categories of assessment, planning, implementation, and evaluation.

Other systems create their own categories; a system might use care planning, care delivery, coordination with other staff, leadership, research, and contribution to the nursing system. Notice that the latter set of categories brings up a question that inevitably arises in the construction of a clinical ladder, to wit: Where does clinical nursing leave off and management begin? This is a difficult question to answer in nursing because the typical clinical nurse has some responsibility for management within the context of her role. Note that with this set of categories, some components (e.g., research) may not arise at all in the early levels of practice.

Once the key responsibilities have been built into the job descriptions, they serve a secondary purpose: They become the categories for evaluation on the measurement tool(s) that judge clinical rank. Even here, the task is not a simple one, for each rank is made up of a constellation of behaviors.

One must make decision rules for the behaviors in the constellation. (1) Must the candidate achieve *all* the behaviors listed for this rank? Most of them? Seventy-five percent? (2) How often must these behaviors be demonstrated? All the time? Most of the time? Seventy-five percent of the time? (3) Are the measurement tools constructed to show whether the candidate *performs* or is *capable of performing* the behaviors? A candidate might submit three excellent nursing care plans for evaluation by a ranking committee, but this is no assurance that she routinely does care plans when on duty. (4) How does one rank a candidate with a mixed performance (e.g., a nurse who performs one-third of the activities on level II, one-third of the activities on level III, and yet another third on level IV)? Decisions such as these must be made before a clinical ladder program is instituted.

Procedures of evaluation also must be considered. Who judges the worth of the candidate? An impartial committee of nurses who have not worked with the nurse? Her own peer work group? Her supervisor? In a mixture of judges, what does each contribute, and how is each one's assessment weighted in the final judgment? Who nominates the candidate in the first place? Is self-nomination required? Must the immediate supervisor recommend the candidate? Is each nurse routinely re-evaluated at some specified time interval?

Methods of evaluation present their own set of problems. Is evaluation by means of some test situation such as a nurse's assignment to three difficult patients while under the eyes of a group of evaluators? Or is evaluation based on the ongoing observation of a nurse's daily work by supervisors and peers? By demonstrations? Or by retrospective reviews? What combination of methods will be used?

The system should relate to the initiation and continuation of employment. At what rank does a new employee begin when her abilities have not yet been assessed? Does everyone begin at the first level until proved more advanced? Or is the beginning rank estimated via years of experience or education? How soon is a change in rank to be done? How much time is allowed for orientation before ranking judgments are made? For continued employment, is routine advancement required? Must one achieve level II within 1 year or be dismissed? Or can one practice at level I for a lifetime, receiving a level I salary?

The procedures for implementing a clinical ladder are as complicated as is the initial building of the ladder and the construction of the measurement tools. The system will fail unless the decision rules for all these system components are determined in advance.

Nevertheless, the clinical ladder is a satisfying concept validating that quality of care delivered actually matters. Most institutions that claim to have a professional model of practice have a clinical ladder.

Administrative Ladder

Some nursing divisions build parallel clinical and administrative ladders. In this case, a single nurse may have two rankings, one clinical and one administrative. Other institutions take an either/or approach; the nurse is ranked either on the clinical ladder or on the administrative ladder. Either approach is defensible.

The administrative ladder has several problems unique to its situation. First, it is not possible to pay someone for administrative acumen not used in the position. One cannot pay an executive's salary to a charge nurse merely because she has the capability to fill that role were she placed in it. This is unlike the clinical situation, in which the nurse is assumed to be able to use all her expertise in her bedside role. The administrative ladder necessarily is tied to the administrative slots available in the given nursing division.

Further, it is difficult to predict the potential for advancement without placing the candidate in the higher role. For example, many excellent head nurses have failed to adapt to the supervisory role. The use of the administrative ladder for assessing advancement potential is somewhat limited. Similarly, although clinical excellence is a prerequisite for an initial management role, in no way does it ensure capability in managerial tasks.

When an individual is ranked simultaneously on both an administrative and a clinical ladder, another complication arises. The long-term administrator often loses some specific clinical skills. For example, one does not expect a nursing vice president to be adept in starting intravenous infusions. How, then, is this loss of clinical skills accounted for in the dual ranking system? Notice that the problem here is one of immediate skill. Obviously, the nurse executive could regain her clinical skills within a short time, but the use of her time is better put to acquiring additional management skills.

An administrative ladder implies a ranking of all nursing administrative/managerial positions in relation to one another. This, in itself, raises some problems. Whose position is higher: the evening supervisor who covers more units but superficially or the day head nurse who covers fewer units but is more accountable for ongoing operations? The ranking of administrative posts inevitably calls for weighing factors of depth versus breadth of responsibility or job scope.

If administrative levels are to be defined in ways that allow one to differentiate among them meaningfully, a strategy is required. Either one may plan and describe the levels independently and then rank the administrative jobs of the division according to where they fall within the levels or one may work backward, cumulating jobs of equivalent responsibility and summarizing them into a level description. The first plan probably is more intellectually satisfying, but the second will pragmatically allow one to relate the administrative levels to the available administrative jobs.

One advantage of having an administrative ladder is that it may be used as a counseling tool for a person who holds a managerial position yet fails to see the full implications of that responsibility. Similarly, such a tool can be used to differentiate management jobs that superficially appear alike, such as the job of a charge nurse of a unit for an 8-hour period versus the job of the head nurse of that unit.

An administrative ladder would make clear to that charge nurse (were she arguing for equal pay for an equal 8-hour shift) the ways in which her responsibilities are more limited than those of the head nurse.

Many institutions also initiate a promotions ladder for other nursing staff such as instructors, aides, and technicians. And some institutions combine staff, instructional staff and administrative staff, on a single ladder.

Job Responsibility Scattergram

Comparing nursing positions regarding overall responsibility is difficult, but the job responsibility scattergram enables one to better grasp the significant differences among jobs. Figure 20–1 illustrates one set of categories that may be used. Figures 20–1 and 20–2 show the contrasts that occur with different jobs.

In the scattergram, responsibilities are listed in relation to size of group: one-to-one relationships, groups rather than single persons, or multiple groups. Normally, these categories would refer to patients, as follows:

RESPONSIBLE FOR	MANAGERIAL TOOLS		
	Self	*Staff*	*Systems*
One			
A group	+	+ x	x x x x x
A total population	+	+ + + +	+ + x x x x x x x x x

Figure 20–1 Job Responsibility Scattergram for a Nurse Executive

- single patient: cares for one patient at a time
- patient group: single team of patients (case manager perhaps)
- total population: several patient groups (supervisor's responsibility) or all patient groups (vice president's responsibility)

These categories are cross-gridded with the major tools used in meeting responsibilities. For example,

- single patient/staff: team leader assignment of aide to Mr. X's care
- single patient/system: arranging for home care for Mr. X using a home care health agency

For certain positions, the groups may refer to staff rather than patients. For example, in looking at staff development work, the following illustrations might pertain:

- single staff member/self: one-to-one educational consultation by a staff development instructor with a staff nurse
- a group of staff members/staff: instructors team teaching a major new procedure to 5 West staff members
- a total staff population/systems: staff development departmental planning for the total program for the year of educational activities

In the scattergram, the greater responsibilities fall toward the lower right-hand box in the dia-

RESPONSIBLE FOR	MANAGERIAL TOOLS		
	Self	*Staff*	*Systems*
One	+	+	x
A group	+ x x	x x x + + x x	x x
A total population	+	+	

Figure 20–2 Job Responsibility Scattergram for a Head Nurse

gram. Further, if each marked item on the grid represents a key job function, then some jobs will have more total xs than others. Hence, the staffing coordinator's job functions will fall primarily in the lower right-hand area, just like the director's functions. In the case of the coordinator, however, she will have fewer xs, representing the limited domain of responsibility. Use of the scattergram in this manner, enables one to reflect both scope of the job (number of total xs) and depth of the job (distribution toward lower right-hand side). If job scattergrams are superimposed on each other, their similarities and differences may be easily reviewed.

PATIENT CLASSIFICATION SYSTEMS

Like staff, patients may be classified along various dimensions of which three are reviewed here: (1) placement on a given patient unit, (2) according to acuity, and (3) assessment through total task quantification systems. Both patient and staff classification systems are used to make a better match of patient needs and staff delivery of care.

Classification by Placement on a Patient Unit

The placement of patients on given geographic units is a major organizing structure, and the nurse executive needs to consider the nature of those placements. Often, the nature of cases mixed on a unit is dictated by size of the population served. For example, a small community hospital may mix diverse patient populations that could be segregated in a larger hospital. Even a large institution must select patient populations large enough to fill a given unit; otherwise, cost-effectiveness will be lost with unfilled beds.

Unit designation usually is a result of past decisions and present power struggles. (Many an institution woos an important cardiologist by promising him his own unit for cardiovascular patients, for example.) Unfortunately, nursing

seldom is considered in such unit-designating activities. This is not a reflection of logic but of power. Indeed, if one were to assign units rationally, it would be on the basis of nursing because it is a 24-hour-a-day ongoing activity, whereas medical care is intermittent and a short-time unit event. Given this logic, the nurse executive should try to influence the unit-designating function.

Nursing once had control of unit designation—in the era of progressive patient care, when nursing divisions designated units according to type or level of nursing care required. When level was the criterion, there were maximal care units, medium care units, and minimal care units. This was the start of the concept of the intensive care unit (maximal care).

A problem with the placement by *level of nursing care* was that the patient was moved from unit to unit as his status changed. This not only caused problems in logistics but also decreased patient satisfaction. Just as a patient finally knew all the staff on one unit and felt comfortable with his surroundings, he was moved.

When type of care rather than level of care was designated, units such as acute care, convalescent care, self-care, and teaching units arose. One still sees long-term care units, for example, as an outgrowth of this placement principle.

There is no single principle on which units should be determined. Many possibilities exist. Fortunately, many of these principles are equally useful to medicine and nursing. Some possibilities include

1. similar patient age (pediatric or adolescent units)
2. similar nursing treatments needed (burn or spinal cord injury units)
3. similar patient needs (recovery rooms, nursery)
4. similar treatments (same-day surgical units, medical units)
5. similar medical specialty (genitourinary, gynecologic units)
6. similar patient behaviors (psychiatry)

Although some of these principles favor nursing and some favor medicine, many represent good compromises. The nurse executive may be able to sell her proposals for unit designation if she can show that such designation promotes better nursing care without impairing medical care. As we move into an age of greater nursing specialization, the control of unit designation will become of even greater significance.

Patient Classification and Task Quantification Systems

Patient classification and task quantification systems are two approaches to the same objective and are discussed together for the sake of comparison. Both systems aim to make some statement concerning the nurse's work load, although they use different methodologies. In a patient classification system, a judgment of patient needs is established and the patient is classified accordingly in one of several categories. (Some systems use as few as three categories; some as many as nine. Most have four to five groups.) Categories are determined in one of two ways. (1) Each category is described generally and reinforced with descriptions of sample patient cases. Given these descriptions, the nurse judges which category comes closest to the patient's status, and he is placed in that category. (2) Critical indices are determined that dictate patient classification.

For example, a system may make absolute statements such as "Any incontinent patient may not be placed lower than category III." Or a system may classify a patient according to several characteristics considered together, stating "If a patient has any two of the following conditions, he belongs in category IV," this statement followed by such characteristics as immobility, intravenous therapy, unable to bathe self, and so forth. In these systems, not all patient characteristics are considered; only those that have been found to have a significant impact on care level or time are elected for review.

A few systems still attempt to account for every act performed for a patient, but these systems are cumbersome, costly to administer, and not much more accurate than those using critical indices.

Whether through a summary judgment or a summarization of specific characteristics, patients are sorted into various classifications, each classification ultimately associated with a normative number of nursing hours required. Hours may vary from shift to shift. For example, a patient who is up and about but learning about a new disability (e.g., diabetes) may need many nursing hours during the day and virtually none related to this variable during the night hours. The hours attributed to physical care of an acutely ill patient, however, might be equal on every shift.

Some patient classification systems actually are patient acuity systems (i.e., based on how sick the patient is). Acuity alone, however, may fail to reflect nursing hours accurately. In the illustration above, the relatively well diabetic will need many nursing hours to learn self-care for his diabetes. Hence, some systems calculate on degree of nursing care required rather than on acuity. Other systems combine these two factors.

When a task quantification system is used, the nursing task rather than the patient need is measured. Here, all required tasks are summarized on average performance time norms. To calculate total nursing hours required, factors are added to build in indirect nursing time. These systems may attempt to account for every nursing task or only for those that make critical differences. For example, some systems eliminate items such as "relief of anxiety," assuming such items will be addressed while accomplishing physical tasks.

One problem arises when tasks are closely associated with staff education level. A throat irrigation, for example, might be assigned to the licensed practical nurse level, with no consideration that the particular patient might be extremely difficult, requiring a registered nurse. As long as one differentiates between specific assignments and typical placement, however, one can use such system data to predict staffing number and mix.

Despite their limitations, task quantification systems give an excellent rough average of the amount of work to be performed on a unit (or for a given patient). Used in the appropriate manner, they are excellent tools for planning the delivery of nursing care.

It is common for these systems to create some form of patient care unit that represents a convenient number of minutes of care. Time norms differ from system to system, especially because some relate only to direct care time and others are factored to include indirect time also.

Whether time norms are cumulated per patient or per nursing unit depends on the use to which they are put. For example, these norms may be used in calculating staffing needs, revising scheduling, setting individual patient fees, determining supply and equipment needs, or developing trend data over time. Not only may data be collected per patient or per patient floor, but they also may be collected per 24-hour time period or per shift. Again, the intended use of the data dictates how often they must be obtained.

Whatever the system that is used to collect data, it should meet the following criteria: (1) simplicity and speed of data collection, (2) accuracy versus ability to manipulate data to one's own ends, and (3) reliability and validity of the format used. Accurate patient or task data enable the nurse executive to relate patient need and nursing care delivery. Such data also reveal instances in which a constant patient population (number) has increasing or decreasing needs for nursing services.

Patients, then, are classified by two different methods. In one case, the classification system relates the patient to some gestalt pattern; he is placed according to his similarity to some prototypical patients. This is usually termed *prototype evaluation*.

The opposite approach is to identify tasks performed for the patient, giving numerical ratings that relate to time or complexity of task. This form of assessment is termed *factor evaluation*. Nor is it unusual to find an assessment tool combining factor-isolating and prototype elements. However, most growth in tools available for purchase has been in the factor systems.

Whatever method is used, the final calculation is one in which the care needs of the patient are estimated (in time required, in level of staff skill required, or both). The classification system becomes a vehicle for estimating staff resources used per patient. Although such systems are not foolproof, they produce important data by which to assess both individual cases and needs of grouped patients (e.g., the patients on a given nursing unit).

One often hears such systems called interchangeably patient acuity or patient classification systems. In truth, most of the systems are more concerned with the time required for care than for the acuity level of the patient. Obviously, there is some correlation between these two factors. The very ill patient is likely to need more care. The correlation is not absolute, however. As indicated earlier, a patient with extensive self-care learning needs might score high in care hours required while not having a high acuity rating.

Most systems, however, do not make differentiations between acuity and care time required. Both acuity and classification systems are used for similar purposes—to make the leap from quality to quantity of nursing care.

Many of the systems derived internally in an organization are based on actual care hours rather than on actual care needs. Hence, a system may reflect the possible rather than the ideal in a given institution.

Whether the system used is purchased or devised internally, it is important that it use valid and reliable tools for data collection. Because such systems are used for calculating staffing requirements, nurses may tend to overrate patients, hoping to acquire additional staff. It is important that all units use identical leniency or strictness in applying system criteria for patient classification. Staff must be educated to the importance of accuracy in making classifications. Nationally used systems have the advantage of large-scale testing and adjustment for validity and reliability. However, homemade tools have the advantage of reflecting more closely the individual institution's situation.

When the same tool is used by multiple institutions, it is possible to collect data on a large scale and also to compare institutions. This advantage probably outweighs the advantage of having a unique tool in each setting. Certainly, any multi-institution corporation would derive greater benefit from the sharing of such tools across institutions than by having separate tools used in each location. Further, the cost of creating such a system is not small.

Classification Systems and Prospective Reimbursement

All patient classification systems allow one to accumulate data concerning nursing effort (use of resources) for a given time period (day or shift). This is the natural unit by which to measure nursing use of resources because patient needs can vary greatly during the course of therapy.

It is important that classification systems be correlated with whatever units are used to determine prospective reimbursement (assuming this is the method of payment). The diagnosis-related group (DRG) system, still used nationally although being replaced in some locations, is based on a medical model: case rather than time as the unit for analysis. This makes difficulties for nursing, because case is not a natural category for estimating use of nursing resources. One patient with a stroke, for example, may have radically different care needs than another case with the same diagnosis.

Nevertheless, because prospective case reimbursement is a fact of life, with or without the DRG system, nursing has no choice but to learn to assess use of nursing resources via prospective case norms, with patients being classified according to categories used for reimbursement decisions. It is imperative that nursing be able to predict and control its costs.

SUMMARY

Both patients and staff may be classified for various purposes: staffing, scheduling, assign-

ing fees, rewarding advanced clinical practices, and collecting data on changes in the health care delivery system. Classification systems are useful if they are reliable, valid, and easy to administer. They allow one to compare interinstitutional data and to account for differences. Such systems increase the data base on which the nurse executive may build and make decisions.

SUGGESTED READINGS

American Nurses Association. 1984. *Career ladders: An approach to professional productivity and job satisfaction.* Washington, D.C.: ANA.

Bost, D., and T.G. Lawler. 1989. Measuring nursing resource consumption. *Nursing Management* 20, no.2:34–35.

Bostrom, J., and M. Mitchel. 1991. Relationship of direct nursing care hours to severity of illness. *Nursing Economics* 9, no.2:105–111.

Carroll, J.G. 1991. *Monitoring with indicators.* Gaithersburg, Md.: Aspen Publishers, Inc.

Cockerill, R., et al. 1993. Measuring nursing workload for case costing. *Nursing Economics* 11, no.6:342–349.

Finnigan, S.A., et al. 1993. Automated patient acuity: Linking nursing systems and quality measurement with patient outcomes. *Journal of Nursing Administration* 23, no.5:62–71.

Hamric, A.B., et al. 1993. Implementing a clinically focused advancement system: One institution's experience. *Journal of Nursing Administration* 23, no.9:20–28.

Jarvis, R., et al. 1991. Implementation of a patient classification system: Using current resources to achieve organizational goals. *Health Care Supervisor* 10, no.1:51–57.

Kelleher, C. 1992. Validated indexes: Key to nursing acuity standardization. *Nursing Economics* 10, no.1:31–37.

Lawson, K.O., et al. 1993. Redefining the purpose of patient classification. *Nursing Economics* 11, no.5:298–302.

Thompson, J.D., and D. Diers. 1988. Management of nursing intensity. *Nursing Clinics of North America* 23, no.3:473–492.

Waltz, C., and O. Strickland. 1991. *Volume IV: Measuring clinical skills and professional development in education and practice.* New York: Springer Publishing Co., Inc.

Part VI
Managing Resources

All management involves managing resources—human, intellectual, material, and fiscal. Therefore, the content in the next group of chapters is extracted artificially from the context of the whole. Nevertheless, the aspects discussed in Part VI concern those aspects of management most often thought of in terms of dollars and cents or concrete resources.

Chapter 21 examines the pricing and productivity of nursing services. Chapter 22 looks at the basics of institutional finance, and Chapter 23 looks at material (physical) resources of the division. These chapters are followed by a discussion of the basics of business planning in Chapter 24.

Business planning is a good example of the problems arising when one focuses on any given aspect of management. Clearly, every business plan has to have a budget that warrants it, yet the budget is only one aspect of a business plan, a justificatory aspect at that. Because attaching a fiscal plan to a business plan is new for some nurse executives, we have elected to place the subject here.

21

Nursing Resources: Pricing and Productivity

Today's ruling principle, whether or not we approve, is that health care is not above price; it is not a value to be delivered at any cost. It is a product, and the level of health care produced relates to the cost. No longer is cost containment enough. Cost reduction has replaced this concept as dollars available for health care delivery shrink. Employers and consumers have experienced the escalating cost of health care, as well as the moves to control costs. Managed care with its emphasis on cost reduction is foremost in this change, forcing everyone to look at costs in new ways.

This chapter looks at nursing as a product of the marketplace. It addresses how one copes with delivery of nursing care in a resource-driven health care economy that is rationing its resources. Nursing can no longer be considered only a service; it is also a business. The cost of this service must continually be evaluated, and new innovative strategies must be developed to meet the cost demands of the marketplace.

A BUSINESS ORIENTATION

In any business, several questions must be answered before the strategies of management are settled. What is the product of the business? What does it cost to manufacture the product? How should the product be priced? Can the product be produced at less cost through greater efficiency?

In the past, nursing's *product* has been loosely identified as quality care for all. This value-laden definition has no reference to quantitative economic considerations. As a definition, it comes closer to expressing a hope than a reality. No longer is it possible to do everything the nurse wants to do for the patient. Instead, controlled quality care must be provided at a cost-effective price. Few organizations have the luxury to provide the ideal product consistently in actual care delivery.

When one asks what it *costs* to manufacture the product, reality sets in. Nursing's product is a service, one whose costs are difficult to extract. Until recently, nursing costs were included with food services, maid functions, and room rent in an undifferentiated daily rate. This rate typically was the same for most patients, regardless of the amount of or level of nursing care received.

Because of greater nursing costs involved, separate fees were usually charged for specialty units such as intensive care or recovery room. Even here, most fees were not set by a logical study of the real costs of nursing care delivered but by arbitrary accounting decisions so that the total health care delivery costs were absorbed and covered by total patient fees.

Now, the health care industry has a real interest in knowing its actual costs, including the cost of providing nursing services. Later in this chapter, methods for calculating nursing service costs are discussed. The question of costs brings up the next business-oriented question: How should the product be priced? It is important to differentiate between costs and price. In business, manufacturing costs are the basis for price setting. In health care, certainly in nursing, that relationship has been tenuous at best.

Health care organizations are now forced by reimbursement plans to function with a bottom-line business orientation in relating cost and fees. Even not-for-profit organizations must stay solvent to provide services and replace capital for the future.

What then can be said about the relationship of costs and price? First, if costs increase, the price of the product must increase if the business is to stay solvent. In nursing (and health care in general), many uncontrolled factors have tended to increase costs. For example, the wages of health care workers have improved in the past two decades. In nursing, the fact that nurses have received better wages has been applauded. Most believe that nurses should be rewarded based on their education and their contribution to society.

Another factor that served to drive up costs until recently was the increased numbers of nurses used because of increasing technology. Until recently, institutions consistently increased their nursing staff ratio to number of patients. Not only did an increased technology demand more nurses, but the technology kept patients alive longer, ultimately requiring more nursing care.

As costs increase in business, the price of the product rises to cover cost plus gain the desired profit. Until the introduction of prospective payment and cost monitoring, health care followed this pattern.

With the advent of managed care, that changed. Now, payers are able to go shopping and demand a lower price because they have a large volume of patients to market. Overnight hospitals can see a major influx of patients or a major loss in patient volume, depending on how successful the institution is in contracting with payers. In many instances, hospitals are operat-

ing at significantly lower margins because they are forced to contract for less and less reimbursement to retain the patient volume.

What occurs when the health care facility loses revenue? Logically, the options are limited:

1. Less of the product can be offered (downsizing) or the quality of the product can be sacrificed.
2. New systems of production must be sought to maintain (or even improve on) the old product.
3. The institution can go out of business, insolvent.

In health care, there is strong preference for trying to find ways to retain the quality of care previously given, by creating new efficiencies and re-engineering delivery methods. This is the source of the present focus on productivity. This chapter looks at general tactics and strategies for increasing productivity, but first it examines the product of nursing and the ideology surrounding it today.

THE NURSING PRODUCT

In this country, the product of nursing has always been defined as quality care (however described). Our nursing traditions have associated professionalism with delivery of the highest level of care that can be envisioned. Our schools have reinforced this ideology by teaching students the care of a limited number of patients (so that they can give each patient that idealized comprehensive care). The ideology has been well ingrained in nurses: Good nursing is synonymous with comprehensive care.

Only a few decades ago, we envisioned a time when we would be able to give this sort of care. The country and its gross national product were expanding; technology was seen as a solution, not a cost; national health insurance was soon to be reality; and all would be bright and beautiful next year if not sooner. In an era that envisioned such a future, the notion of ideal nursing care fit. Missing was an emphasis on productivity and delivering the quality at the lowest possible cost.

There were, however, some flaws in the design of that era. For example, few institutions were ever able to live up to the ideal. We experienced phenomena such as Schmalenberg and Kramer's (1979) "reality shock," a signpost to the disjuncture between ideology and practice. Usually, nurses proposed that the answer to reality shock was to change the reality, not to question the ideology. Indeed, chief nursing officers were often set up as obstructionists who willfully prevented such ideal care from taking place. Sometimes, they were given the benefit of the doubt and merely judged to be inept. The practicing nurse, unschooled in the intricacies of the financial management of health care, remained naive about such matters.

This same era had a matching managerial ideology, solving problems by a system of management by objectives (MBO). MBO and total nursing care had much in common. For both systems, one could identify the same method of operation:

- Set the goals.
- Decide how to achieve them.
- Procure the resources.
- Put the plan into effect.
- Evaluate success in reaching the goal.

Nothing is inherently wrong with this system; it works well in some circumstances. Indeed, this is the goal-driven model described in Chapter 2, a goal-driven model whether it refers to MBO in nursing management or comprehensive care in patient care. It begins with the setting of goals, and those goals dictate the rest of the model's application.

The problems with this model occur in an environment that is less than ideal (i.e., one that will not provide the resources one needs to procure). As indicated in Chapter 2, the goal-driven model fails in a financially restrictive environment.

The paradigm of health care is changing. We can no longer depend on passing costs on to the payer or shifting the cost of care to groups of payers with more resources. We must revise the model so that it becomes resource-driven rather than goal-driven. The reader will remember the steps from Chapter 2:

- Assess the resources.
- Prioritize the number and types of goals that one can take on, given the resources.
- Determine the most feasible methods.
- Put the plan into effect.
- Evaluate.

The resource-driven model, despite its complexity, avoids the chief flaw in the goal-driven model, for here one can succeed (or fail) in any given environment. In a resource-scarce situation, one's success rests in the talented selection and prioritizing of goals to be achieved.

However, the resource-driven model, used alone, has no fail-safe mechanism; nursing care resources can reach a critical deficit. Although selecting more efficient methods increases productivity, it is not true that this principle can compensate forever. An institution using a resource-driven model for management and nursing care needs to have baseline goal-driven safety nets (i.e., predetermined standards that must be achieved to secure patient safety). One must be able to recognize when an emergency state exists, using such management and nursing criteria as have been set in advance.

When we look at nursing as a product, we see that it is not necessary to equate nursing with total nursing care; the product can be defined in another way. With a resource-driven model, it is possible to define different levels of patient care if that is desired. The model is compatible with some of the extant changes coming about in nursing and health care. The old goal-driven model of nursing is clearly not compatible with a productivity model of scarce resources. It is in conflict with the environment of cost reductions and resource limitation that dominates today.

PRODUCTIVITY

Productivity is the ratio between input and output. In nursing, input primarily is measured in man-hours, but it also may involve supplies, equipment, and use of space. Output is the unit of service rendered. The appropriate output measure might be different for different services. For example, a clinic might identify the number of patient visits, whereas an acute care unit might have a measure based on a summative number of patient care units (PCUs) derived from its patient classification system.

Productivity is increased if the ratio of input falls in relation to the measure of output or if the measure of output increases in relation to the input. *Effectiveness* is the achievement of one's objectives, and *efficiency* is the achievement of those objectives with the greatest possible economy. The latter combines notions of quality (attaining objectives) and quantity (least cost).

In contrast to the definition of efficiency used here, many authors view productivity aside from an assessment of quality. For example, one might determine the productivity of a nurse-run clinic by comparing the number of clients served in a day (output) to the number of nurse man-hours spent in the clinic that day. In this strictly quantitative calculation, nothing is said concerning whether the clients received good or poor care.

Deniston and colleagues (1973) noted the need to consider both effectiveness and efficiency simultaneously. To that end, they proposed several ratios. The ratios of effectiveness included:

1. AO:PO (attainment of objectives: proposed objectives)
2. AA:PA (actual activities performed: planned activities to be performed)
3. AR:PR (actual resource expenditure: planned resource expenditure) (pp. 444–455)

In contrast, they identified the following efficiency ratios:

1. AO:AR (attainment of objectives: actual resource expenditure)
2. AA:AR (actual activities performed: actual resource expenditure)
3. AO:AA (attainment of objectives: actual activities performed) (pp. 444–455)

As these authors noted, additional equations would allow one to interrelate effectiveness and efficiency ratios.

Indices

For nursing, the next major task related to productivity is to select (or create) indices for measuring it. Census data combined with acuity data give important information. Data on nursing staff man-hours can be more refined if the level of nursing staff (skill mix) is factored into the equation. (This is the staff equivalent of the acuity modification for patient census.)

Simple indices for activity levels are important in making day-to-day adjustments in resources. For example, one might explore whether the use of 4×4s or intravenous pumps are good indices for level of patient care activity on surgical units. Or one might explore whether use of patient underpads reflects the level of activity on long-term care units. The simpler the index, the less work is needed to extrapolate nursing productivity.

These simple indices do not preclude the need for more detailed long-term collection of data. However, they may be of pragmatic assistance in day-to-day management, and they are available before more complex staffing/patient acuity calculations are made. The simpler the index, the more use it will be in practice. Finding productivity indices requires a ready eye to correlations. What is a likely index of something else (when that something else is complex to measure in itself)?

Productivity Tactics

There are many tactics whereby the nurse executive can encourage productivity among the staff. Chief among them is the creation of a philosophy of productivity throughout the institution. Staff must be cognizant of the need for productivity and encouraged to seek new ways to achieve it.

Many practices and attitudes fly in the face of productivity. For example, the nurse who resists being sent to another floor after "finishing" her assigned patients shows an attitude that perceives the original day's assignment as the rightful amount of work. Additions to that work load are seen as infringements on the worker's time. Hourly workers must be made to understand that they are paid for an entire shift, not for completing an initial assignment.

An attitude that a worker owes the employer his services for the entire shift is not encouraged when workers are expected to stay overtime without remuneration if they have not finished their assigned work load. Indeed, some institutions have high productivity due to giving workers unusually heavy work assignments and expecting the work to be performed, however long it takes.

Such a practice may create high productivity temporarily, but a price will be paid in worker fallout. However, there are places where workers run unusually high overtime costs simply because oncoming shifts do not accept that they are to pick up unfinished work of the last shift.

In each case, it is essential to create a high-performance and high-productivity culture. The newly graduated nurse, for example, cannot perceive of the work arena simply as a place for self-actualization but a place where one is paid in return for valuable service that can be measured in both quantity and quality.

A second productivity tactic is the careful use of skills at the fitting level. In industry, this is an easier concept to apply. One can say that a registered nurse (RN) should not do a nurses' aide level task, but the problem is more complex than the factory-line image would indicate. For a given patient, a typical "aide-level" task may be more complex because of intervening patient factors. Nevertheless, one can aim for appropriate fit of tasks and employee skill level.

Productivity also may be achieved through standardization. When procedures are routinized, time is not lost in resolving the same old problems. Uniformity in practices, procedures, and policies throughout an institution or in multi-institution corporations produces efficiency. Even here, the answer is not simple. Too much standardization may thwart the nurse's professional autonomy. There is a fine line to be

drawn between standardization and freedom of professional practice.

There are many situations in which standardization does not fit the work of the nursing unit. For example, two patients with the same diagnosis may require quite different critical paths because of individual contingencies. Even here, however, productivity may be enhanced by building these different care plans on the framework of a standard care plan and/or critical path map.

In other instances, one must ask which saves time: standardization or individualization? Consider, for example, whether one saves time by reviewing which patients on a unit require morning vital signs and which do not. Is more time saved by only checking selected patients? Or is more time saved by not making the decision concerning who should be monitored? On a unit where most patients require monitoring, the savings might be made by standardization (i.e., simply taking all vital signs for all patients indiscriminately). On another unit, where few patients need monitoring of vital signs, the opposite tactic would be more productive.

Productivity is encouraged by streamlining routine patterns of care. Are assignment methods those most efficient for the given unit? Efficiency and effectiveness, as well as patient and staff satisfaction, must be considered simultaneously. Systems should be reviewed. Are frequently used supplies kept at a convenient storage center? Are traffic patterns simplified? Can events be staggered throughout the day to avoid peaks and valleys of work? Can non-nursing systems be redesigned to relieve periods of non-productivity on the nursing unit? Are functions duplicated by two professional groups? Do nursing assessments gather data that will not be used? Are nurses' notes designed for quick recording while still capturing vital information and recording it where it will be read? All systems, nursing and interfacing ones, can be reviewed for efficiency.

Feedback to the nursing unit concerning its productivity encourages improvement. Feedback should include recognition of persons who think of ideas that improve efficiency. However, if productivity becomes a fetish, it can be counterproductive. Staff must not feel that they are eternally driven to work faster and harder. Such a perception leads to burnout. Instead, staff should appreciate that productivity helps find easier ways to do the work.

Any measure that contains costs necessarily improves productivity (by lessening the input in the productivity ratio). Economies of scale, for example, improve productivity. If one makes purchases in bulk, at a reduced price, then the input costs are lower in relation to output. Formal corporations and informal consortia take advantage of group efforts—not only in purchasing economies but in joint program efforts. For example, neighboring institutions may join staff for selected inservice education, pooling expert resources, allowing their respective staff development departments to save on costs. Multi-institution corporations further save by transferring personnel as needed from one institution to another, improving flexibility in the use of human resources.

Productivity in Use of Personnel

Because nursing is labor-intensive, the best way to contain costs is the frugal use of personnel. Some management policies increase productivity by optimizing on the output of each employee. Effective formulation of policies regulating illness, tardiness, and leaves is critical. Policies designed to discourage use of sick time and those deducting salary for tardiness increase efficiency. One also must scrutinize policies concerning paid leaves. What is gained and what is lost in such policies?

Overtime policies also come under scrutiny. Is overtime used in excess? Is it really required if oncoming shifts assume unfinished tasks? Is overtime so frequent that it would be cheaper to increase the staff complement? On-call policies need the same sort of financial analysis.

The nurse executive also will want to eliminate flaws from the hire–fire policies. Suppose that a head nurse knows she will lose a position if she fails to fill it immediately. In that case, she may hire a replacement that she really does not

need during a slack period. All policies should be reviewed to see whether they encourage cost saving or force managers and staff into costly patterns of behavior. Once nurse managers understand and are evaluated by cost per unit of service and other productivity standards, this kind of gaming stops.

One of the greatest costs in staff time is use of nurses on committees. Every hour in committee work is an hour not given for patient care. Much committee work is important, but often committees are larger than necessary. Many committees actually function better if their membership is lean.

Every employee's performance must count. One cannot carry a nonproductive employee on the hope that he will improve. Evaluation, discipline, and—when needed—removal from employment must follow inferior performance. Evaluation and discipline systems should be refined so that such actions do not drag out over an unnecessarily long period. Obviously, an employee must be given a chance to improve, but if improvement does not occur or does not last, then action is required.

One also must examine employee educational benefits. For example, should an institution pay for an employee to attend education programs not related to his arena of work? Even if such classes are internal, they are not "free" if the employee is sitting in class instead of giving service on duty time.

An institution may need to examine its reimbursement policies for formal education programs. Does the institution need such policies to attract capable nurses? Does the beneficiary give anything in return? Does she agree to remain on staff for a given time period or else refund the educational support? Some institutions pay full tuition for nurses completing advanced degrees when they have no openings for nurses with those degrees. In essence, this practice pays an employee to prepare to leave his position.

Nursing management must be careful to maintain its managerial flexibility in negotiating labor contracts. If a nurse executive gives up the right to move nurses from one unit to another, she necessarily increases personnel costs. Expensive management practices such as shift differentials, extra money for critical care, and use of agency nurses will have to be examined. Major savings in the nursing division can result from improved staffing practices. It often takes money to save money; an adequate and well-supervised orientation period for personnel costs more than does a hasty orientation, for example, but the investment is recovered in higher retention of personnel. Inadequate orientation followed by too much responsibility too soon is a major cause of premature resignation. Turnover is a major expense in nursing.

When staffing is excessively short, another false economy occurs. When staff are unable to cover normal deviations in the work load because they have been pared too thin, the costs of overtime and staff replacement are far greater than the amount saved by inadequate staffing. Such staffing also leads to resignations and increased recruitment and orientation costs.

Finally, nursing management must look close at hand. Is the management staff excessive for the size of the nursing operation? Many institutions have already flattened their organizations, sometimes removing whole layers of nursing management. Is there really a full complement of work for every nurse manager?

A nurse executive can also make relationships with outside institutions productive. The facility providing clinical placement for students, for example, can request reciprocal services from faculty (e.g., staff education programs).

Internally, does the nurse executive optimize on all services? Does the volunteer department have people who could be trained to do more and different tasks? Nurse executives sometimes think only of volunteers who wish to work with patients. Retired executives may be helpful in business planning; volunteer secretarial services may be great additions. Often, volunteers are overlooked because they are seen as ill-trained for work in a health care institution. Although they may lack medical and nursing knowledge, one often finds volunteers with expertise concerning publicity campaigns or in staging major social events. The director of a volunteer department should have a ready analysis of the skills of all present volunteers. When a specific skill is desired, the director may be pressed to search for the right volunteer from the community.

Cost Containment in Material

Although savings may not be so great on material (equipment and supplies) as on personnel, there is enough potential to merit concern.

One main source of loss is theft by staff—nursing, medical, or other. (A recent advertisement showing interns on a picnic in scrubs testifies to the general acceptance of the problem.) The nurse executive will want to consider the systems for management of equipment and supplies. Is accountability built in? Is it possible to determine who has missing equipment? What accounting systems monitor supplies? Do these systems function to protect supplies without frustrating staff who need them?

Often, discount purchases available to staff will preserve those items that might otherwise be stolen. Scrubs, scissors, stethoscopes, and sphygmomanometers head the list. Each institution has a good idea of its primary theft items. One should focus on development of fail-safe systems for managing these supplies.

However, common sense must reign. A theft prevention system that costs hundreds of hours of staff time filling out vouchers and reports may cost more than it saves. Nor should pettiness over trivial expenses be mistaken for frugality. If staff perceive that changes have more to do with cheapness, they will find ways to subvert the purported savings.

The nursing division can save on personnel and material costs by a careful review of its systems. It may be useful to hire a systems analyst if none is on staff. The systems of the divisions may be examined for streamlining potential and for standardizing where economies of scale may be gained.

The nurse executive should not be overconcerned with every minor system; concentration should be on the big systems, those where there is potential for significant savings. No system is entirely fail-safe, but many systems can be improved with a little work.

Sometimes, the employees who know them best are good analysts of systems. Most institutions find that a small bonus for cost-saving ideas is well worth the investment.

The nurse executive will want to examine the budgetary system of the institution for procedures that encourage or discourage cost saving. For example, a nurse executive may be buying some equipment (perhaps bedside tables) in small numbers, month by month, because they can be slipped into the operational budget in this manner. However, if the budgetary system would allow her to make one major purchase in a year, it might be possible to get a big discount on the tables, a discount that is unavailable if purchased a few at a time.

Similarly—unless cash flow is in a critical state—if a nurse executive waits to purchase an expensive item in a later budget period (when an increase in price is expected), this is wasteful, especially if the money for the item has already been budgeted.

The quality of equipment and supplies requires scrutiny. Some people explore use of vendors outside of the usual hospital suppliers. Items of furniture, for example, are lower priced when purchased this way. The process is risky, however, for many such items simply are not made for the hard wear received in an institutional setting.

It is important to specify exactly when ordering supplies through a purchasing department. Otherwise, in its own attempts to save, the purchasing department may buy an inferior product that does not meet the specifications for the task for which the item is purchased. The nursing division and the purchasing department must cooperate for both cost saving and appropriate purchases.

COSTING OUT NURSING SERVICES

One of the first requirements for judging productivity is a clear idea of actual costs (input).

Further, input costs are essential for pricing of services. Whether or not an institution tracks separate charges for nursing services, it is incumbent on the nurse executive to know what it costs to deliver those nursing services.

In a resource-limited system, knowledge of real costs becomes critical. When the nurse executive is fighting to receive a fair share of a shrinking budget, she must be able to judge what sort of care can be delivered for what level of funding.

One logical way to determine nursing costs is to use the patient acuity system as a base. Because nursing is a labor-intensive practice, the closest reflection of cost is that of nursing hours per patient per day. The patient acuity (classification) system should be designed to give that estimate. For units where use of supplies also is a major variant, separate charges can be devised for expensive items. Although an amalgam of charging for supplies and charging by acuity classification is imperfect, it is one solution for estimating costs in nursing.

A more accurate cost can be obtained using a time and task analysis, recording exact care times and exact costs of all equipment and supplies used per patient. The problem with this method is the large number of administrative costs (i.e., the time spent in recording all the data). For this reason, it is seldom done, except in initial cost studies. Normally, one sacrifices some accuracy in cost accounting so as not to incur even more costs in excessive administrative record keeping.

No complete cost system can be calculated only using direct costs of nursing care hours plus use of equipment and supplies. Indirect costs must be considered (i.e., costs of nursing administrative salaries, nursing education, and other divisionally distributed nursing functions). All cost systems, therefore, are extractions from the best available data.

The best unit for calculation of nursing costs, given nursing's labor intensity, is the nursing hours per patient day (or shift). Such a measure allows for the changes in care level that come about during a patient's hospitalization. In this sense, community health visits or clinic services have simple units to calculate, because they may allow routine time periods per client. In acute care, however, it is generally the case that hours of care relate closely to acuity status.

Unfortunately, the nationally used Medicare reimbursement (diagnosis-related group [DRG]) system does not use a time-dependent unit. The reimbursement is per case, not per day or shift. This creates great difficulties for nursing because care per case is not a natural measurement.

It is, however, no accident that the way in which an institution profits is by decreasing length of stay for each case. Length of stay reflects the time-dependent nursing variable.

In using a patient acuity system to calculate man-hour costs, the nurse executive will need to decide whether the system norms are to be devised based on what patients in each class *need* in the way of nursing hours or whether the norms are to be based on the average care hours actually *given* per acuity level in the institution. Obviously, these two figures may or may not coincide.

Most systems today measure what is actually given, not what is deemed to be required. If the system merely measures the norm, it is important that it be recognized as such. Such norms will need to be retested periodically, especially if nursing staffing or patient acuity change.

There are at least four approaches to costing out nursing services. The first is based on a patient acuity system. A second approach using a nursing task-oriented tracking system is perhaps more accurate but involves more data collection. The third uses a case management projection; the fourth is similar, using the DRG system (or equivalent) as its base.

Costing Out by Patient Classification

The first costing method uses the institution's patient classification system as a base by calculating the average cost of nursing associated with each patient category per day or by calculating costs averaged for patients who fall within predetermined ranges of numerical scores (if the system uses quantitative tallies instead of patient categories).

Once costs per category per day have been established, then total costs are easily calculated based on acuity and census data. The original costs may be determined by a study of actual nursing time and tasks, relating those tasks back to nursing personnel and their salary rates in the institution. These data then are related to the classification plan to complete the system.

In all systems of costing out nursing, administrative costs of the nursing division must be distributed over nursing units according to the institution's policy. What gets labeled as an administrative cost varies from institution to institution.

A simpler calculation system involves a mathematical extrapolation from prior cost data if available on a unit basis. Here, one works backward, extracting administrative overhead and redistributing remaining costs over patient categories. Usually, the accounting department will assist in applying this method.

Costing Out Nursing by Time and Motion Studies

The second proposed method of costing out nursing relies on time and motion studies of actual nursing tasks performed. Here, all the nursing procedures of the institution are timed and norms established for each task. The average level of the worker doing the task also may be determined. When the average time of each procedure and the average level of the worker performing the task are known, direct costs of labor are determined and added to cost of materials.

Calculations can then be made by knowing the specific tasks performed on a unit on a given day. Charges can be averaged out over a selected time period for unit data, or items may be tracked on a patient-by-patient basis. Again, it is necessary to add in administrative overhead to reach a reasonable cost.

After the initial costs are determined for all nursing tasks, a checklist approach can calculate costs for each patient per day, for each unit per week or month (whatever base is desired). This system gives relatively accurate cost figures.

Costing Out Nursing by Case or DRG

The third and fourth methods associate costs with care patterns expressed in case management maps or tied to DRG categories. Whichever basis, the cost estimates can be set as described earlier, but then costs are calculated per case (map or DRG) rather than per day.

Acuity-based, task-based, and case-based systems all have advantages and disadvantages. In using patient classifications, the system is as equitable as the classification is accurate. One critical question to be answered in these cost systems is how often the patient is reclassified. Each shift? Each day? Obviously, a patient condition can change dramatically even during a single shift, thereby throwing off the accuracy of estimated data.

A task-based system has the advantage of avoiding the acuity analysis but encounters the difficulty of demanding more details than any other system. Nor do tasks, no matter how many are specified, directly reflect all costs.

When a case-based method is used, problems occur when assigning costs for a patient whose illness does not follow a typical trajectory. Not all patients in a defined category have similar care needs nor similar convalescence trajectories. In all these cases, the methods are better at establishing norms than at reflecting the real costs of any actual patient.

However achieved, costing out nursing services is the first step in resource management and judging productivity. It is also essential for building a realistic pricing strategy in which the fees for nursing services are set independently.

Fee Structures

Once one knows the cost of providing nursing services, one can reflect on fee structure. In a free market, there are two basic approaches to pricing (fee setting). First, one can find out what it costs to produce the goods or service, then set a price designed to break even or reach a predetermined profit level, or even give charitable services at an affordable subsidized loss. The pricing strategy selected depends on one's

goals. Under older cost-based reimbursement systems, hospitals could set price based on cost or cost-plus and pass the price, however high, on to the payer. Without competitive bidding, the incentives to keep cost down were missing.

The second pricing strategy begins with the price rather than with the product. In this case, one determines the price or fee, then decides what costs can be incurred in making the product. Here, what costs are acceptable depends on the financial goals for the enterprise.

To illustrate this second mode of pricing, suppose that a car manufacturer decides to provide a model for a new market—those who previously purchased used autos. The manufacturer might research this population and come up with a price that would entice a large enough market to warrant production of a car. From this determined price, he would calculate the profit margin and, deducting this, arrive at what he could afford for production costs. In this design, the final quality and nature of the product are necessarily influenced by the dictate that it be produced at a set cost.

In prior eras of health care, as was indicated, the first model was used. Care was delivered; then insurance companies were billed for whatever it cost. In other words, cost determined price.

Most nursing situations today come closer to the second pricing strategy. One starts with the price (i.e., the institution's reimbursement expectation) rather than with the product. Most reimbursement is set in advance by insurers. Institutions are paid set fees such as DRG payments or negotiated reimbursement rates for managed care contracts. If the costs of providing services outstrip the fee structure, an institution bears the loss.

The move to prospective reimbursement (preset fees) was engendered by the lack of cost control in the old model. In a free market, a manufacturer can charge any price he pleases for his product, but an exorbitant pricing structure limits the number of customers. Health care, in contrast, has no built-in restraint. When people are sick enough, they seek help first and worry about cost later.

In the old system, indifference to cost was encouraged by the fact that customers paid through a third party, an insurer. In this system, there was little need for the consumer to care what it cost, little motivation for the provider to monitor costs. Whatever costs were incurred would be reimbursed.

Today, most but not all health care institutions derive a large portion of their income from prospective payments. In this case, like the car manufacturer, one starts with the price. The most common prospective payment system in effect today is the DRG system that controls federal reimbursements of Medicare. Whether DRGs last or not, it is likely that other insurers will continue with prospective payment plans. Managed care companies already negotiate per diem rates per case and capitation payments in addition to discounted prices. The prospective payment in all its forms essentially dominates reimbursement nationally.

When payments are both prospective and reduced over past funding, nursing is in competition within the institution for its fair share of that reduced funding. If nursing can attest to its real costs, then requested support can be substantiated.

Whatever system is used to fund nursing, it must be interfaced with nursing's system for determining costs. For example, if a large part of the funding of an institution depends on DRG reimbursements, then the director needs to determine nursing costs per DRG classification.

The nurse executive, then, has the following tasks to complete for accurate financial management of her division:

- Determine the real resources used in providing nursing care to patients (by actual data on use per patient or estimated use).
- Use data to deduce direct costs and to prorate indirect costs.
- Calculate costs for each patient's care.
- Use cost figures as a base for fee setting if a fee structure is used.
- If nursing costs are not separately accounted in the billing system, the cost data can be used to make a case for resources needed within the nursing division as allotted by the institutional budget.
- Collect trend data relating costs to significant variables. For example, a nurse executive might want to substantiate whether costs increase or decrease given certain nursing care protocols.

Diagnosis-Related Groups

The DRGs were derived from the *International Classification of Diseases (Adapted)*. These medical diagnoses were related in groups according to their use of institutional resources. Hence, diseases and conditions were linked in a single group if they used similar amounts of resources, no matter what their clinical similarities or dissimilarities. The notion of resources encompassed all items of cost, including nursing. The original system made no attempt to isolate costs for nursing or other professional services. The unit of analysis was the whole patient time of hospitalization (i.e., his total case).

The nursing literature is replete with excellent descriptions of the DRG system. The summaries given in this book provide only a brief outline. Unless a nurse executive is in a state exempted from the DRG system, she will want more information than is presented here. Furthermore, the system is undergoing change and evolution. Hence, a general picture suffices for this presentation.

Certain systems were designed to cope with the unusual DRG case (e.g., a patient who has an excessively long stay because of complications). Adjustments and ways to use them are still being made in the system. Because patients use more resources the longer they are hospitalized, the chief way to increase income over expense is to discharge the patient as soon as possible. Not surprisingly, this may mean approaches are used that (1) get him well faster, (2) prepare the family to cope with him sooner, or (3) shift him to another institution or agency faster.

Other ways to increase income involve manipulating the system. And for each new manipulation that is discovered, the regulators design a counter-move designed to control and prevent the manipulation. Only two examples are given here as illustrations. Because certain DRG categories pay higher reimbursement levels, it is not surprising that some institutions tried to classify patients with multiple conditions according to the diagnoses with the greatest financial payoff ("DRG creep"), even if these were not the basic presenting conditions.

The second illustration of system manipulation involves selective admission of patients with preferred diagnoses. Most institutions, because of their unique circumstances or because of flaws in the reimbursement scheme, found that certain diagnoses paid better than others. After this discovery, attempts were made by various institutions to admit more patients with better paying classifications (DRG skimming) and to discourage admission of patients in financially losing classifications.

The objective underlying the move to DRGs, or more correctly to prospective payment, involves controlling cost through purposeful use of competition. Reimbursement rates are set low to start, so even without competition an institution must be frugal to survive financially. And every institution is in competition with others in its neighborhood concerning the kind of care that can be offered (a productivity factor).

With new tracking systems in place, institutions also could assess which physicians used more or less resources in their patterns of practice. Those who use excessive resources are encouraged to change practice patterns or leave. In essence, the hospital is forced into the business of modifying physician behavior toward cost efficiency.

Institutional behavior (patterns, procedures, practices) also is modified in this cost-conscious system. With the unending search for cost savings, the institution has incentive for continuous modification and streamlining.

SUMMARY

Massive system revisions are underway to decrease health care costs. Those changes involve putting fewer resources into the system and changing the system to improve productivity. Nursing must understand these changes and how they operate. This is especially difficult for all professionals (including nursing) who tend to work from idealized models of care in which all persons are entitled to the best professional care possible. It is an age of great challenge to nursing management.

REFERENCES

Deniston, O.L., et al. 1973. Evaluation of program efficiency. In *Health care administration: A managerial perspective*, ed. S. Levey and N.P. Loomba, 444–455. Philadelphia: J.B. Lippincott Co.

Schmalenberg, C., and M. Kramer. 1979. *Coping with reality shock: The voices of experience.* Wakefield, Mass.: Nursing Resources.

SUGGESTED READINGS

Allen, G.S. 1993. How much does absenteeism cost? *Journal of Human Resources* 18, no.3:379–394.

Eckhart, J.G. 1993. Costing out nursing services: Examining the research. *Nursing Economics* 11, no.2:91–98.

Felteau, A.L. 1993. Tools and techniques to effect budget neutrality. *Nursing Administration Quarterly* 17, no.4:59–64.

Finkler, S.A. 1991. Variance analysis, part II: The use of computers. *Journal of Nursing Administration* 21, no.9:9–15.

Gardner, K.G., and M. Tilbury. 1991. A longitudinal cost analysis of primary and team nursing. *Nursing Economics* 9, no.2:97–104.

Johnson, M. 1989. Perspectives on costing nursing. *Nursing Administration Quarterly* 14, no.1:65–71.

McNeese-Smith, D. 1992. The impact of leadership upon productivity. *Nursing Economics* 10, no.6:393–396.

22

Institutional Finance and Nursing Management

To be an effective administrator, the nurse executive must have an excellent grasp of the financial side of management for the entire facility, not just the nursing division. The chief nursing officer is not only accountable for a large share of the expenses and revenue in a health care organization, but he must also accept accountability for the financial health of the entire institution.

The financial management of health care is so integrally entwined throughout a facility that it is impossible to be effective while having tunnel vision and looking only at the financial health of one's own department. Nursing has an effect on many budgets. For example, the wastage of medications has an effect on the pharmacy budget, and the supply budget is affected by the way the nursing staff use supplies. The nurse executive must see the big picture, not only of institutional finance but also of health care financing.

One of the most important tasks of a nurse executive is to infuse the entire division with an entrepreneurial attitude in which nurses view their work unit as their own business. Nurses will make sound financial decisions if they treat the finances of the work unit as they would the finances of their own business.

The staff must learn to see the impact of their actions on other departments and to focus on the larger perspective of the financial needs of the patient and of society, especially now that many patients have to face larger copayments and businesses are faced with severe economic challenges. The nurse executive must infuse this sense of responsibility and accountability for the cost of health care throughout the nursing division. By helping the staff to understand health care finance and how to manage the limited dollars, nurses will reach beyond their circumscribed domain to affect the larger world of financing and cost.

Before accepting a position, a chief nursing officer must examine the financial accounting and the managerial accounting within the organization. With the proper analysis, financial statements will provide a picture of the financial health of the organization. After a nurse executive accepts the job, the financial statement becomes a barometer or benchmark for determining the ongoing financial health of the organization. By using ratio analysis to compare the relationships presented on the financial statement of the organization, he may track the health of that organization over time.

The nurse executive must understand ratio analysis as a method of gauging the financial success of programs. In a financially healthy organization with good management, ratios should improve over time. There are also industry standards available to compare the organization's performance with others. For example, a consortium of teaching hospitals or a religiously affiliated group of hospitals will have a comparative data base available for their member institutions.

This chapter reviews several important aspects of health care finance including institutional finance and budgeting, nursing division budgeting, and mechanisms of cost accounting that can be used for accountability and divisional decision making.

INSTITUTIONAL FINANCE

The financial system of a health care organization is headed by the chief financial officer (CFO), sometimes called the director of finance or sometimes the controller. Whatever his title, the CFO oversees the following functions and/ or departments:

- *Financial planning and auditing:* This unit prepares and administers the institutional budget and audits funds; it provides ongoing fiscal reports to the nurse executive. If the nursing department has its own financial manager, the financial planning officer will closely coordinate with him.
- *Accounting services:* This unit controls and administers payroll, accounts payable, cash control, and taxes following prescribed protocols or decision rules.
- *Reimbursement and fiscal projects:* This unit handles external regulatory impacts on finance; it deals with Medicare, Medicaid, and other third-party payers such as Blue Cross, Blue Shield, and Major Medical. It also handles managed care plans and the cost reports required by external agencies to ensure reimbursement.
- *Data processing:* This unit collects data that affect finance, such as census, patient days, admissions and discharges, and patient usage of various clinics and services. What data are collected depends on executive dictates and the capabilities of the collection systems used.
- *Patient financial services:* This unit handles patient billing, credit and collection of fees, and the cashier function following set decision rules. The complexity of this function is reflected in the fact that the average hospital has 20 to 30 independent revenue centers and approximately 2,000 billable items. This number is growing as many institutions attempt to more closely associate actual costs and fees.

Rate Structure

One main policy issue in financial management of a health care institution involves establishing rates and charges. The decisions here involve negotiating contracts with managed care firms, funding unprofitable departments, and adjusting financial policies to the demands of the environment.

Establishing a rate structure and charges is a difficult balancing act. The rate is set to achieve financing above the break-even line, even in institutions that are not for profit. This is to offset loss on uncollected debts, Medicare, or other prospective/risk-engendering reimbursement plans and to fund future needs of the facility and, in a for-profit setting, to provide for a return to investors.

At one stage, institutional finance was managed as an entirety, with unprofitable services financed through a generalized rate structure high enough to cover such losses. In essence, the total institutional billing was adequate to cover costs plus, but the bill for any given patient was not closely related to the specific costs incurred by her. Cost shifting occurred as higher rates were set to cover those who do not pay their share of cost (e.g., patients covered by Medicare).

Changes taking place in reimbursement designs make it essential that an institution have accurate data on what costs are actually incurred by individual patients and separate departments. Knowledge of real costs has led to many institutional changes including variable billing based on real cost and, in some institutions, closure of departments identified as financial losers. (Community protest has often accompanied unpopular decisions made strictly on financial criteria rather than on a survey of community needs.)

In the past, many patients came to the health care institution because they were directed to do so by their physician or on the basis of their personal preference. Today, their choices may be limited to those institutions approved by their insurers. The managed care organizations negotiate with individual hospitals for a discounted rate in exchange for directing large volumes of patients and their physicians (usually linked in health maintenance organizations, independent practice associations, independent practice organizations, or some other organizational format) to the particular health care facility.

It is imperative that the hospital know the costs of delivering care so that enlightened contracting with managed care firms can be done, preserving the financial health of the organization. Hospitals lacking sophisticated financial costing systems have not been able to compete effectively in the managed care market. If they cannot determine their costs accurately, the discounted price that they offered to contractors may prove to be set too low, threatening the financial viability of the organization.

Physician Influence on Costs

Hospitals have a new perspective on the relationship between physicians and costs, as well as the data on which to base their conclusions. At one time, the physician staff could win most arguments concerning the need for new equipment and services by threats to the economic security of the institution. The ultimate physician threat was that of taking their patients elsewhere. At that stage, the physician was viewed as the chief (and only) source of revenue—via bringing in patients.

Now, "economic credentialing" is being discussed as a method to ensure that, in addition to the quality of his clinical care, the physician is achieving stated financial outcomes. Although economic credentialing is controversial, the misuse of finite and dwindling economic resources has become acute. No longer can hospitals afford physicians who are not cost conscious in their delivery of patient care.

With new systems that differentiate costs, institutions are able to tell which physicians do or do not contribute to the financial health of the institution. The realistic assessment of costs incurred by physician practice changes the nature of the relationship between a physician and administration. No longer are the admissions of every physician desirable. When a physician's pattern of practice incurs excessive cost, pressures are brought to encourage him to modify his practices.

In managed care, even cost-effective physicians have lost some power to manipulate the institution. No longer do they have the choice of institution; they must admit patients where the payer has contracts. The power shifts from the physician to the managed care firm that can bring and take away large volumes of patients.

Fiscal Decisions

Management of cash flow is another financial problem for the health care institution. Cash flow becomes a problem when patients and third-party insurers are slow to pay. Not only does slowed payment cost an institution because of inflation, but it also limits funds available for operational costs. Cash flow problems make the idea of prospective reimbursement desirable. If one can receive or count on given reimbursements in advance, it is possible to do more long-range institutional planning. If the payments are ensured to arrive in a timely fashion, then many frustrations of management can be avoided.

Another problem for the CFO is to determine a depreciation strategy that will be financially advantageous to the institution. Straight-line depreciation allows for the same amount of depreciation every year until an item has been fully depreciated. Accelerated depreciation allows for a larger deduction in the first years. Depending on the third-party payment arrangements, one plan may be preferable over the other. A typical solution is to arrive at a mixed strategy that reflects the types of coverage held by the average patient population. For example, what is allowable under a Medicaid or Medicare plan may be different from what is allowable under private third-party payment. The depreciation strategy would reflect the type of payment most used by the institution's clients.

NURSING DIVISION BUDGETING

Generating and controlling a nursing divisional budget is a major responsibility of the nurse executive. The budget, a major operating document of the nursing division, can best be thought of as a third-level statement of the division's activities. The first level is the statement of basic objectives of the nursing division and the elaboration of those objectives into departmental and unit objectives. The second-level statement is the translation of those objectives into specific, identified activities that will accomplish the objectives. The third-level statement, the budget, is the financial description of those activities.

However, in a resource-driven model, the course of these activities is often reversed. In capitated payments, a top-down dollar amount is given around which all activities must be organized. Per diem rates also are fixed regardless of resources consumed. Gone are the days when a health care organization could first determine the expenses and then request increases in reimbursements to cover them. Increasingly, as health care dollars constrict, the resource-driven model will dictate budgets, often with decreasing funds available.

To predict budget expenses for any anticipated period of time, the nurse executive first needs to identify the financial resources available, the present activities of the division, the activity plans to be instituted during the projected financial period, and those activities to be deleted during the projected period. With reimbursement shrinking every year through government-financed programs and managed care, it is common to be confronted with the challenge of doing more with less.

The planned activities may be partly dependent on events occasioned by others: the opening of a new patient unit, a new surgical physicians' group in the community, or a medical research project that will require extra nursing hours. As a starting point, the nurse executive will require the financial records from prior financial periods as a basis for planning. Also, he must know the available dollars. Budget plan-

ning can be only as good as the institution's accounting system permits.

Cost Centers

The nurse executive needs to identify cost centers. A cost center is the smallest functional unit for which cost control and accountability can be assigned under the existing accounting system. Ideally, each separate functional unit in the nursing division should have its separate account for expenses. For example, a nursing service budget should make it possible to charge each separate patient floor for the actual supplies used on that single unit. Logically, a head nurse cannot be held responsible for costs on her unit unless they are identified and separated from costs accrued by other nursing units.

Some institutions put out financial statements in which they allocate costs by formula rather than by actual usage. They may buy supplies in bulk quantity and allocate the cost of these items among nursing units based on bed count or patient occupancy figures. Such distribution of costs by formula does not reflect the actual use of supplies on the units. Just because a financial statement shows the nursing units as "cost centers" it does not necessarily follow that the nursing unit is, in fact, the cost center.

Accounting objectives and nursing objectives often conflict on establishment of cost centers. For example, an accounting department may be very willing to make a ten-crib nursery a separate cost center (because its supplies are different from those of other cost centers); the same accounting department may resist separating accounts for several 30-bed medical units that use similar supplies. On items such as this, the needs of the nurse executive for appropriate management have to be weighed against the capacities of the institution's accounting department.

The problem of traditionally established cost centers failing to coincide with management centers makes financial management of a large division extremely difficult. To match accounting cost centers to management centers is usually a priority of a nurse executive. When such matching requires a change in accounting systems, the nurse executive must be aware that the change requires increased manpower hours on the part of the accounting department and may require the keeping of double books until the new system is firmly established. Such a change is a long-term project. When cost centers already coincide with management centers, fiscal responsibility can be more easily shared with lower nursing management levels.

Divisional Income and Expenses

Most nursing budgets are expense budgets, reflecting only what the nursing division spends; they often fail to indicate the income resulting from department services rendered. Often, income generated by nursing is undifferentiated from other income. The psychology of this form of budgeting is disastrous because other managers and often nursing managers themselves come to think of the nursing division as non-income producing—in contrast to the X-ray department, or pharmacy, or other departments in which patient fees are carried over in the billing.

Crediting revenues to departments can be misleading, too. In the present environment, for example, many payers fail to pay the full price. As an illustration, Medicare contracturals (the difference between what the institution charges and the reimbursement provided by Medicare) are seldom to the institution's benefit. And the discount-off-charges negotiated with managed care firms and certain other charges that are generated but for which certain payers will not pay place actual income far below the established rates. These deviations must be reflected in the revenue statements of individual departments to create a valid statement of revenues.

Sometimes, the staff of a nursing unit may believe that their revenues are increasing as they charge patients for nursing procedures such as patient teaching and nursing consultation. However, under closer scrutiny, it is apparent that even though the patient has been "charged" and this appears as a revenue on the nursing budget, no one has actually paid these charges. Ironically, the nursing unit may show less actual revenue if they insist on expanding the number of procedures performed when there is no actual reimbursement available.

Other departments are also confronted with this issue. As more plans are capitated, fewer payers pay for drug or physical therapy charges. Therefore, more hospitals are looking at these provider departments as expense-generating and not revenue-generating.

Line-Item Budgets

The nursing budget usually is a line-item budget, with items budgeted according to specific departments or units. Another form of budgeting—planned program budgeting discussed later in this chapter—allocates expenses per activity or project rather than by department or division. This discussion concerns itself with the line-item budget.

In determining the content of a nursing budget, it is not feasible to rely merely on a review of items that seem to belong to the nursing budget. All items that are, in fact, presently charged to the division must be identified.

Because most accounting departments group like expenditures in their financial statements, the nurse executive needs to learn what individual items are included in each grouping. There often is no clear-cut logic as to which items are charged against nursing accounts and which are charged against other divisions, so this step of identifying each separate charge item is unavoidable. Much equipment, for example, is shared by nursing and respiratory therapy, but usually only one of these departments bears purchase and upkeep expenses.

Clear explanation of all line-by-line items makes the nurse executive aware of expenses that were not anticipated, such as depreciation costs, service contracts, and in-house service charges. Once he has a clear understanding of those items charged to the budget, the nurse executive can plan for reallocation of expenses to other divisions if needed.

Manpower Budgets

In generating a budget, most institutions project costs of activities in three categories: manpower costs, operational costs, and capital expenses. As mentioned earlier, the manpower (personnel) budget is usually the largest single expense in a nursing budget. Planning this budget requires determining the number of persons needed in each job category for the planned fiscal period.

A baseline for this prediction can be established by first determining if the present manpower is adequate for the current divisional activities. The first step in this process is to obtain an exact accounting of employees on the nursing payroll. Only persons directly responsible to the nursing division should be on this account. Once the nurse executive knows which employees are charged to the division, he can adjust this figure on the basis of the planned alterations in divisional activities for the proposed fiscal period.

Adjustments in personnel may involve raising or lowering the skill mix and changing the number of persons in each job category as well as increasing or decreasing the total number of employees. For control of staffing decisions during any proposed fiscal period, the nurse executive must know if manpower funds are regulated by position control or by budget allocations. In the first instance, the positions identified in the budget serve as the criterion for hiring of new personnel. In the second instance, the nurse executive is free to change positions if desired but is restricted to the original budgeted total salary figure.

Indicators for needed adjustment in manpower in nursing service would include such items as increasing or decreasing rates of patient occupancy, change in the complexity of patient cases handled, functional changes in role expectations, or addition of new departments and functions.

The nurse executive who is new to budget making is cautioned to make sure that extra manpower hours for vacations, illness, education time, and overtime are included. It is a good idea to review the overtime of the prior financial period. If it is a large expense, then overtime costs may need to be weighed against the cost of creating new positions. Usually three types of staff need funding: regular staffing, anticipated replacement staffing, and emergency situation replacement staffing.

In addition to actual salary expenses, employee fringe benefits usually are charged to the division. In most institutions, a formula using a set percentage of the gross salary is used to calculate fringe benefits. Anticipated increments in wages also must be calculated for the proposed financial period. The personnel department usually can supply the estimates for both fringe benefit costs and anticipated raises.

Employee turnover must be considered in estimating manpower costs. Recruitment costs such as advertising and agency fees often are charged to the division seeking to hire new personnel. Orientation costs also should be calculated as should retirement benefits.

Often the nurse executive builds flexibility into the personnel budget by requesting funds to cover *all* positions in the staffing plan. If some periods then occur when some positions are vacant, this builds in unused funds that may be applied to any overlap of staff (e.g., when a new employee is being oriented for a position not yet vacated).

When, instead, the nurse executive is on a tight position control system, funds that were allotted to unfilled positions may be immediately withdrawn. When possible, the nurse executive will want to control these monies. Some institutions decrease the nursing manpower budgets this way, assuming that the nurse executive will be unable to fill vacant positions at once.

The nurse executive should inquire as to where funds for unemployment compensation are charged: The nursing division may have to pay these costs if an employee is discharged rather than resigns.

In planning a manpower budget, it is useful to work with estimates for each class of worker. Except in a very small institution, the time spent in calculating to the penny each yearly salary for each employee is unnecessary work. Such exacting calculation for the coming year is wasted effort because unexpected resignations and changes within the staff will alter the picture. A budget requires only an estimate.

It is more important, for example, to know the turnover rate for each class of employee than to know individual salary details. The turnover affects the budget for the coming year because newly hired personnel are likely to be hired at a lower pay rate than that received by the longer-tenured staff whom they replace. This savings, however, may be lost to the cost of recruitment and orientation.

Operational Budgets

The operational budget finances the equipment and supplies needed for divisional activities. Most institutions have a financial cut-off point above which purchases of equipment and supplies are termed *capital* instead of operational expenditures. The nurse executive will need to know which budget, operational or capital, should be used when bulk purchase of like items presents a total cost over the cut-off point for operational expenditure. For example, if the nurse executive plans to buy 50 dressing carts at $100 each, one will need to know whether to consider them ten items for the operational budget or one $5,000 item for the capital budget (assuming the capital budget kicked in at this figure).

The starting point for operational budget planning is review of the cost of the division's activities during its last fiscal period. Next, projected increases, decreases, or alterations in divisional activities and resources available are calculated. In addition to actual changes in the activities, the influence of technological or methodological changes on the use of operational supplies and equipment is reviewed. Planned changes in manpower will affect the need for selected supplies and equipment as well as changes in the anticipated number and acuity of patients.

Notice that this whole process can be put in reverse when funds are limited. One can start with the funds and calculate backward, determining what activities and what staff may be afforded.

The nurse executive also should review the major grants and contracts in effect for the upcoming budget period. Often physicians (and sometimes nurses) propose and receive funding for grants without taking into account their effect on nursing division costs. This may involve manpower, operational budgets, or both. Grantees are notorious for failing to calculate the expenses involved in providing the additional nursing equipment or nursing hours needed to carry out the work funded by the grant. If the institution has significant outside funding, then the nursing division should have the right of review on all such grants to prevent miscalculations concerning the impact of projects on nursing costs.

In addition to reviewing the cost of operations during the last financial period, it is important that the nurse executive identify each operational item in his past accounts to preclude mistakes of omission or commission in future planning. There is usually no way to predict logically which charges are made directly to the patient and which to the nursing unit. Similarly, nursing support equipment may be charged either to the nursing division or to the supplying division. The nurse executive must find out what is and what is not charged to his division.

Among the many problems in budgeting is coordination with the medical staff. Do new equipment requests from medicine come out of the nursing budget? Physicians often request purchases when new products or conveniences come on the market. Such items are frequently used by both the physician and nurse, so there must be a clear understanding of the budgetary procedures for such items. Unanticipated changes in physicians' modes of therapy also can tax the nursing budget and may affect the manpower budget as well as the operational budget.

Nursing interacts not only with medicine but with many other divisions and departments. Changes in management of equipment and supplies, for example, can affect operational and manpower budgets of nursing. Therefore, interdivisional discussion and comparison of objectives and projected activities for the planned financial period are essential.

Many unseen elements enter into the operational budget. Inflation is perhaps the most insidious. Anticipated price changes usually are available from the institution's purchasing agent or from product salesmen. Another unseen cost is depreciation. How is it handled in the institution? Also to be considered are repair and renovation costs, both those handled within the institution and those for services and contracts with outside agencies. Repair contracts for intensive care and coronary care equipment, for example, are major expenses. Are these items charged to the nursing division? The nurse executive must know.

Besides ongoing supply costs, there are such sporadic costs as recreation (e.g., Christmas parties, retirement teas), consultation and education fees, accreditation expenses, and travel expenses. Administrative overhead also should be added, including such indirect costs as plant maintenance, heat, light, housekeeping, and general administration. Many institutions add allocated administrative overhead later to the total organizational budget instead of calculating it by division. Again, the nurse executive will have to know if he is accountable for allocated overhead in the budget.

Finally, even when equipment is donated or originally purchased by another division, there are costs of upkeep to consider. A simple gift piece of equipment may cost hundreds of dollars a year if it uses supplies and needs servicing.

Capital Budgets

The capital budget is the projection of costs for major purchases or projects. Each institution has its own definition of what qualifies as a capital expense. Two common criteria are that the item be above a certain baseline cost and that the expected life span of the item be longer than a set time period. For example, an institution might decide that all items more than $5,000 in cost with a life span of at least 3 years are capital expenses. Under that definition, a $6,000 purchase of admission kits expected to last 1 year would not be considered a capital purchase, whereas a $5,500 resuscitation system with a 7-year life expectancy would be considered a capital purchase. Capital items usually include major architectural renovations as well as discrete items.

One major problem the nurse executive has in preparing a capital budget for a technologically oriented environment is the inability to predict what new major equipment is coming on the market during the projected financial period. This problem may be averted somewhat if the nurse executive is allowed to trade off items originally budgeted for unanticipated technologically advanced equipment if it becomes available. Another problem is forecasting what capital items need to be replaced and when.

Capital purchases can involve unseen costs. Operational and manpower budgets will require adjustment if planned capital purchases involve special upkeep, supplies, or man-hours. Also, projected inflation must be considered when pricing items that will not be purchased for 6 months to 1 year. Either the accounting department or the purchasing department usually can advise what percentage inflation to expect on individual capital items.

In preparing a capital budget, the nurse executive is required to document the need for all items. When the purchase will partly pay for itself over a period of time (because it will mean decreased man-hours or decreased use of supplies), the potential savings is calculated and included in documentation. For example, if the nurse executive wants "nurse server" cabinets in every patient room on a unit undergoing renovation, part of the supporting documentation should include an estimate of anticipated nursing hours saved by this convenience.

How purchase requests from physicians are handled affects both the capital budget and the operational budget. The chief problem here is that physicians are likely to request capital items during rather than before the planned fiscal period. It is sometimes difficult to get a large staff of entrepreneurial physicians to plan ahead as a body.

The difficulty is accentuated when new items appear on the market at unexpected times. However, if nurse–physician collaborative committees are in place, the capital items are more likely to be identified prospectively. In some institutions, physician-initiated requests for capital expenses go through other channels, even if the equipment will also be used by nurses. Total cost becomes important in a resource-driven model, and these collaborative projects are excellent ways to reach agreement not only on capital equipment but on outcomes sought.

Relating the Nursing and the Institutional Budgets

The health care institution prepares several types of budgets simultaneously. These include the operating budget, the capital budget, the cash budget, the balance sheet, and the master budget. Nursing typically participates in the operating and capital budgets. The *operating budget* includes the revenue budget and the expense budget. The expense budget has two components: personnel (manpower) and operational (equipment and supplies). The nursing division usually completes both parts of the expense budget but seldom submits a revenue budget.

The *cash budget* deals only with resources that are available or required in negotiable form. It balances cash disbursements against cash receipts. The cash budget does not consider resources such as land, buildings, or other items that would have to undergo conversion into financial revenues. The *balance sheet,* however, includes all the institution's assets and liabilities. Assets include cash available, buildings and equipment owned, and the portfolio of investment. Liabilities might include debt service, payroll owed, capital layouts, and outstanding debts. The *master budget* is the summary of all these budgets taken together—manpower, operating, capital, cash budgets, together with the balance sheet.

It is important that all divisions come together to discuss their proposed divisional budgets before a total budget is prepared, because actions in one division may have an effect on planned budgets of other divisions. The final summarized budget is taken to the trustees of the institution for approval.

Financial Control

Once a budget has been approved and implemented, it becomes a control system. Reports are distributed to each division periodically, usually monthly or 4-weekly, comparing actual to budgeted figures. In this way, the nurse executive can quickly determine if the budget is on target, overspent, or underspent. When cost centers and managerial centers coincide, departmental or unit budget reports are shared with the subordinate managers responsible for these areas. These managers should be able to explain any variance from the expected expenditures.

Not all overages are indices of poor management. For example, an increase in patient occupancy figures will increase expenditures. (However, this increase in patients is paying for itself in increased revenue.) Nevertheless, it is the responsibility of the nurse executive to track budget variances and to have clear explanations for them.

In some instances, funds may be moved from one line-item category to another to cover overexpenditures. The nurse executive needs to know what manipulations are allowable within his budget. The ideal budget is flexible enough to allow such movement of funds from one category to another. Because a budget is a prediction, it is not logical to expect absolute correspondence between the actual and the predicted expenditures.

Alternate System: Planned Program Budgeting

Planned program budgeting is an alternative to the line-item budget. With this method, every service program is viewed as a separate entity, with a separate budget cutting across traditional divisional lines. For example, an emergency department service would be one program, and its budget would include items previously charged to nursing, to medicine, to materials management, and to various other divisions.

The objective of a planned program budget is to put an accurate price tag on each program so that a realistic comparison of cost and income can be calculated. The institution can then accurately identify the true costs of any specific service program. A primary advantage of planned program budgeting is evident when funds are limited.

In typical budget cutting of the traditional divisional budget, a nursing division (or any other division) simply is given less money with which to manage the division's proposed activities. The nurse executive, then, is forced to decide which activities to curtail. His ability to make such decisions, however, is closely tied to the planned activities of other divisions. For example, how far can the nurse executive reduce the staffing in the operating rooms without impairing the activities of the surgical staff?

When heavy cuts are demanded in a divisional nursing budget, departments having less interaction with patients or other divisions become "targets of opportunity." The staff development department may be singled out because its involvement in patient care is indirect. Corporate nursing headquarters is sometimes a target for an uncreative president with his back to the wall.

The planned program budget avoids this sacrifice of quality. All programs offered by the institution are budgeted separately and given priorities. Then, if budget cuts are required, total programs of low priority are eliminated, ensuring adequate funding for the quality programs that remain.

Planned program budgeting is not without its flaws. Computation of salaries of individuals who work in several programs is tedious. Calculating program costs is also difficult and often requires exacting care.

As nursing develops more self-supporting activities, it is not unusual for the nurse executive to have self-contained budgets for special programs outside the regular line-item budget. For example, a nursing division may have elected to run a health advisement program for a local industry. Such an item would be likely to have its own program-type budget.

It is not at all unusual, then, that today's nurse executive may have diverse kinds of budgets to manage simultaneously. Program budgeting is most often limited to those specialty programs that are expected to be fiscally self-sufficient.

Whatever the budgeting and accounting systems of the institution, the nurse executive has responsibility for careful fiscal management. In large institutions, the executive may have accountants within the nursing division to help in financial planning and control. In smaller institutions, the nurse executive may not have this advantage but still may be responsible for managing millions of dollars.

COST ACCOUNTING

The nurse executive often needs to know the basics of cost accounting, as when assigning costs for nursing services or in assigning fees for services. He may need cost accounting skills when arranging conventions or working on other mass-attended events in relation to his professional organization responsibilities as well as when arranging large events for his own institution. Grantsmanship also requires the ability to put a price tag on an event or series of events or projects.

Accurate cost accounting enables the nurse executive to associate costs with the purposes for which they are incurred. When the nurse executive has an accurate idea of the cost of a given project, he can determine when the cost/benefit ratio is reasonable. He may determine if the cost per client served, in a proposed clinic for alcoholics, for example, may be warranted in the expected benefit. Cost accounting will enable him to compare proposed programs when he does not have sufficient resources for all desired projects. For example, cost accounting would enable the executive to compare the costs/benefits of the proposed alcoholic care clinic to the costs/benefits of a proposed birth control clinic.

In business, the *cost/benefit ratio* is usually a financial one, with input costs identified and compared with expected profits. In nursing, it may not always be meaningful to state the ratio of cost to benefit in financial terms. Consider the situation in which a nurse executive is adding a home visit program for patients discharged from the hospital after strokes. Let us assume that the financial benefits are not equal to the input costs. Yet, the real benefit may be in the number of senior citizens who are able to manage on their own without being placed in nursing homes.

However, one might extrapolate a financial gain—in years lived independently versus years in a nursing home—if one could calculate the financial differences in life style and multiply those costs by life expectancies of persons in and not in the home program. In nursing, it often makes sense to identify the benefit in human terms rather than merely in dollars and cents. It is difficult to put a price tag on improved quality of life—on increased comfort, security, independence, or self-control. These explanations can accompany financial statements to help others understand the calculations.

In addition to calculating cost/benefit ratios for programs and projects, the nurse executive may calculate *cost-effectiveness ratios*. In this construct, cost is related to the achievement of given, specified objectives. If the objective of a nurse executive is to prepare ten staff nurses to give updated coronary care to patients in the coronary care unit, then one may compare the cost of two or more programs for reaching that goal. For example, the nurse executive may calculate the cost of having the staff development department offer a course versus the cost of sending the staff members to a program of similar education elsewhere.

In calculating such costs for program decisions, there are several terms with which the nurse executive should be familiar. A *sunk cost* is an investment in some particular equipment or system that encourages further investments compatible with it. For example, if a nursing division has a sunk cost in a given bedside computer system, it is unlikely to buy software that is incompatible with the system. A sunk cost weighs heavily in future administrative decisions; indeed, the sunk cost requires ongoing related funding/purchases if it is to be justified.

A *fixed cost* is one not related to volume of business. For example, the salary of the head nurse is "fixed" (i.e., invariant, no matter how large or small the unit's patient load). A *proportional cost* reflects the volume of business: the cost of 4×4s on a surgical unit reflects the num-

ber of patients on the unit or the number of surgeries performed. A *step cost* reflects volume of business as does a proportional cost, but instead of rising or falling at a steady rate, it increases or decreases at critical levels. For example, the staffing of an emergency department will not be readjusted based on a minor increase in patient traffic, but if traffic is accelerated for a sustained period, staff may be added, reflecting a step cost. Both the proportional cost and the step cost are *variable costs* as opposed to fixed costs (i.e., they are related to some measure of volume).

Besides knowing the nature of each cost, the nurse executive may want to differentiate *controllable costs* from *real costs* before making managerial decisions. The *real cost* of a project will include all the labor, materials, and administrative overhead required for the project's enactment. In contrast, the *controllable* costs are those that would not exist if the project were eliminated.

Suppose, for example, that the nurse executive and the staff development director create a case management nursing education project. Suppose that the secretary for the staff development department devotes one-fifth working time to the project; also assume that one regular instructor is assigned for 50 percent time to the project. The project will include 10 hours of lecture by an outside expert and the distribution of materials on case management to program attendees. It is anticipated that the program will be offered to 40 nurses on work hours, for a total of 30 hours by each nurse for the total course.

In this example, real costs would include distributed materials, salaries (proportional) of the secretary and the staff development instructor, time of the staff development director, and the total time of the outside expert. Real costs also would include salaries of the employees for the hours that they are attending the program, administrative overhead (proportion of overhead charged to the staff development department), and depreciation of any audio-visual equipment used in the classroom. Charges also might be calculated for use of a classroom.

Many of these costs would be eliminated if the executive only considers controllable costs. For example, if the in-house instructor were a full-time employee, her salary would have been paid even if she were not involved in this project; the same is true for the secretary and the staff development director. Only the fees of the outside expert would be listed as controllable costs. Cost of materials are also controllable costs, but salaries of employees attending the course only would be counted if they actually were replaced on their units for the time of class learning. Similarly, if the classroom belonged to the staff development department and did not need to be rented from another source, then its cost would not be considered.

It is important that the nurse executive have a good idea of both real and controllable costs for major projects in the division. Real costs in some cases and controllable costs in other cases will be dominant in the decision making. At other times, the nurse executive will wish to compare these costs. Some nurse executives repeatedly lose money on projects because they forget some real costs involved. For example, if a nurse executive contracts to run a new clinic on funds sufficient only for controllable costs, then he will have to find support for administrative overhead elsewhere. Such expenses, if not considered when a budget is set, may make a funded project a major expense to the organization in terms of real costs.

For some projects, it is important to have a *unit cost* as well as a *total* project cost. A unit cost tells what it will cost to turn out a single "unit" of production. What comprises the unit of production will vary from circumstance to circumstance. For example, the absolute cost of running a labor and delivery function may not tell the executive as much as would a figure that describes average cost per delivery. Similarly, cost per clinic visit and cost per employee hired may have more significance than the report of a total cost. A *unit cost* is one that is reported in terms of one unit of production, whether that unit be a patient, a surgical experience, a student, a visit, or any other item determined to be appropriate to the subject under consideration.

It is particularly important to calculate unit costs if fees are to be associated with costs. In this way, it is possible to determine what to charge the clinic patient per visit, what to charge the nurse for attending a continuing education course, or what to charge the patient for use of the surgical suite. In the resource-driven model with the reality of decreasing resources, the cost-per-unit-of-service methodology is an excellent productivity measure for benchmarking. As the volume goes up, the challenge is to hold cost as stable as possible. Similarly, when the volume drops, the challenge is to maintain the cost per unit of service and not to let the ratio of costs to unit of service escalate. Therefore, this measure is significant for assessing productivity.

The nurse executive will discover that some unit costs vary depending on the volume. It becomes expensive to staff an emergency department with two nurses if few patients wander in; costs of their salaries are covered if there is a high or normal volume of emergency department traffic. Costs per unit of production usually go down as volume increases, although the relation may not be exact. (Step or proportional costs may be involved.)

Often, there is a critical volume at which costs invested in the project are recovered, and it is important that such volumes be determined. For example, the fee for a staff development offering to outsiders may be determined based on a certain volume of attendees. If that volume is not achieved, the program may lose money. Certainly, the staff development director will need to learn how to calculate break-even costs, as will any other nurse manager who is involved in fee setting when volume affects profit or loss.

Managing the Department of Nursing Finances

Unfortunately, the management of the finances of the nursing department has often been highly centralized. A few years ago, the only person who knew the budget for the nursing department was the nurse executive. As the roles of other nurse managers expanded, they have been brought into full partnership with the nurse executive in developing and managing the finances of the department.

Unfortunately, staff nurses often have been left out of this process. Yet, the success of financial management of the division is in their hands. Staff nurses consume most supplies, and they can run up costs by inefficient nursing practices. Executives only have themselves to blame when this happens. It makes no sense to tell staff nurses that they are responsible for cost containment if they are not made aware of the cost of supplies and labor. One cannot expect staff to make good decisions about what practices are cost-effective if they have no information on which to make such judgments.

This practice is similar to giving someone a checkbook to use but not telling them the balance in the account. Uninformed staff nurses cannot be expected to participate in cost containment and revenue generation. Many staff nurses come from schools of nursing offering no preparation in financial management. Yet, to be a full professional, the nurse must understand the costs of clinical care as well as the management of illness and maintenance of health. Nurse executives must see that financial management of nursing care is taught to the staff to control successfully the nursing budget. Staff nurses must become full participants in this process and must be credentialed in financial management. They must be supplied with the proper tools and techniques to manage effectively.

As we move into models of shared governance and self-managed teams, it is even more essential that the staff have the knowledge base to manage the cost of their practice. There is no self-governance when there is no acceptance of accountability for resource consumption.

In addition to being informed, staff must buy into the philosophy of cost control. The challenge for the nurse executive is to build a culture in which excellence in the financial performance of the unit is as exciting as the excellence of achieving clinical outcomes. Consideration of cost must become a natural part of work planning on every level of the nursing organization. It must be integrated into the role expectations.

The barrier to staff nurses learning about financial management is often the language used.

For example, full-time equivalent is not a common expression for most staff nurses. Simple terms, those describing expenses and revenues, are not always familiar. Each facility has its own language of financial management. The first step is to develop programs that explain the common financial terms, breaking them down into easily understood concepts. Staff nurses also should be taught how to interpret the monthly fiscal reports. The reports should be summarized in meaningful ways so that this is a reasonable expectation.

It is also critical that staff nurses learn the cost of routine supplies. Many health care facilities now have supplies labeled with costs so that the nurse can make an informed decision about the cheaper product to use. When nurses know, for example, the cost of dietary supplies sent to the unit for patient use, they become concerned when they see cost overruns incurred by nursing staff and other professionals helping themselves to these dietary items.

When staff nurses know the overall budget within which their unit must operate, they become very proud and excited to participate in reaching the fiscal targets. Indeed, competitiveness arises concerning whose unit is the most cost-effective in the facility. For example, when staff understand the effect of excessive absenteeism on their budget, they begin to assert pressures against the worst offenders.

Nurses must feel a sense of ownership in the unit and their budget. They must have a say in the management of the finances to feel a real professional status. When the cost of health care is "owned" by the staff nurses, effective financial management of the unit happens.

In shared governance structures, it is becoming more common to share information with the staff concerning the cost of supplies as they relate to patient care. In case management/outcomes management protocols, it is now more common to see the cost of supplies, procedures, rooms rates, etc., on the critical path, so clinicians have better information on which to base their clinical judgments.

Although it is usually not appropriate to disclose individual salary information, standard salary scales can be used to help staff understand the costs of the human resources involved in delivering the care.

In some health care facilities, there is disagreement about the appropriateness of sharing the financial information with the staff. The fear is that this information will be taken to competitive facilities that will then use the information to their own advantage, especially in managed care contracting. Although this is an important concern, it is virtually impossible to help the staff to manage costs unless they know the parameters around which they can operate.

It is important to separate price from cost. It is fairly easy to determine a facility's price because this shows up on any patient's bill. It is more common that a facility share the price of supplies with the staff rather than the actual cost. In reality, as indicated earlier, the price sometimes has no relationship to the cost because the facility marks some supplies up much higher than the others. Even so, price at least gives the clinicians a range for managing the finances of the unit.

As we move to self-managed units and to more professional models, it is imperative to devise ways for the staff to manage the cost of providing care in addition to managing the quality of care. The trend is to share financial information with the staff rather than keeping it the exclusive domain of the nurse executive and other nurse managers.

SUMMARY

In budgeting or other financial matters, the nurse executive must have a good idea of accounting methods and of systems for accounting used in his own institution. If the nurse executive has a large division, he may have an accountant on his own staff. He should expect that the employer provide data and keep records—not to substitute for the nurse executive's decision making but to enlighten it.

When the nurse executive does not have a financial staff, he will need to work intimately with the CFO of the institution. The nurse executive can neither ignore nor be intimidated by the financial aspects of management. A brief course in basic accounting may be a big help to the nurse executive who is unsure in the financial side of management.

SUGGESTED READINGS

Barron, J., et al. 1992. Cost reduction, part 2: An organization culture perspective. *Nursing Economics* 10, no.6:402–405.

Blancett, S.S. 1991. Finance for nurse managers: A software package. *Journal of Nursing Administration* 21, no.11:11.

Finkler, S.A. 1991. Performance budgeting. *Nursing Economics* 9, no.6:401–408.

Gilbert, R.L. 1992. Director of nursing planning and finance: A new role. *Nursing Management* 23, no.2:50–52.

Hollander, S.F., et al. 1992. Cost reduction, part 1: An operations improvement process. *Nursing Economics* 10, no.5:325–330.

Holzemer, W.L. 1990. Quality and cost of nursing care: Is anybody out there listening? *Nursing and Health Care* 11, no.8:412–415.

Kerfoot, K.M., and B.J. Vigh. 1991. Staff nurse financial management committees—The nurse manager's guide to effective financial performance. *Nursing Economics* 9, no.4:287–289.

Lubin, B.S., and T. Powell. 1991. Pressure sores and specialty beds: Cost containment and ensurance of quality care. *Journal of ET Nursing* 18, no.6:190–197.

Nicoll, L.H., and N.B. Niman. 1991. Deficit reduction and healthcare expenditures. *Journal of Nursing Administration* 21, no.6:35–39.

Patterson, C. 1992. The economic value of nursing. *Nursing Economics* 10, no.3:193–204.

Porter-O'Grady, T. 1987. *Nursing finance: Budgeting strategies for a new age.* Gaithersburg, Md.: Aspen Publishers, Inc.

Poteet, G.W., et al.1991. Financial responsibilities of preparation of chief nurse executives. *Nursing Economics* 9, no.5:305–309.

Pruitt, R.H., and A.K. Jacox. 1991. Looking above the bottom line: Decisions in economic evaluation. *Nursing Economics* 9, no.2:87–91.

Sherman, J.J. 1990. Costing nursing care: A review. *Nursing Administration Quarterly* 14, no.3:11–17.

Wong, R., et al. 1993. A cost analysis of a professional practice model for nursing. *Nursing Economics* 11, no.5:292–297.

Zembala, S.A. 1993. Managing the costs of nursing care delivery. *Nursing Administration Quarterly* 17, no.4:74–79.

23

Material Resources of Nursing Management

The material resources of nursing management include the supplies, equipment, and facilities of the division as they are distributed over space and time. This chapter focuses on two main elements of this distribution: the design of facilities for patient care, and the design of logistic systems to supply material within the health care facility.

DESIGN OF FACILITIES

Design of space for patient care involves both planning for new facilities and reorganizing extant facilities for new purposes. Whenever new facilities are planned for the health care institution, be they patient care units or other structures, the nurse executive and her staff should be actively in on the planning. There are few aspects of a building that do not have an effect on nursing, even on non-nursing turf.

The nurse executive should be in on facilities planning *from the start*. If not consulted until late in the process, it may be too late to make revisions in plans without incurring great expense. Often, only late in the planning do others think to include the nurse executive; she should not wait for an invitation but should request to participate the moment any building plans are proposed.

Because facilities planning involves a special domain of knowledge, the nurse executive will want to become knowledgeable about this domain or else appoint a nurse specialist to work on renovation and construction projects. If a major building project is involved, someone in the nursing division should work permanently on the planning. There are nurses who have made a career specialization of design as it relates to patient care and architecture. Many firms specializing in health care architecture employ nurses to bring considerations of patients and staff to design.

All too often, plans have been made without the input of the users. Staff who will work in these areas every day can quickly critique what will and will not work and should be consulted at all phases of development. Significant costs can be saved by developing teams of these front-line people.

Now, we recognize the importance of patient input in the design of space. No longer do we design without considering the impact of the space on the patient. Everyone who will have to live within the space should be allowed to express his or her opinion.

Process of Building

There are several discrete stages in facilities building. The first is long-range planning. Here, the goals and needs of the community and the organization itself are considered, and future needs are projected. This part of the planning involves both long-range goal setting and the gathering of much demographic and other data to support the legitimacy of those goals.

Demographic data will describe the service area of the planned facility. It will also discuss subsidiary service areas expected to develop as the facility comes into being. Shifts in populations served may be due to changes in the community's population or due to an institution's plan to appeal to new groups within a community.

Changes in health manpower capabilities of the community (physician, nurse, technician, other) and growth or decline of other health service agencies in the community also need to be factored into the decision. Data concerning financing for the planned new facilities also must be gathered.

At the end of the planning phase, the institution is ready to make a knowledgeable decision as to whether the construction is feasible and logical. Typically, a certificate of need is required to build, and the data identified above provide the basis for this request.

The institution that hopes to put up new buildings also must deal with the community. Does the community want it? Are there groups that will contest it? Good relations with a community often make the difference between a building plan progressing smoothly or meeting insurmountable obstacles. Once an institution has determined to build, a good marketing plan usually is the next step: selling the notion to all potential interest groups.

In a resource-driven health care model, extensive financial analysis is necessary to ensure that the additional costs can be covered in an economically restrained environment. Revenue per square foot analysis is becoming as important to health care facilities as it is to retail stores. Overages can be reduced if the architecture can be turned into revenue generating space. This usually means that space is conserved; broad-scale plans are pared back. It makes no sense in this economy to bring more space onto the books if the space cannot generate the revenue to pay for itself over time.

While legal, political, and financial forces are being handled, the first phase of building involves development of a master site plan. This plan should take into account all foreseeable expansion, now and in the future. The site plan inter-relates all lands owned by the institution, be they in geographic proximity or separated. Many institutions with tunnel vision have failed to acquire adequate land for expansion. In heavily built-up areas, it may be impossible to count on geographic expansion later, so that most planning will have to involve expensive vertical rather than horizontal extension.

An institution often walks a fine line with a community; although the community may want medical facilities to expand, it may balk at such a project if it involves the displacement of community residents or businesses. Now, many communities see new buildings as a symbol of escalating health care costs and actively oppose building programs.

The third phase begins the actual design of facilities. First, block schematics are drawn to show how major areas to be built will relate to each other, both horizontally and vertically. Figure 23–1 is a simplified block drawing. In an actual block drawing, the scale would be indicated. Computer-generated schematics allow planners to consider many different designs and design changes over a short period of time. In block schematics, the nurse executive must be careful to note the common pathways by which patients flow from one department to another.

An ideal structure would allow all departments immediate access to all other departments; unfortunately, the realities of space do not easily allow such construction. Any block design is a compromise, placing in close proximity those departments that most require it. For

	Parking Lot	
X-ray Department	Dietary Kitchen	Emergency Room
Pharmacy	Cafeteria	Conference Rooms
	Lobby	

Figure 23–1 Block Schematic for the First Floor of a Hospital

example, it makes sense if the recovery room is near the operating rooms, the nursery near post-partum, and so forth. On one set of block schematics, a nurse executive pointed out that the only way in which emergency department patients could be taken to the X-ray department was by moving them through the cafeteria or the front lobby (as in Figure 23–1).

In the next phase of planning, single-line sketches are composed for all areas to be constructed. Actual space constraints such as internal columns, elevators, and corridors are drawn to scale, and rooms are designed with beds and room equipment also drawn to scale. Entrances and exits are indicated in the single-line drawings. The finished single-line drawings reveal the configuration of each unit, the size and shape of planned spaces, and the functional relationships (horizontal and vertical connections) between planned units.

Design development drawings are refinements of the single-line sketches. These drawings include such things as structural, mechanical, electrical systems, as well as built-in equipment. By the time the architects reach this stage of development, they are hesitant to make changes, and changes will cost significant amounts of money for the organization. The final planning stage is the development of blueprints—a refinement of the design development drawings.

Construction of facilities always is a compromise between what an institution wants and what it can afford. Few nurse executives have the privilege of having a building designed just as they desire. The nurse executive must beware of building savings that will cost money in the long run. For example, if the institution will have to pay extra nursing salaries over the next 20 or more years, a plan may end up costing far more than was saved by some architectural shortcut.

Suppose elevator service was limited because elevators are expensive to install: Thousands of nursing hours may be lost in waiting time. Similarly, if a work area is too small, nurses may have to wait until other nurses vacate an area. Nurse executives are successful in getting architectural plans changed by pointing out potential inefficiencies with cost benefit analysis data.

It is amazing how often the managerial needs of a nursing unit are overlooked by planners if nurses are not adequately represented on the planning committees. Head nurses' offices and conference rooms certainly should be included in any modern design, but even basics can be forgotten without nursing input.

One nursing vice president told of an institution that attempted to save money by hiring an architectural firm that had never worked on hospital designs previously. In the single-line sketch stage, she asked where the nurses' bathrooms were to be located, only to find that the architects had given thorough attention to patients' bathrooms but had totally forgotten that nurses might require such facilities. The architects argued in vain that the large nurses' bathroom in the basement locker facility would be adequate.

The nurse executive will need to be especially careful in the design of patient units. Many architectural horror stories are told by nurse executives. One moved into a new facility only to discover the door proportions somehow had been changed, making it impossible to roll a bed directly into a room; thousands of nursing hours would be spent in unnecessary stretcher-to-bed transfers.

Another new facility had bathrooms in which the patient had to be a healthy contortionist to use the bowl. Another had nurses' stations in a niche that could not be watched from the hall that led to patients' rooms. Worse, it was directly accessible to an elevator used by the public. Hundreds of dollars worth of equipment "walked off" before this nursing station was restructured.

Another, a critical care unit, had half partitions so that nurses could watch patients above the newest monitoring equipment installed in the lower portion. The only problem was that the heights were perfect for the average man, but many of the female nurses had to jump if they wanted to see over the partition. The area soon became cluttered with boxes, stools, and other contraptions for the shorter nurses.

Although common sense will prevent some errors of this sort, more refinement of judgment is required to do a good planning job. The nurse in charge of planning should know such things as the legal requirements for space usage, the norms of space footage for various facilities, state regulations and accreditation standards, and other tricks of facilities planning. If there is no one with such expertise in the nursing division, it may be wise to use a nurse consultant who is an expert in this area.

After blueprints receive final approval, the building phase is initiated. By then, it usually is too late for any changes unless a catastrophic error is discovered. If a major error is discovered at this late date, it means that the nurse executive did not give enough attention to the project at an earlier stage and costly revisions will be necessary.

Even with the best of planning, it is possible to become the victim of planning that fails to predict changes. For example, one facility was designed specially to keep the nurses at the bedside. One element in the building design illustrated this principle. A large 50-bed intensive care unit was designed around pods of three patients each. In each pod, the nursing station was centered among three highly visible patient rooms. The atmosphere was excellent; the latest of monitoring equipment was relayed to the mini-nursing stations. There was only one problem with the design; no pod had easy access to another pod. The stations were designed for separate staffing for each pod. The designer did not anticipate a time when costs would dictate reduced nursing staff. Now, this facility cannot safely afford to use this unit for intensive care, because it cannot afford to staff all these architecturally isolated pods.

Many buildings that applied the Friesen principle had similar problems. In this plan, all care equipment and records are kept adjoining the patient's room. The design was planned to allow the nurse to stay at the bedside. Many plans reinforced this method by eliminating the central nursing station. In most cases, however, nurses soon created their own nurses' station in halls, in treatment rooms, wherever a central meeting place could be created, however haphazardly. The designer simply failed to predict that nurses would not enjoy functioning in isolation. He failed to recognize the need for professional communication and consultation.

Many errors in design involve a failure to anticipate the security systems required today. One building, for example, was designed with large numbers of entry doors to facilitate traffic patterns. Now, because of security needs, most of these exits are locked. The resultant traffic patterns require great inconvenience on the part of many. And one can say without possibility of contradiction that no facility yet built has predicted how soon the planned number of elevators and parking spaces would be inadequate.

During the planning phases, the nurse executive will need to consider the architect's plan for (1) flow patterns for patients, staff, and visitors; (2) security needs of the facility; (3) facilities' proximity needs; (4) movement of equipment and supplies; (5) placement of nursing offices and managerial space as they relate to the space of other key managers; (6) educational and conference space needs; and (7) patients' convenience in use of the facilities.

Basic Plans for Patient Units

The design of patient care units needs special attention. The oldest and least satisfactory design is the single-corridor design, in which patient rooms as well as nurses' stations, treatment rooms, and other service areas all branch off the same long hall. Such a long-hall construction incurs many more man-hours spent in walking than is the case with the more compact designs. (Figure 23–2 is an illustration of this design. Here and in subsequent illustrations, the dark areas indicate nurses' stations and other work areas.)

In the double-corridor design (Figure 23–3), patient rooms branch off halls located on both sides of a central core containing the work areas of the unit. Advocates of this design claim walking time is cut nearly by half compared with a long corridor with the same number of patient

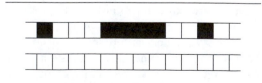

Figure 23–2 Single-Corridor Patient Unit (Dark areas indicate nurses' stations and other staff work areas.)

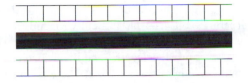

Figure 23–3 Double-Corridor Patient Unit (Dark areas indicate nurses' stations and other staff work areas.)

rooms. However, this design cuts down visibility of hall activities because only one-half of the unit can be seen at any one time.

Each variation in unit design has advantages and limitations. The triangle, circle, and square designs usually simplify walking but may devote more space to central work areas than is necessary (Figures 23–4 through 23–6). T-shaped units attempt to solve this problem while still shortening the length of any given corridor (Figure 23–7).

When deciding on the shape of nursing units, the nurse executive will want to consult people

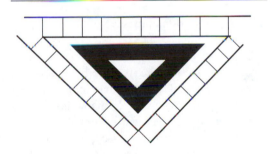

Figure 23–4 Triangular Patient Unit (Dark areas indicate nurses' stations and other staff work areas.)

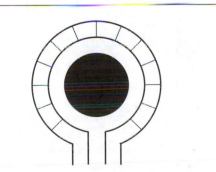

Figure 23–5 Circular Patient Unit (Dark areas indicate nurses' stations and other staff work areas.)

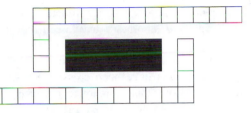

Figure 23–6 Square Patient Unit (Dark areas indicate nurses' stations and other staff work areas.)

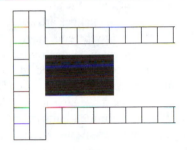

Figure 23–7 T-shaped Patient Unit (Dark areas indicate nurses' stations and other staff work areas.)

who have lived with the designs under consideration. Some of the newer designs may look attractive and efficient but contain subtle flaws. No one can anticipate how it is to inhabit a structure without visiting one and asking those who have worked there whether they like it and how it works.

Census is another issue. Builders generally prefer large-census patient units because they are less expensive to construct than small-census ones. The nurse executive will want a size compatible with the assignment system used. However, assignments systems change as other circumstances change.

Many nurse executives have managed to get smaller-census units or better designed facilities by quantifying the staffing costs incurred by the inferior design. A chief executive officer who favors a cheaper design because of cost factors is likely to be amenable to analyses that predict greater ultimate cost savings. If a building design causes the need for additional nursing staff, an institution will pay for a false economy many times over, every year that the building is in use.

A new initiative in many hospitals is to bring care to the patient instead of transporting the patient all over the health care facility for tests and procedures. In some settings, functions such as radiology and laboratory have been moved to the unit in an attempt to decrease transportation time and increase patient satisfaction. People on individual units have been cross-trained to do many functions that were once performed by people in centralized departments. In some cases this patient-focused redesign creates major renovation programs (e.g., when functions such as radiology are moved to the unit).

When architectural changes are *not* made but functions are moved to the unit, many hospitals must redesign. For example, centralized nursing stations have been replaced by bedside computers, and functions such as recording electrocardiographs have been moved to the bedside to be performed by cross-trained unit-based staff. In some facilities, this has meant overcrowding on the unit as more functions, people, and support equipment move there from formerly centralized departments.

In an attempt to move patients less often, some health care facilities are experimenting with rooms that can be upgraded to an intensive care unit or downgraded to a step-down or acute care unit, depending on the needs of the patient and the acuity. The concepts of patient-focused redesign force us to think in terms of designing care programs around the patient and not around the staff or personnel. As more functions are brought to the bedside, more creativity is demanded to create the support systems for these new patient care delivery models through innovation in architectural design.

Interior design also may present problems. Typically, the closet area in patients' rooms is inadequate. Another common fault is lack of counter space in bathrooms. Both of these problems arise out of attempts to save space, usually to increase the number of private over shared patient rooms. Another question in interior design is whether to go for built-in versus mobile equipment. Flexibility is maintained with mobile equipment, but such equipment typically needs more care and tending.

Carpeting is another issue that is usually debated in relation to patient rooms. Arguments *for* carpeting include aesthetic pleasure, noise reduction, fewer injuries in patient falls, and psychological satisfaction. Arguments against carpeting concern the difficulty of infection control, problems with moving stock such as stretchers and wheelchairs, and the difficulty of cleaning spills of various sorts. There is no single satisfactory answer, although the type of carpet used may make a radical difference in how satisfactory it is in patient rooms.

Interior design of the nurses' stations deserves attention; typically, these areas lack enough seating space. The need is greatest when physicians and nurses share the same space. As more professionals become unit-based, the need for writing, thinking, and conferencing space becomes critical.

Again, if the nurse executive or one of her staff has not had considerable experience in interior design, it is probably a good idea to hire a nurse consultant who specializes in this area. There are just too many possibilities of making mistakes that must be lived with for inordinately long times.

Redesign of Old Facilities

In an era when the nation is overbedded, a nurse executive is more likely to be involved in redesigning extant facilities than in the building of new ones. Indeed, with many institutions branching out into vertical integration of services, it is common that unused acute units be converted to other purposes. Adapting an old facility to a different purpose is probably even more challenging than designing a new facility.

One constructive way to begin such a challenge is to identify the requirements that one would have if a new facility were built. This forces one to identify the purposes of the proposed unit. Once these desirable traits have been identified, then one asks how or to what extent they can be realized in the redesign of the old facility.

Suppose, for example, that two old acute care hospital units are to be turned into a skilled nursing facility for long-term care patients. If one just rearranges without an overall plan, the results are likely to be bleak. With this haphazard method, one asks things such as, "Now where will I put the television room?" With the advised plan, instead, one starts with questions such as, "What are the requirements of persons who will make this facility their home for a sustained period? What are their abilities, their disabilities?"

Once one has identified the ideal arrangements, then one needs a realistic notion of what can and cannot be done with the old facility. This involves two aspects: what can be done from the point of view of cost, and what can be done given the architecture of the facility. Perhaps the most important questions involve what walls are weight-bearing and cannot be removed and what plumbing and service lines are permanent. When one has an idea of what cannot be changed, then it is easier to remember that all else becomes open to revision (at least within a feasible budget). When deficits cannot be cured by revising space, then interior design becomes the challenge.

One should never underestimate the effect of architecture and the arrangement of space on human activities and perceptions. For example, in one hospital renovated into a nursing home, residents were simply placed in rooms as the acute care patients before them had been. The nurses, not surprisingly, were treating the residents much as if they were acute care patients. The pull of the old facilities led to old behavior patterns, and the residents were treated as if they were ill.

Traffic patterns constitute another major consideration in redesigning facilities. In the nursing home example, the planners failed to recognize that permanent residents would be trafficking the halls far more than the previous inhabitants. Nor did the designers consider all aspects of mobility of the elderly well who would live there. Bright-colored handrails were put in, lining the halls for the walking elderly. Although these were useful, the planners failed to think about placement of communal rooms. These rooms were placed at the farthest ends of long corridors, making the walking distance formidable for many residents even with rails lining the corridors.

This mistake would not have been made if the planners had started with the needs of the resi-

dents. Instead, they asked, how can we use what is already here?

Esthetics are especially important in redesigning facilities. When the logistics may involve making do with less than ideal architectural designs, the environment can be made pleasant.

A HEALING HEALTH CARE ENVIRONMENT

As more information has become available from the field of environmental psychology, the positive and negative influence of design on people's emotional state has become apparent. Studies in environmental psychology have shown that properly designed areas can create a sense of well-being, nurturing, relaxation, and comfort. The use of color, lighting, furnishing, the use of nature, art, music, and the sense of smell all help to create a concept of the health care facility as a healing environment.

As more information has become available about the interaction of mind and illness, it has become imperative for us to turn our high-tech facilities into centers of healing with as much high touch, sensitivity, nurturing, and compassion integrated into patient care as possible. Unfortunately, many of our health care facilities have become nothing more than the machine shops where patients come to have high-tech things done to them in noisy, frightening environments that have been built for the convenience of the staff. The effect of this design on patients and their families was not considered.

Florence Nightingale (1859) knew about the effect of environment on healing and wrote in *Notes on Nursing,* "The symptoms or the sufferings generally considered to be inevitable and incident to the disease are very often not symptoms of the disease at all, they are something quite different—the want of fresh air, or of light, or of warmth, or of quiet, or of cleanliness, or of punctuality of care in the administration of diet, or of all of these" (p. 25).

Before there was cure, cultures embraced healing by using healing temples, baths, cathedral-like infirmaries, light therapy, music therapy, nutrition, and herbs to create an atmosphere of confidence, serenity, spirituality, and strength. When high tech became such an important part of health care, we abandoned many of these traditional practices, instead treating our patients in stressful, nonsupportive, and often inhumane facilities.

Color can effect musculature, brainwave activity, heart, and respiration and can influence moods and lift spirits and make space seem more restful and cheerful. Colors that are warm or cool can be chosen for special effects and can be used not only to foster desired feelings among patients and their families but also to create a sense of more or less space. Light is also an important variable. For example, we know that natural light and views of nature create desirable impacts in patients and families. Not only does the cycle of natural light regulate many of the bodily processes, it also creates a sense of healing.

Nor is it unusual for someone in a health care facility to be bombarded with many obnoxious scents. With altered conditions resulting from illness and treatments, many patients are affected by smells. Pregnancy and chemotherapy are two examples of how alterations in the body can cause alterations in smell and consequent nausea. Good air quality control is essential.

Noise levels in a hospital are often disturbing to patients and their families. Overhead speakers, pagers, telephones, alarms from monitors, and sounds from noisy equipment all serve to create a stressful environment. Acoustic design is part of any good architectural plan and so is sensitivity training in human thoughtfulness. Of all the noise pollution, patients are most stressed by loud staff because this source rightfully is taken as a basic lack of consideration. Consumer satisfaction programs work on the latter problem while acoustic engineering as well as sensible selection and maintenance of equipment mitigates the former.

In addition to thoughtfully using the concepts of environmental psychology to design areas, the nurse executive should be cognizant of how music, art, humor, therapeutic massage, and other interventions can help the patients and their families cope better because they are sup-

ported in their healing process. Health care facilities are now installing relaxation channels on the closed-circuit televisions and also humor channels so that patients and their families may receive the therapeutic effects of techniques shown to positively alter endorphins and other hormones.

Programs that feature rotating displays of visual art and programs in the performing arts are also useful for humanizing the health care environment and can be instituted at very little cost. A program as simple as an art cart (in which volunteers ask patients and their families to choose which pictures they would like to hang on their hospital wall) are significant for individualizing health care and making the hospital as homelike and stress-free as possible.

Caregivers must also be nurtured for them to complete effectively their business of caring. They need a therapeutic place to retreat and relax so that they may return to the front line of working intensely with patients and their families.

Caregivers come in two classes: families and staff. Both tend to be overlooked in architectural planning and interior decorating. Few health care institutions, for example, provide space for family caregivers. In today's minimalist approach to staffing, family often remain with a patient night and day, requiring two sorts of consideration. First, there should be comfortable chairs and sleeping arrangements in the patient's room or in near proximity.

Second, a comfortable family lounge provides for temporary retreat from a tense situation as well as a place to wait, other than the hall, when therapies are being administered. A lounge also provides a place where nurses can talk freely to a family member.

Concern for the caregiver has become a matter of interest to nursing as it applies to caregivers in the community. Indeed, programs for these family members are beginning to arise in community facilities around the nation. At the same time, little consideration is given to the family member who accompanies the patient to a health care facility. Whether involving the family in a patient's care stems from philosophic convictions or from staffing pressures, family have virtually become additional staff.

But they are helpers under acute stress, needing and receptive to a comfortable environment.

Staff comprise the other group of often-neglected caregivers. They, too, have needs for space and periodic relief. The best assigned spaces to which staff may retreat are those that they design themselves. They know what kind of lounges work best for them. They also know what support systems they need to help them reduce stress and gain the strength to continue in their very intensive interactions.

Hence, architecture must not only supply space for patients that is healing, it must also design space that sustains and nurtures staff. Much turnover in hospitals occurs because staff literally cannot continue the high level of interaction necessary in today's health care facilities without respite. When the facilities ignore these needs, it gives a demotivating message to staff.

LOGISTIC SYSTEMS TO SUPPLY MATERIAL

There are two major types of supply systems in the health care institution, those that match supplies or services on a one-to-one basis with requests, and those that supply items or services in accordance with usage norms. The dietary and pharmacy departments usually have the first type of supply system. Patient trays and drugs are supplied on the basis of specific requests. Some leeway may be established by maintaining stock and emergency drugs on a patient unit or by holding some stock food supplies on the unit.

On the whole, resource problems with departments, divisions, or sections that supply goods and services on request turn out to be problems of timing or communication. Because the supplier and the user both are involved in the logistic system, it is useful to examine a defective system rather than to try to place blame for its failures. Many health institutions hire systems analysts or have a department of operations research just for the purpose of handling such problems.

When assistance is not available, the nurse executive or the nursing management staff involved in the systems breakdown may undertake an analysis. A flowchart may reveal system defects and suggest solutions to the manager's problem. Consider the flowchart analysis in Figure 23–8, which describes the problem of a

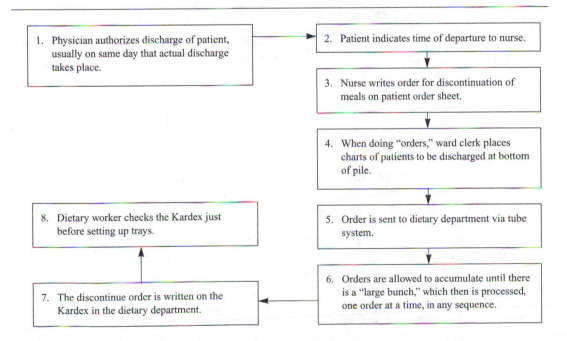

Figure 23–8 Flowchart Analysis of the Problem of Unneeded Dietary Trays

nursing unit that chronically received and had to send back to the dietary department trays for patients who had already been discharged.

Clearly, the problem is one of timing. The flowchart demonstrates at least two deficits. First, there is a slowdown at step 4. The ward clerk who delays handling of charts of patients to be discharged might be re-educated to sequence her tasks differently; alternatively, the nurse might use a different system for issuing stop orders on meals. On the dietary side of the system, a slowdown occurs at step 6. Because orders are ignored until a large batch have accumulated, those that arrive during a relatively inactive period are delayed. A reorganization in which orders are attended to every 15 or 30 minutes no matter how many or how few have accumulated would decrease the slowdown. Systems analysis is a rational approach to supply problems that works to the advantage of all parties, acquainting each manager with the problems and goals of the other.

A second type of supply system in a health care institution is one that works on usage norms rather than on individual requests. The laundry service is an example of this sort of system. When problems arise in a system based on usage norms, the manager needs to inquire how the norms are set. For example, the laundry might calculate linen supply according to number of beds per unit, daily census, average yearly or monthly census, or past linen usage practices of a unit.

However, a unit of 30 patients who are less critical will require fewer linens than a unit of 30 critical patients; hence, even an accurate census is not a direct predictor of linen usage. Perhaps this system problem could be solved by deriving linen requirements on the basis of the patient classification system rather than the census. In other words, some systems problems can be solved by establishing a norm that is more reflective of the supply in question.

Any system based on norms should have a means of flexibility built into it for instances when the units being supplied are above or below the norm. Often, a flowchart will show that the norms are acceptable but that the system lacks flexibility.

When dealing with the delivery system, the nurse executive must ensure, through the necessary negotiations with others, that the right equipment and supplies are where they are needed when they are needed. The systems that control movements of material must be efficient, economical, and designed to control accountability. When these systems are efficient, huge productivity and financial savings can be the result.

Re-engineering and process improvement are methods as well as the standard total quality management methods that have evolved to make supply systems more effective and more cost-effective. Great efficiencies can be obtained through analysis of how quotas are derived and materials distributed.

SUMMARY

Whether one looks at physical space, its decor, or the supplies and systems that flow through it, all these factors deserve careful thought. Streamlining systems and creating a positive atmosphere are equally important. Both need to consider human goals and sensitivities, as well as organizational goals and requisite activities.

REFERENCE

Nightingale, F. 1859. *Notes on nursing*. Philadelphia: Edward Stern & Co., Inc. 1992. Reissued in Philadelphia: J.B. Lippincott Co.

SUGGESTED READINGS

Achterberg, J. 1985. *Imagery in healing*. Boston: New Science Library, Shambhala Publications.

Birren, F. 1978. *Color and human response*. New York: Van Nostrand Reinhold.

Bush-Brown, A., and D. Davis. 1992. *Hospital design for healthcare and senior communities*. New York: Van Nostrand Reinhold.

Collins, D.F. 1984. Skilled nursing unit fashioned from acute care space. *Hospitals* 58, no.4:100.

Haack, J.L. 1981. Ambulatory care addition honors local tradition. *Hospitals* 55, no.4:97, 99.

Hammer, M., and J. Champy. 1993. *Reengineering the corporation*. New York: Harper Business.

Harju, M. 1984. Who's responsible for hospital equipment and product purchasing decisions? *Hospitals* 58, no.13:70–71.

Johnson, D. 1982. Circular tower cuts staffing needs, increases patients' sense of security. *Modern Healthcare* 12, no.2:102–104, 106.

Klettner, S.J. 1981. Hospital design is geared toward patients with sensory impairments. *Hospitals* 55, no.4:103–104.

MacDonald, M.R., et al. 1981. ICU nurses rate their work places. *Hospitals* 55, no.2:115–116, 118.

Mazer, S., and D. Smith. In press. *Sing a song for the sick and tense*. South Lake Tahoe, Calif.: Healthcare Systems.

Miller, M.A. 1983. The nurse as builder: Getting form to follow function. *Nursing Management* 14, no.11:42–44.

Swenson, B., et al. 1984. Effectively employing support services: The key for increasing nursing personnel productivity. *Modern Healthcare* 14, no.16:101–102.

Turner, W.A., and T. Carney. 1984. Circular nursing units and two-bed rooms keep patients in touch. *Hospitals* 58, no.4:122.

Ulrich, R.S. 1992. How design impacts wellness. *Healthcare Forum Journal* 35, no.5:20–25.

Updike, P. 1990. Music therapy results for ICU patients. *Dimensions of Critical Care Nursing* 9, no.1:39–45.

Vernolia, C. 1988. *Creating healing environments*. Berkeley, Calif.: Celestial Arts.

24

Business Planning

Today, nurse executives and even nurse managers are required to develop business plans for new programs or products for which they are requesting funding from the organization. In some situations, the annual budgeting process also involves developing a comprehensive business plan for the next year or for a prescribed period.

Business plans have always been used by entrepreneurs to secure financing from investors. The same process is now being applied to ventures in health care. Typically, the person writing the plan is the one attempting to get the project approved. This assumption is made in the following discussion.

Even though a formal business plan might not be required in every facility, the nurse executive should know how to derive such a plan. Formatting a new program within the structure of the business plan helps the nurse executive to think through the different nuances and loopholes that might stand in the way of gaining approval.

If the nurse executive is reviewing competitive requests from subordinates, having them all presented in the same format allows her to compare requests more easily, selecting those with the most likely payoffs. Some institutions create a single business plan format so that all requests can be compared with greater facility; other institutions allow writers more freedom, providing the general principles of a business plan are followed.

A business plan helps the project director herself (whether she be the nurse executive or a subordinate manager) because the plan provides a defined model by which to frame not only the request but the project itself. Often, it is in composing the plan that the author first thinks through all the complexities and pitfalls that are involved in the project. In other words, it helps the writer consolidate the idea. The author ends up with a comprehensive plan that is likely both to be easily understood and to obtain its objectives if enacted.

Obviously, no matter how skillfully a plan is written, it cannot guarantee acceptance of the plan. Plans are rejected because they are bad ideas, because they cost too much, because they are competing with even better ideas for scarce funds, or because they were politically out of step with major decision makers. Nevertheless, a good idea can be lost because of a deficient business plan. That alone is reason for an author working diligently to produce a superior document.

In the health care setting, a business plan may support a proposed program, project, or product. Usually a product is supported by a business plan only when its cost is formidable, the product is new and relatively untested, or the product is to be manufactured as part of the plan. Sometimes, the manufacture or use of a product is part of a more comprehensive project.

The business plan can take many forms, and different facilities emphasize different aspects of it. Business plans need to be tailored to the mission, philosophy, and culture of the organization. If an organization has its own format, it should be followed. That said, the basic components of any business plan are presented here.

BUSINESS PLAN DEVELOPMENT

A business plan begins with a brief *executive summary*, (i.e., a terse overview of one or two pages summarizing the highlights of sections of the plan that follow). This allows the reader to quickly refresh her mind concerning the project should she be dealing with numerous plans at the same time.

The body of the plan starts by describing the *present situation* and the need for change. This serves as a basic orientation for anyone unfamiliar with the underlying problem or opportunity. For example, a nurse executive's business plan to start a community nursing center might be presented to hospital trustees unfamiliar with the immediate neighborhood situation. Describing this community and its needs would lay the basis for the proposal to follow.

In setting the scene, the author hopes to sidestep objections and general resistance to change. She hopes that the reader will start to unfreeze his thinking about the situation if a negative mind set is anticipated. Nevertheless, this is a business plan, not a white paper, so the author should be terse and to the point.

This introduction is followed by a *description of the new program* or product. Details of the plan or a description of the product take up much of this section. The description is followed by statements about how the plan will improve the present problematic situation or take advantage of a competitive opportunity. An overview of the accomplishments to be expected from the program is appropriate. Some formats identify this section of the form as a *program goal* statement, preferring that it precede the description of the new program.

The next section usually presents the *market analysis*, explaining why market forces will lead to this program's success. Commonly, this is performed by looking at the threats and opportunities that exist in the marketplace as they pertain to this particular project or product.

Statistical data are often used in this section to support assertions. When such measures are not available or sufficient, quality measures such as focused interviews and surveys can provide important support. Population demographics or data from internal resources that lend light to the project are included.

Once a case has been established for the project in relation to market forces, the next step is to describe how this program (or product) will be designed to be attractive to the designated customers/consumers. Some plans call this the *product value* section. In this section, the business plan outlines in detail how the product will be constructed and used or how the program will be constituted with the market in mind.

Next, in the *description of operations,* the business plan describes how the program will be produced, priced if applicable, put in place, and marketed. In health care, rather than bringing a product to the market often the plan involves getting a new project started on a patient care unit or clinic.

An easy way to think of this section is that it concerns the strategies and tactics involved in bringing the plan to life. For many projects, the required operations are dual. First, there are the strategies and tactics of preparing the staff who will work with the project or product. Second, there are the strategies and tactics required to bring the plan successfully to the prospective consumer/user.

Some business plans consider these two elements together, some separate them. For some products, there will only be one of these two elements present. Let us take an example of one such plan, a patient-focused redesign project for a pediatric unit. Here, the staff to be involved and the "consumer" are the same people. In this presentation, the operations section might address how acceptance would be sought among the staff, how the program would be introduced, how staff would be trained, and how the program would be initiated. In other words, this section of the plan describes the strategy and

212 THE NURSE AS EXECUTIVE

tactics for putting the project or product in place and functioning.

This involves staff and any changes in staffing, the orientation and training time, and the overall organizational modifications that will support the achievement of this plan.

Another business plan might involve the application of a piece of capital equipment (e.g., a new computer software product) rather than a project. Here, the plan would demonstrate how staff could be sold on changing from the old software (or substituting the software for manual systems), how they could be trained, and how the equipment could be interfaced with in-place systems.

For some projects, the author also must consider the strategies to be used in marketing and distributing the product or program to a target audience. In health care, this might involve a new dialysis center, for example. In addition to saying how the center and its staff would be put in place, the business plan delineates how this facility will be marketed to consumers and how the marketing plan will bring in business. The plan also designates who will be responsible for doing what aspects of this marketing.

An *evaluation* section is included in the plan. This is where the author of the business plan tells how she will track and evaluate the program as it is put in place and into operation. This brings the plan full cycle, comparing the outcome to the project goals. It may also indicate what is to happen if the plan fails to measure up. Will it be discontinued? How soon? Will it be studied and modified? What will be the outcome if a plan fails? If possible, evaluation forms should be included with the plan.

The final section of the business plan is the *financial presentation*. This section may come last, but it is one of the most important. Board members and executives often leaf ahead to this section before reading all the front matter. A good financial plan gives both the costs of the plan and the fiscal benefits anticipated, if any.

In presenting costs, the plan must be comprehensive and exacting. In the case of a project, this involves the cost of staff, including the orientation and developmental time, and the cost of the overall organizational plan to put the

project in place. The cost of additional material, equipment, and supplies, is included. If a product must be purchased or manufactured, these costs are displayed. When costs will be incurred over different time periods, this data should be given. Projections should include both start-up and maintenance costs.

Where appropriate, costs are distributed (prorated) over time. If the project will pay for itself or partially pay for itself, these projections are included. A good presentation is sophisticated in terms of trend analysis; it may present cost/benefit data, cost/effectiveness data, or both. Obviously, a plan that has the benefit of supporting itself (sooner or later) will be looked on with favor over one that incurs continuing costs, albeit for good human outcomes.

PROCESSING BUSINESS PLANS

An effective business plan demonstrates that the project merits attention. The documentation of the plan is critical, but equally important is the presenter's ability to argue her case. Whether the idea is discussed one-on-one or with a wide audience, she must be able to demonstrate presentation skills and effective display and use of data from the business plan.

In some settings, the business plan is merely submitted, and there is little opportunity for presentation or discussion. In many settings, however, it is expected that a written report will be supported by an oral presentation. The latter case gives the author an opportunity to enhance her case with graphic presentations of data as well as with informal explanations and examples.

Depending on the audience, a business presentation can be very formal or informal and can be followed by no discussion or by extensive discussion. What is important is that the presenter know what to expect and plan accordingly.

Audiences have various needs when business plans are presented. It is essential, therefore, to know who will be present to hear the plan. When more than one person is involved in the plan, it is important to choose the right person to present the business plan. One selects the person with the best public presentation skills, one who has the best chance of influencing the group.

Presentation of self is important in these meetings. In one such meeting, a head nurse presenter arrived directly from her unit, in uniform, a stethoscope around her neck. She gave a good presentation, but the board was less attentive to her than to the other presenters. All the others (mostly from non-nursing departments) were in business suits, looking crisp and businesslike. The head nurse missed an opportunity to present her proposal in the best possible light.

Presentation of a business plan is more than an exercise in logic; it involves politics, too. It is not uncommon that an excellent business plan, with all the correct technical support, fails to be accepted because the author is not well connected with those in charge of the approval process. The nurse executive, for example, cannot count on well-developed business plans and quality presentation skills alone. Her ongoing relationships with important decision makers are just as important.

SUMMARY

Today, most health care facilities must function like businesses. This means that they are adopting the techniques of business, including formal presentations of business plans for major proposed changes in products and programs.

The nurse executive will require skills in three domains to push through her plans. First, she must learn to compose a business plan skillfully. Second, she must learn the skills of making a business presentation. Finally, she must make sure that the politics of communication and influence are brought to bear on those who will make the final decisions.

For her own internal management, the nurse executive is wise to require that subordinate staff prepare business plans for recommended changes. Not only does this give the executive the information she needs for decision making, but it serves as an education for her staff.

SUGGESTED READINGS

Alward, R.R., and C. Camunas. 1991. *The nurse's guide to marketing.* Albany, N.Y.: Delmar Publishers, Inc.

Krentz, S.E., and S.M. Pilskaln. 1988. Product life cycle: Still a valid framework for business planning. *Topics in Health Care Financing* 15, no.1:40–48.

McLaughlin, H. 1985. *Building a business plan.* New York: John Wiley & Sons, Inc.

Silvester, J.L. 1984. *How to start in finance and operate your own business.* Secaucus, N.J.: Lyle-Stewart.

Summers, P.M., et al. 1988. Quality management: Program design—An interdisciplinary approach. *Nursing Clinics of North America* 23, no.3:665–670.

Worthem, J.C. 1992. Business planning: Who, what, when where, why, and how. *Topics in Health Care Financing* 18, no.3:1–8.

Part VII

Achieving Quality Outcomes

One could argue that the most radical change in health care in recent times is the focus on patient outcomes, including controlling and improving them. Several forces came together to produce this trend. First came a natural outgrowth of the health care professions' growing sophistication in quality measurement.

One could argue that nursing was more involved with formalized quality measurement sooner than any other health care professions. And we experimented our way through the quality management system, initially—like the accrediting agencies of the time—focusing on structure standards, mostly the state of the organization. Then, we moved on to process standards, typically the actions of the nurse. We were getting sophisticated about outcome standards, mostly of patient states, when other groups, including accreditors, discovered them.

This "discovery" occurred just about the same time that the diagnosis-related group system made everyone aware that the patient's length of stay was the most critical factor in how much his care cost. The obvious implication was that to discharge patients sooner, one had to work at getting them well faster, and that meant identifying the outcomes that marked wellness (or a given level of recovery) and working every day toward those end goals.

At first glance, it appears logical to say that if the desired patient outcomes are met, the structure and the processes that achieve them matter little. Yet economy and efficiency rest in the processes and structures. Yes, we must achieve the desired outcomes as quickly as possible, but whether we succeed in so doing may depend on our processes and structures. And in today's world, we cannot always afford the most luxurious processes and structures. Indeed, a new set of desired fiscal outcomes competes with care outcomes for the nurse executive's attention. Balancing cost and care outcomes is today's special challenge.

The current focus on outcomes, therefore, should be seen as completing the circle, complementing the other components of quality management rather than supplanting them. Structure, process, *and* outcome goals are directed toward many subject matters, including organizations, groups, and individuals.

Outcomes management is no longer limited to patient outcomes, as is seen in the upcoming chapters. Nursing administration has its own outcomes, including outcomes for financial achievement and staff performance. This section of the book, therefore, looks at outcomes from three perspectives, that of patient, staff, and organization.

25

Managing Outcomes

The nurse executive's success or failure depends on her ability to accept accountability for and to achieve results in financial and quality outcomes. Some nurse executives are very nice people but have no track record for achieving these outcomes. By contrast, other nurse executives have a clearly outlined program that is integrated with the organization's vision, and the desired outcomes actually do happen.

RESULTS-ORIENTED MANAGEMENT

Results-oriented is a term that describes these nurse executives. They have clearly defined outcomes and achieve them within stated periods. Not only can these nurse executives get things done within the department, but they can achieve the integration with other departments that is essential in achieving their initiatives. Results-oriented nurse executives are people who can clearly define the outcomes and then control the processes to achieve them successfully.

As the competitive forces heat up in health care, the results-oriented nurse executive is in much greater demand, because she can achieve the desired quality and financial objectives of the organization and can quickly turn the organization in a different direction if the environment suddenly changes.

Health care organizations cannot tolerate much variability in results. The room for error in either quality or financial outcomes has become much narrower. Variations in the achievement of quality outcomes can result in multimillion dollar lawsuits that can deal a crushing financial blow to the health care facility.

The inability to achieve sustained high performance in financial outcomes also can bring devastation to the organization. When a nursing budget has large positive or negative variances, the whole health care institution is affected.

If the tolerable financial variances have grown narrow, so have allowable variances in quality of care. A major shift in the thinking of nurse executives and their bosses warns us that just having a given care outcome program in place is not good enough. No longer, for example, can a hospital simply have a fall prevention program. Instead, the nurse executive is accountable for the outcomes of such a program. In other words, these programs must show results in terms of outcomes—the progressive decrease in the number and severity of falls.

Indeed, many would argue that we have passed the place where continuous quality improvement is adequate. As consumers demand more of us, it is no longer acceptable to keep negative outcomes such as falls under a certain threshold. The fact that one person fell, even though the total number of falls is under the designated threshold, is no longer good enough.

Not only can the one who falls suffer unnecessarily, but the facility can suffer dramatically in terms of exposure to a lawsuit.

The general public no longer tolerates the notion that hospitals are dangerous places; they refuse to accept the fact that we have medication errors, falls, and other negative outcomes of hospitalization. For example, an orthopedic patient with a hip replacement expects that he will not be subjected to any medication errors, infections, or procedures done to him that were ordered for another patient. Patients expect that their length of stay will not increase because of any complications, and their payers expect care to be delivered within a reasonable, often predetermined cost.

The nurse executive is responsible for obtaining these nurse-sensitive outcomes. Indeed, she is mandated to be results-oriented and to pursue outcomes aggressively that produce excellence in terms of quality and financial performance. Results-driven nurse executives hold themselves and their staff members accountable for outcomes such as these as well as achieving regulatory standards and all the other complex outcomes that are necessary for today's standards.

One sign of this new perspective is that our language has been changing from goal-directed to outcome-oriented. In keeping with the new concept, Russell Ackoff (1986) first developed the concept of "managing backward." He believed that we should imagine the ideal, develop the outcomes that we want, and manage backward from that. He believed that if we start from where we are, we just move forward with imperfect systems. If, however, we imagine the ideal and work backward, we can make the ideal happen. In fact, we will be managing the idealized outcome. The nurse executive who operates from this model will achieve the outcomes necessary to achieve financial and quality objectives.

RESEARCH-BASED PRACTICE AND OUTCOMES

Nurse executives must be committed to providing the best care based on the latest in research-based outcomes and on the latest information available for developing financially sound practices. It is not only unethical but also unwise to expose oneself to legal action by failing to incorporate the latest findings into practice.

However, using the latest research in practice is often easier said than done. If one is not practicing in an academic institution, the availability of the people who have research training and who can analyze published nursing research may be limited.

The nurse executive must develop a research surveillance system so that new data is continually assessed and, when valid, implemented in practice. The staff in charge of the various specialty units within the division must be aware of the latest findings presented at national meetings and published in nursing journals. The practice of these units must incorporate the implications drawn from this research. Only through use of research can the nurse executive guarantee that the appropriate care and financial outcomes will be achieved.

Integrating research into the practice culture will become a reality when nursing units become places where information about nursing practice is readily available (through articles or computer-based on-line systems). Research-based staff development programs reinforce this pattern.

The culture is fostered when all unit-based programs are research-based and when talking about the latest research becomes the norm of nurse behavior. Research-based practice occurs when nurses become vitally interested in searching out how to care for patients better through continual updating of their knowledge base.

A departmental newsletter that describes new research, references pertinent articles, and reports on news presented at meetings throughout the nation encourages a research-based practice. All this is not merely nice but essential. Managing outcomes and achieving quality can only be done through developing a research-based practice.

PERCEPTION OF QUALITY

The nurse executive is obligated to develop excellence in clinical and financial outcomes as indicated by professional standards, regulatory standards, and standards that are dictated by research. However, there are also other perceptions of quality that must be managed and achieved.

There are a variety of customers in the health care system who define quality differently from the nurse executive. If their definitions of quality are not met and their perception of quality is not achieved, they will think that quality care does not exist.

Patients, for example, can have very different standards of quality than does the nurse executive. For example, although some nurse executive might define quality as a very low rate of medication errors, the patient expects that his safety will be assured 100 percent of the time and that he will never be subject to a medication error.

Patients also define quality care in terms of staff helpfulness and a caring concern demonstrated on the part of the nursing staff: The patient expects to find a supportive environment. Even if the best clinical outcomes are achieved but these expectations of quality are not met, the patient will believe he received poor care.

Payers also have specific perceptions of quality—ones that can be described by cost per case, length of stay, and other measurable criteria. Physicians have definitions of the quality of care that might be subsumed under the category of the efficiency with which the unit is run. They are not aware of all the silent work of surveillance and assessment that is part of the nurse's work; they see the unit as it facilitates or hinders their interaction with patients.

Organizations such as the Joint Commission on the Accreditation of Healthcare Organizations and Medicare also have set expectations about quality that must be met. These are just a few of the customers that the nurse executive has to address in looking at diverse definitions of quality and the need to have nursing achieve these customer expectations.

To achieve quality outcomes, the nurse executive must carefully and thoughtfully "manage backward," determining the outcomes that must be achieved, her own objectives as well as those of all the other customers and regulatory agencies that define quality. The nurse executive can then design the structure to achieve these outcomes through the nursing administration control system, the quality control system, and the performance appraisal system, as well as many other parts of the nursing program that contribute to the achievement of quality outcomes.

EVALUATING PROCESSES THAT MANAGE OUTCOMES

Aiming at the right outcomes alone is not enough. Systems must be put in place to measure accurately one's achievements in reaching defined outcomes. Evaluation is an essential part, the feedback loop, of every system of outcomes management. Evaluation, however, must be followed by system correction when the results indicate the need.

In the chapters that follow, attention is given to setting in place the systems whereby outcomes may be measured, as well as looking at how such feedback is used in making system alterations.

As more information becomes available about outcomes and the management of outcomes, more will be expected of the nurse executive. As with other research, it is expected that the nurse executive will incorporate outcomes research into her practice.

SUMMARY

Outcomes management is the name of today's health care game. One can see the nurse executive's role as managing many outcomes simultaneously—hers as well those expected by other major consumers and evaluators of nursing services.

One of the main changes in outcomes management is the notion of total compliance rather than the older perspective of continuous improvement toward one's targets. Outcomes management involves outcomes of many types, designed to meet the expectations of many consumer groups. The nurse executive's effectiveness (and how effective others perceive her to be) rests heavily on outcomes management.

REFERENCE

Ackoff, R. 1986. *Management in small doses*. New York: John Wiley & Sons, Inc.

SUGGESTED READINGS

Cesta, T.G. 1993. The link between continuous quality improvement and case management. *Journal of Nursing Administration* 23, no.6:55–61.

Daly, B.J., et al. 1991. A nurse-managed special care unit. *Journal of Nursing Administration* 21, no.7–8:31–38.

Erkel, E.A. 1993. The impact of case management in preventive services. *Journal of Nursing Administration* 23, no.1:27–32.

Goodwin, D.R. 1992. Critical pathways in home healthcare. *Journal of Nursing Administration* 22, no.2:35–40.

Hampton, D.C. 1993. Implementing a managed care framework through care maps. *Journal of Nursing Administration* 23, no.5:21–27.

Hegyvary, S.T. 1993. The shift of focus from provider processes to population outcomes. *Nursing Administration Quarterly* 17, no.3:viii–ix.

Kirk, R. 1992. The big picture: Total quality management and continuous quality improvement. *Journal of Nursing Administration* 22, no.4:24–31.

Marschke, P., and M.T. Nolan. 1993. Research related to case management. *Nursing Administration Quarterly* 17, no.3:16–21.

Sandhu, B., et al. 1992. Nursing assignment patterns and patient outcomes. *Journal of Nursing Administration* 5, no.3:14–19.

Trella, R.S. 1993. A multidisciplinary approach to case management of frail, hospitalized older adults. *Journal of Nursing Administration* 23, no.2:20–26.

26

Nursing Administration Control System

Achieving outcomes calls for the conscious planned application of resources, processes, and structures by the nurse executive to the achievement of desired outcomes. These outcomes include obtaining the desired patient health outcomes, implementing effective and efficient patterns of organization, and reaching fiscal targets. To evaluate success in achieving nursing outcomes, it is necessary to devise mechanisms for feedback of results and the consequent adjustment of resources, processes, and structures when necessary to better achieve goals. These two mechanisms, feedback and adjustment, comprise the corrective element of the nursing management control system.

SYSTEMS MODEL

Because it is useful in explaining control phenomena, a systems model is used as the basic theme of this chapter. A system is a set of interrelated and interdependent parts (e.g., nursing's resources, processes, and structures) designed to achieve an outcome or set of goals. The goal dictates the system's central processes (i.e., the activities that turn the raw material [input] into the finished product [output]). In Figure 26–1, the system gets its raw materials from the surrounding environment and returns its finished product to that environment.

A system is differentiated from its environment and that which is external to its environ-

ment. A system's environment surrounds the system, and the system interacts with it. An element is part of the environment, not of the system, when the system can do relatively little about the element's characteristics or behavior, and when the element determines, in part, how the system performs. That which is external to the system has no interaction with it. Some systems are closed (i.e., they do not interact with an environment). Such systems supply their own energy for continuation. Because closed systems are rarely seen in the nursing division, the reader may assume that subsequent discussion refers to open systems that interact with their environments.

Virtually any phenomenon can be viewed from the systems approach. Indeed, a component of one system may itself be viewed as a system or as a subsystem of the larger system. Within the total system of the nursing division, one can identify subsystems for patient care, employee performance, administration, education, and fiscal management. It is possible to relate these subsystems to each other by viewing the nursing system as a whole, thus producing a better mechanism for control of outcomes in the nursing division.

It is logical to assume that patient care is the major subsystem of the nursing division. Improved patient health may be assumed to be the major nursing goal, with ill persons as the system input, well or improved patients as the out-

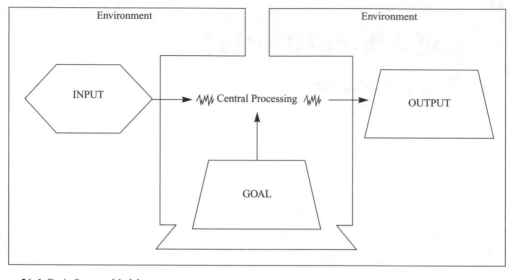

Figure 26–1 Basic Systems Model

put, and the nursing actions that affect the change as central processing, sometimes called thruput. Figure 26–2 is an illustration of the patient care system.

Other nursing goals for other nursing subject matter may be viewed similarly in a systems model. Figure 26–3 illustrates an instance when staff behavior is taken as the subject matter.

An effective systems model requires still another component—a cybernetic loop to estab-

lish communication and control (Figure 26–4). The properties of a cybernetic system can be summarized as follows:

1. *The system has the capacity to sense departures from the desired outcome.* For this to happen, the system first must know what output is desired. A clear description or measure of the goal is necessary to have a basis for comparison. Second, the

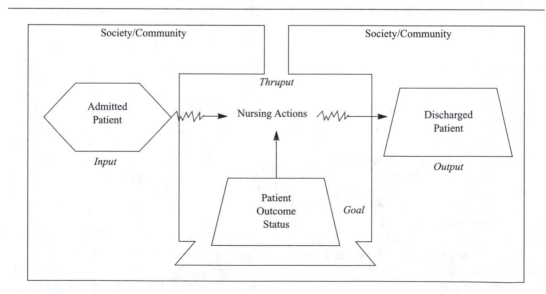

Figure 26–2 Patient As Input to the Nursing System

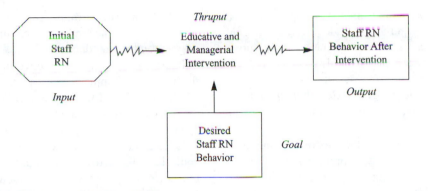

Figure 26–3 Staff As Input to the Systems Model

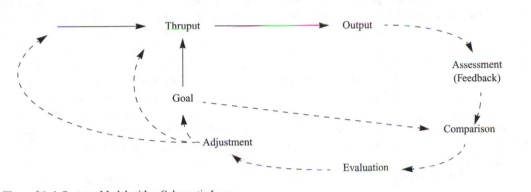

Figure 26–4 Systems Model with a Cybernetic Loop

product of the system must be assessed, measured, or described in a similar manner. If the product cannot be characterized in the same way as the goal, there is no way to compare them. Finally, one must be able to tell how the two items (goal and product) differ.

2. *The system is able to prescribe action to correct deficiencies in the product.* When differences between the product and the goal can be identified, the system must be able to determine or hypothesize the source of that difference, and it must formulate a decision strategy to correct the disparity. In other words, the system must relate the outcome to the processes (central processing or thruput) that caused it. The cybernetic system, therefore, prescribes corrective actions. In some cases, those actions may be obvious; in others, the system may have to explore proposed

alternative actions until successful ones are discovered.

3. *The system allocates resources and efforts to implement the proposed corrective actions.* The proposed corrective actions must be feasible, and they must be implemented. Otherwise, the prescription is meaningless.

4. *The system has the capacity to sense results of the change in processing.* Here, one is back to the first step, for the system again measures output (the new output) against the original goal.

Notice in Figure 26–4 that control can be exercised to make the product and goal correspond in three different ways: (1) The thruput may be altered to produce a product as desired, (2) the goal itself may be altered to resemble the product more closely (this might be done if it were determined that a goal originally had been set too high or too low), and (3) the input may be altered so it responds more adequately to the available processes. As an illustration, only nurses' aides of a certain IQ would be admitted to a training program if those with lower IQs habitually failed the program. Hereafter, illustrations deal with the most common condition: alteration of thruput.

One may illustrate the cybernetic function in relation to a staff development education program. Suppose that a given patient outcome, such as safe use of crutches, is measured by numbers of falls and accidents suffered by patients while using crutches. Suppose, also, that the set standard has been exceeded: More falls and injuries are occurring than should be tolerated. The cause has been diagnosed as staff ignorance of procedures for safe use of crutches. The relevant systems model, including a cybernetic loop, might look like Figure 26–5.

In this example, the change in central processing (offering an educational program) improved the output but did not succeed in causing the goal to be met. Hence, the cybernetic system calls for still further changes in the central processing. Still assuming the problem is educa-

tional, the instructor might change the content of her course or the method of instruction or she might monitor attendance.

If these steps prove ineffective in decreasing the number of injuries on crutches, then she would consider further factors of education or other factors unrelated to education (perhaps some factor in the environment contributes to falls [e.g., poorly kept crutches]). Also, the staff could have learned the procedure satisfactorily but failed to apply the safe technique (a factor of motivation rather than education).

Another example illustrates alternate paths, different modifications of the central processing component of the system. Suppose that two head nurses in a nursing home are finding an unacceptable number of geriatric patients falling out of bed and suffering injury at night. One head nurse might choose to reduce injuries by requiring that siderails be in place and elevated for every geriatric patient every night. She might combine this requirement with a request for increased frequency of nightly rounds by the nurse in charge.

The second head nurse might try a different process alteration: having carpet installed in pa-

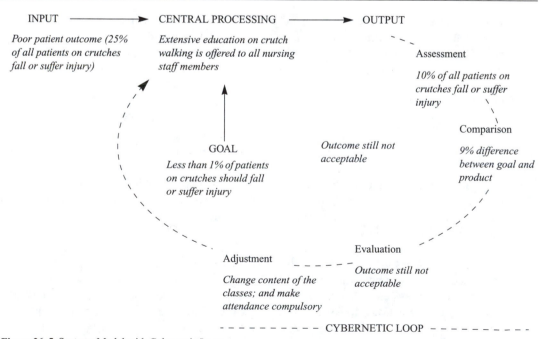

Figure 26–5 Systems Model with Cybernetic Loop

tients' rooms, lowering each bed nightly, and using few if any siderails. Obviously, this head nurse is hypothesizing that many falls are due to confused patients trying to climb over siderails. She further hypothesizes that lower beds and carpeting will reduce incidence of injury in such cases. The first head nurse is working toward the goal from different premises, trying to prevent falls rather than to lessen their impact.

Suppose that both head nurses bring their injury rate down to the acceptable level. How does one judge which approach was best? Other values, both human values and managerial, will serve as criteria for the judgment. If one places a high value on human autonomy, the solution that restrains fewer patients will be selected. If, however, the expense of carpeting is an imposing cost, economy may be the deciding factor. Further considerations might include the kinds of patients admitted to the two units. Perhaps the solution for one unit would be unsuccessful when applied to the patient population of the other unit.

This incident describes an important fluctuation in a systems model. When the input differs, the processes also must differ to reach the same output goals. Figure 26–6 illustrates this point.

Suppose that the goal is the same (e.g., no development of hypostatic pneumonia after surgery). Suppose, however, that patient A is a 95-year-old man admitted from a nursing home with a pathologic fracture of the hip. Suppose patient B is a 17-year-old man who sustained

his hip fracture during participation in a football game. Medical therapy for both patients involved surgical hip pinning. Obviously, neither patient should fail to meet the standard (no hypostatic pneumonia), but the nursing care (thruput) probably will not be the same, one patient needing more special care than the other for achievement of the same standard.

These examples illustrate the use of a systems model with cybernetic controls in nursing management. Such a model enables the manager to relate outcomes to central processing in a significant way. If the central processes are unsuccessful in producing the goals, they are systematically modified until a sequence of processes is found that achieves the desired outcome.

When the desired goal has been achieved, the management job still is not complete. Even when nursing values have been satisfied and the goal has been effectively reached, management values of efficiency and economy still must be addressed. The manager now applies the same model, asking in each case whether the product (the desired goal) can be achieved with less expense, fewer resources, or in a shorter time. When two processes are equally successful in achieving the desired goal, the less costly process usually is to be preferred.

Figure 26–7 illustrates an instance in which the same input is handled in diverse ways to produce the same goal. Suppose some staff learn by attending a class whereas others learn by view-

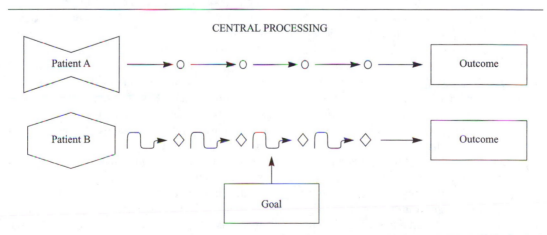

Figure 26–6 Different Central Processing To Assure Same Product When Input Varies Significantly

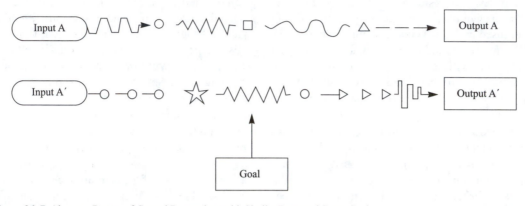

Figure 26–7 Alternate Routes of Central Processing, with Similar Input and Same Goal

ing an audiovisual tape. Or the alternate path model might represent two different nursing plans to achieve the same patient health outcome for similar patients. In this case, the deviation might be due to different resources available at two different points in time.

SYSTEM ERRORS

A systems model is useless if any part of the system is missing or inaccurate. The success of the system can be ensured only by careful design of the elements. What can go wrong with the components? It is useful to consider each element separately.

First, what can go wrong in setting *goals*? A goal is useless if it is set too high. A goal that cannot be met makes staff members feel like failures. Similarly, if a goal is set too low, it is meaningless. If everyone reaches the goal as a matter of course, it hardly can be directive for practice. Also, goals may be inappropriate or just plain wrong for this system at this time or in this setting. Goals set for matters not within the control of the nursing division are also useless, not to mention frustrating.

A good goal is one that represents the best realistic outcome that can be achieved through the influence of nursing care or nursing administrative processes in a given institution. It is a sign of institutional health when the nursing division is able to identify realistic goals for all its activities.

This said, there are times when the standards set by accreditors must be taken as the goal.

Also bear in mind that what might be realistic for expected outcomes of nursing care might not be acceptable to patients. Although a medication error rate less than .05 percent might be acceptable to the nursing division, it will not be acceptable under any circumstances to the patient receiving the wrong drug. The goal must be the aggressive elimination of mistakes by mistake-proofing the process of drug administration. This chapter, however, does not deal with the merits of the standards set. The purpose here is simply to show how a system with feedback/control mechanisms works.

What about *input*? The level of control over input may vary radically among nursing systems. For example, when the patient is the system input, the nursing division may perceive that it has no control because it does not regulate patient admissions to the institution. In other cases, however, nursing may have total control over input. For example, the nurse executive may set her own standards for each class of employee hired in her division, and she may refuse input of a candidate who does not meet the qualifications. Sometimes, the nursing division may wish to control the input to one system by acts in another system. For example, a home care program may decrease the numbers of admissions of geriatric patients who have limitations in self-care abilities.

Figure 26–8 illustrates another important relationship: the one between *input* and *environment*. In this instance, the input is the battered child. Because the system in this model only covers hospitalized care, it cannot be totally successful in managing the problem. It is obvious that the environmental effects are self-defeating. In this illustration, the system reaches the desired output (a child with physical injuries healed), only to have the environment return that output to its original detrimental state. Obviously, one could construct an image of a larger system, one that includes the aspects labeled environment, the parents, and home situation along with the hospitalization segment of the system. The output desired of this larger system would be more comprehensive than the more narrow goals of the limited hospital system.

What about *central processing?* Errors here tend to be those of traditionalism, clinging to a process that either does not achieve the goals or is unrelated to goals or achieves goals at too great a cost. Another error in nursing related to central processing is that of covert processing. When nurses fail to identify and keep records of the plan of nursing care, it is not even possible to know the processes and hence never possible to make reasonable judgments concerning what processes are effective in producing what outcomes.

What about the *feedback* and *comparison* phases of control? What can go wrong in the control process? Clearly, control cannot succeed unless the goals can be operationalized to lend themselves to careful and consistent measurement. Similarly, control will fail if for some reason there is no way to apply these operationalized measurements to the output. Feedback and comparison are not enough if one cannot make a judgment as to whether the reality has missed or conformed with the goal. Usually, this means that the system sets mini-max levels of acceptable conformity, but one must know when that leeway has been overextended.

Feedback and comparison are only as good as the tools that allow one to collect and analyze the data. Hence, if a format is devised to meas-

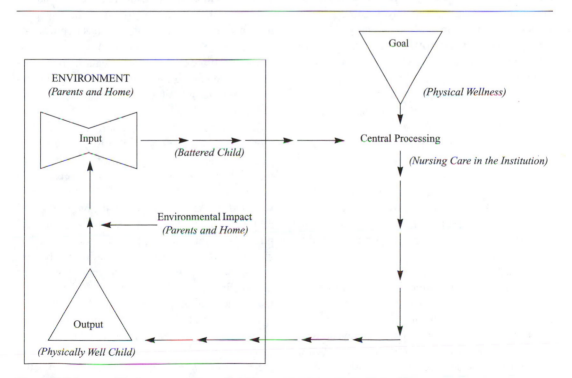

Figure 26–8 Impact of Environment on System Output

ure a given output, it is important that the form be both valid and reliable. A tool is valid if it measures what it purports to measure, reliable if it measures with consistency. As an illustration of validity, a tool to measure mental status of patients in a psychiatric unit, for example, would not have questions dealing with the patient's physical status, unless those items could be related directly to mental status.

A tool lacks reliability if different persons using the same tool come up with different ratings or scores on the same subject matter. Suppose a quality control tool asks nurses to judge the muscle strength of patients yet fails to give adequate criteria to make such a judgment. If the tool just says to rate muscle strength as excellent, good, fair, or poor, these terms are not definitive and are too subjective to ensure that any group of nurses would rate a group of patients similarly.

Another deficit in reliability occurs when a tool can call forth different responses from the same rater at different times. A supervisor using the same evaluation tool she used a month or more ago to rate an employee whose performance has not changed in any significant way should not come up with a radically different score. If the tool did not help the supervisor to interpret a similar performance in a similar manner, then that tool lacks reliability.

What about the *adjustment* element of the control system? What can go wrong in making adjustments? There can be no intelligible adjustment if the processes (thruput) and the output have not been properly associated. Hence, if the thruput varies from day to day, there is no way to establish correlations between thruput and output nor to control thruput for a systematic change. Thruput, then, must be known and repetitive before one is ready to make any adjustment in it.

The adjustment component must allow for a reasoned change. In some systems, the needed change will be evident. In other systems, the nurse executive may postulate and test alternatives. And in some cases, change may be trial and error—or nearly that—until a successful methodology is discovered. Obviously, this aspect is where nursing research and nursing ad-

ministrative research fit in. Research becomes the adjustment phase when one is unsure of the proper changes to make in a system to produce the desired goals.

The adjustment component also requires an environment in which controlled change is possible. When rigidities in the nursing division prevent the adjustment phase, it is a waste of time to evaluate carefully; evaluation for its own sake produces no improvement in patient care. Adjustment must be possible for a systems model to work.

Stability after an adjustment is essential if the worth of the adjustment is to be assessed. Many people make the mistake of measuring an adjustment before it is fully integrated into the norms of the system. Judgment of a given adjustment should not be made until it has become part of the standard operating procedure.

What errors can be made in the *output* of the system? Many of the potential problems already have been discussed in looking at how the goal relates to the output. One additional element may be mentioned, however. Many people determine to measure all aspects of the output for a system. Every nurse executive has seen at least one measurement tool that has hundreds of standards for many parts of a given output. Often, such a detailed tool defeats its own purpose. If the testing mechanism involved in measuring the output is too complex, it is not likely to be used for long.

Instead of aiming for comprehensiveness in measurement, the nurse executive will be wise to encourage the development of measurements that address the critical elements of a given output, ignoring the less essential elements. In this way, indices are developed that give quick and relatively accurate information on a given output. A critical index approach to diabetic hygiene might concentrate on status of the patient's foot care. Although foot care is only part of the care required by a diabetic, it is assumed that if the feet are properly cared for, it is likely that the rest of the body will be in a similar state. The foot has been picked as the index because of its vulnerability; if there is a deficit in the body or its care, it is likely to be reflected first in the foot.

DIVERSE NURSING SYSTEMS

The systems model may be applied to diverse phenomena in the nursing division (for several major applications, see Table 26–1). Notice that each of these major systems deals with one model of quality management, controlling quality of patient outcomes, of staff behavior, of organizational effectiveness, of educational output, or of financial management.

In each case, the system must be developed as a totality if it is to be effective. Standards (or outcomes) must be determined, methods selected for implementation, feedback information collected and analyzed, and adjustment in the thruput must be made when results differ from goals set. To activate a control system, the nurse executive must see that three steps are followed for each system:

1. setting standards/defining expected outcomes
2. developing or selecting measuring tools and/or indices
3. developing a surveillance process to carry out measurements, analyze data, recommend or implement corrective actions

How then does the nurse executive establish control over the multiple and diverse components of her division? The control function may be divided into internal and external control subsystems. External control are those standards that originate outside of the nursing division itself; internal controls are originated as part of self-regulation within the division.

External controls are federal, state, local, and professional standards imposed on the health care institution (including its nursing division). The nurse executive, accountable for meeting these expected outcomes, must have mechanisms in place to monitor and evaluate compliance with these standards. Federal control rests primarily with the Social Security Administration, which sets institutional qualifications for receipt of Medicare and Medicaid payments. One can choose to ignore the required standards only at the price of being denied payments for Medicare and Medicaid patients. Other federal regulations and controls are imposed by the Fair Labor Standards Act and the Occupational Safety and Health Act. National and state constitutional and contractual law also acts to regulate the institution and the nursing division.

Because the state is the organ of government that licenses health care organizations, each state has developed various codes and requirements. State board of health regulations represent one application of such codes. Local units of government may add additional constraints and regulations to institutions within their borders.

As is the case with federal regulation, an institution does not have to accede to accreditation review by the Joint Commission on Accreditation of Healthcare Organizations (JCAHO), but the benefits associated with such accreditation usually make it more than advantageous to acquiesce. Furthermore, most other evaluating groups will accept JCAHO approval in lieu of their own accrediting visits.

At present, the nursing professional organization does not have an accreditation program for nursing divisions. But it does have published standards, and the effective nurse executive administrator will feel a professional obligation to conform to these basic standards. In addition to publishing standards for nursing service, the American Nurses Association (ANA) publishes standards for individual nursing practice and for practice in a wide variety of nursing specializations. Several of these standards are cited in the Suggested Readings for this chapter. The ANA also has certification programs for individuals who wish to testify to their advanced practice. The first certification examinations for nursing service administrators were offered late in 1979. Specialty organizations also may offer either accreditation or credentials in conjunction with ANA or separately.

Within the institution, yet external to the nursing division, the nurse executive will be subjected to corporate control systems. The nurse executive will be expected to report activities and administrative decisions through a yearly or twice-yearly report. The formulation of such a report deserves careful consideration. Not only does it report the activities of the division for the period, but it serves as a history of accomplishments.

Table 26-1 Major Systems of the Nursing Division

System	Input	Thruput	Goal	Output	Feedback	Adjustment
Patient care	Individual patients	Nursing interventions	Set in care plan	Meets goals, patients satisfied	Case assessments	Care plan modification
	Patient groups (by need, problem, DRG, or disease category)	Nursing interventions	Patient care standards Quality management criteria ANA standards	Meets goals, patients satisfied	Patient opinionnaires Quality audits	Change in nursing interventions
Employee performance	Employee skills Knowledge Attitudes Actions	Supervision Self-assessment Inservice education	Job descriptions Quality criteria Policies/procedures ANA standards	Nursing acts	Supervisor's observation, appraisal	Coaching and counseling Education
Nursing division	Organization structures/ processes Division structures/ processes	Nursing management	Own objectives External standards (JCAHO, ANA)	Direction and control of division	Summaries of performance of major nursing systems	Reorganization Changes in system
Staff development	Staff ignorance or lack of skills	Education Orientation Departmental programs/projects	Divisional/ departmental objectives Quality management standards Job functions	Knowledge Skills Attitudes	Quality control audits Performance appraisals Tests subsequent to education	Education Orientation Information Job functions
Budget	Fiscal needs/demands	Actual expenditures	Projected budget	Budget variances	Variance analysis Ratio analysis	Budget revision Meeting one's budget

The nurse executive can prepare for the writing of these reports by systematically accumulating data. Without this preparation, if she merely tries to remember at one sitting what she has accomplished during the past year, she is likely to miss some of the most important accomplishments. An ongoing record to refresh her mind is essential.

This report serves several secondary functions, and all or part of the report may be communicated to nursing managers and staff. When staff are constantly involved in the change process, it is easy for them to forget the achievements of the past. The yearly report serves as a pleasant reminder of these achievements. Moreover, copies of their yearly reports have been known to help more than one nurse executive obtain a desired position. The ability to put together a clear, organized coherent annual report impresses a prospective employer almost as much as its content.

Interdivisional feedback for the administration control system comes from diverse sources: results of quality measurement from patient care, summaries of performance appraisals, feedback concerning inservice education offerings and attendance, incident/accident reports, personnel files, reports of patient census and classification, staffing and scheduling data, budget reports including variance analyses, and weekly (or less frequent) reports from subordinate managers.

All these sources provide information for control activities. It is important that the nurse executive determine what information should be sought and communicated for each of these feedback systems. The nature of that information will direct activities within the division. Nurses and managers spend time on what is seen as important by their superiors; by requiring data on a given subject, the nurse executive is signaling its importance.

INTEGRATED NURSING MANAGEMENT SYSTEM

At this stage in the development of nursing management, most nurse executives are building an integrated nursing management system, whereby performance of subsystems can be correlated and interfaced. The systems to be correlated include quality measurement/control systems, patient classification system, staffing and scheduling systems, diagnosis-related group (DRG) system if applicable, productivity measures, the performance appraisal system, nursing resource use measurements, any existing billing systems for nursing, budget reports, and other nursing staff demographics.

An effective system for correlating data among and between these subsystems probably requires the use of a computerized information system. Also, it is necessary that cumulative results of measurements in all these systems be quantified for comparison and correlational purposes. Once such a system is in place, one should be able to ask questions such as

1. At what level of staffing do the quality control reports show negative changes in patient outcomes?
2. At what level of staffing does the productivity ratio fall or stabilize?
3. How do staff performance appraisals relate to quality control scores for patient outcomes?
4. How do patient costs per DRG relate to nursing hours per DRG?
5. Does improvement on quality control measures correlate with increased staff development education hours?
6. Does an increasing productivity level correlate with shifts in quality assurance measures?
7. How do budget cuts affect quality measures?
8. What factors explain budget variances?

A well-designed nursing information system performs nursing service administration research on all sorts of questions. Also, it suggests cures for identified deficiencies. For example, if staffing ratios are found to correlate with quality assurance reports, falling scores in the latter would indicate a need for more nurses.

It is important that the nursing management system be able to correlate managerial and clinical data. It also is useful if the nursing computerized system interfaces with the other systems of the institution. These systems, depending on their capacity, may hold patient data for orders and billing, personnel management systems, inventories of various sorts, and clinical data. Obviously, the more interactions that are possible, the more useful the system is to the nurse executive.

One problem with a sophisticated computerized system may be that it is capable of delivering information overload. The nurse executive may receive so many reports on so many aspects of institutional and divisional operations that it is difficult to get to them all, let alone make appropriate interpretations. When the system produces this sort of overload, the nurse executive will be wise to arrange for data to be processed for her consumption, with summative data, important correlations, and unusual data (management-by-exception) brought to her attention.

When the nursing division lacks its own systems specialist, it is useful to appoint a managerial communications committee to determine answers to the following questions:

1. What information do we need?
2. How can it be programmed into the computerized systems? If it can't be computerized, how else can it be gathered?
3. How should it be processed? Who should get what reports? At what intervals?
4. How should the data be summarized?
5. What evaluations should be made in relation to the data?

Another major problem with a computerized information system is control of access. The system must be designed so that only those who have a right to have the information are able to retrieve it. Issues of patient confidentiality (and staff record confidentiality) are of major concern in designing a system.

The nurse executive will need expert help in learning what can and what cannot be performed by computerized information systems. Essentially, they can handle and correlate easily quantifiable variables of the nurse executive's choosing. Not all computer systems have similar capabilities, so the nurse executive will have to have generalized knowledge about computer systems and also information concerning the specific capabilities of the system in her institution.

If installation of a new computer system is being planned, it is imperative that the nursing division be part of the planning. Otherwise, it is unlikely that anyone will consider the nursing needs that can be served by the system. A computer system is a good example of a sunk cost; once a given system is installed, it is often too late to get services that were not considered when the system was selected. Nursing must plan for its needs and make its requests long before computer purchases or leases are finalized.

Noncomputerized Information System

Not all official communications channels are computerized in the typical nursing division. Other channels include supervisors' reports, head nurses' reports, change-of-shift reports, managers' verbal reports, and whatever other documents are devised in a given nursing system to manage the ongoing work. The importance of these channels for control by nursing management often is overlooked. Even the verbal exchanges can direct activities of subordinates. Let us consider both informal and formal communications channels as they relate to control issues.

The manager controls the perceptions of subordinates by regulating the flow of information that they receive. Even the nurse executive's vocabulary is attention-directing and cue-establishing. The same is true of the corporate lingo. These verbal aspects of the corporate culture and its officers maintain an employee mind-set by supplying the accepted categories and classifications of thought. Attention-directing and cue-establishing communications are unobtrusive but effective means for control.

The manager does not have to change the individual to change his behavior. The manager need change only the premises for the decisions of others. If promotions and other rewards go to those who have the right perspective, for example, the ambitious members will soon adopt the desired perspective.

One way to establish the desired mind-set is the directive use of the questioning technique. Staff members take on the purposes of their managers, not through the philosophy of nursing espoused but through the requirements that are impressed on them in the work situation. The informal use of the question is one of the best devices for establishing desired work and thought patterns. The nurse executive who asks a supervisor, "How are things going?" misses a valuable opportunity for influence. She has lost the chance to convey to the supervisor the kinds of things to be thinking about and acting on in her supervisory role. A question such as "What are you doing about the teaching needs of your Spanish-speaking patients?" is directive.

The nurse executive also can use communication channels for promulgating her philosophy of management and of nursing. Routine report forms provide an excellent set for thinking patterns. For example, the nurse executive who wishes to promote problem solving among her supervisors might structure her weekly supervisory report form as shown in Figure 26–9. However, the nurse executive who is trying to encourage management by objectives (MBO) might use a weekly report form to encourage that mind-set (Figure 26–10). Before the nurse executive has said a word, her required report

systems have directed staff managers into the desired thought patterns. When structured reports are used only at the highest administrative level, one soon finds supervisors using similar forms for input from lower-level staff.

Both the directive question and the carefully constructed communications form control the work that gets performed. Both can be used to establish a mind-set that will reinforce the decisions of the nurse executive.

SUMMARY

This chapter has focused on the nursing administration control system—on the data that are routinely collected, interpreted, and communicated within the nursing division. Collection of data structures the nursing division in that it points out which elements of the environment are considered significant, and that data, once interpreted, initiate changes in the nursing systems. Major sources of administrative control data include patient information, personnel data, reports and records of movements of material, managerial status reports, routine interdivisional communication systems, and financial reports.

SUPERVISOR'S WEEKLY REPORT OF ACTIVITIES		
Problem Situation	Solutions Considered	Present Status of Problem Solving

Figure 26–9 Problem-Oriented Supervisory Report

SUPERVISOR'S WEEKLY REPORT OF ACTIVITIES			
Objective	Planned Activities	Present Status	Evaluation

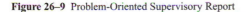

Figure 26–10 MBO-Oriented Supervisory Report

In determining what data to collect, the nurse executive may apply the following criteria:

1. Data are relatively easy to collect.
2. Data are meaningful and necessary to the nursing operations.
3. Data actually are used in making improvements in the nursing system.

What are the purposes of the nursing administration control system? All the following are included:

1. to improve patient care
2. to evaluate the effectiveness of the division as a managerial unit
3. to meet demands of licensure, accreditation, and review by other legal or quasi-legal bodies
4. to protect employees and employer
5. to implement nursing research by identifying deficiencies meriting serious inquiry
6. to facilitate the work process
7. to regulate costs

The nurse executive and her top management staff assume responsibility for maintaining the view of the whole. One way that this responsibility is fulfilled is through careful monitoring of the division's major control systems, which should be organized to provide meaningful feedback on the state of the organization.

The systems should be organized for action, so that corrective measures are determined and implemented when a deficit is identified by the control system. The nurse executive will want to balance her activities over the major control systems of the division in such a way that attention is given to each system in proportion to its significance to the whole. Top management also must consider the performance of the major nursing systems as they relate to each other. This synthesis of data and response is one of the main responsibilities of executive management.

SUGGESTED READINGS

Alexander, J.W., and B. Mark. 1990. Technology and structure of nursing organizations. *Nursing and Health Care* 11, no.4:194–199.

American Nurses Association. 1977. *Standards of rehabilitation nursing practice.* Washington, D.C.: ANA.

American Nurses Association. 1980. *A statement on the scope of medical-surgical nursing practice.* Washington, D.C.: ANA.

American Nurses Association. 1981. *Standards of cardiovascular nursing practice.* Washington, D.C.: ANA.

American Nurses Association. 1981. *Standards of perioperative nursing practice.* Washington, D.C.: ANA.

American Nurses Association. 1985. *The scope of practice of the primary health care nurse practitioner.* Washington, D.C.: ANA.

American Nurses Association. 1985. *Standards of child and adolescent psychiatric and mental health nursing practice.* Washington, D.C.: ANA.

American Nurses Association. 1986. *The role of the clinical nurse specialist.* Washington, D.C.: ANA.

American Nurses Association. 1987. *The scope of nursing practice.* Washington, D.C.: ANA.

American Nurses Association. 1987. *Standards of addictions nursing practice with selected diagnoses and criteria.* Washington, D.C.: ANA.

American Nurses Association. 1987. *Standards of oncology nursing practice.* Washington, D.C.: ANA.

American Nurses Association. 1988. *Computer design criteria for systems that support the nursing process.* Washington, D.C.: ANA.

American Nurses Association. 1990. *Standards of psychiatric consultation-liaison nursing practice.* Washington, D.C.: ANA.

American Nurses Association. 1991. *Standards of clinical nursing practice.* Washington, D.C.: ANA.

American Nurses Association. 1993. *The scope of cardiac rehabilitation nursing practice.* Washington, D.C.: ANA.

Arnold, J.M., and G.A. Pearson. 1993. *Computer applications in nursing education and practice.* New York: National League for Nursing.

Beckham, J. 1993. The architecture of integration. *Healthcare Forum Journal* 36, no.5:56–63.

Benjamin, R., and E. Levinson. 1993. A framework for managing IT change. *Sloan Management Review* 34, no.3:23–34.

Ernst, D.F. 1994. Total quality management in the hospital setting. *Journal of Nursing Care Quality* 8, no.2:1–8.

Flarey, D.L. 1993. Quality improvement through data analysis: Concepts and applications. *Journal of Nursing Administration* 23, no.12:21–37.

Heyden, R., et al. 1990. Development of management for nursing administration. *Nursing and Health Care* 11, no.4:178–182.

Johnson, K., and E.F. Morrison. 1993. Control or negotiation: A health care challenge. *Nursing Administration Quarterly* 17, no.4:27–33.

Jones-Schenk, J., and P. Hartley. 1993. Organizing for communication and integration. *Journal of Nursing Administration* 23, no.10:30–37.

Masters, M.L., and R.J. Masters. 1993. Building total quality management into nursing management. *Nursing Economics* 11, no.5:274–278.

Mathews, J., and K. Zadak. 1993. Managerial decisions for computerized patient care planning. *Nursing Management* 24, no.7:54–56.

Mitchell, P. H. 1993. Perspectives on outcome-oriented care systems. *Nursing Administration Quarterly* 17, no.3:1–7.

Snowdon, A.W., and D. Rajacich. 1993. The challenge of accountability in nursing. *Nursing Forum* 28, no.1:5–11.

27

Quality Management

A quality management system in nursing administration resembles a quality control system for any other field, occupation, or subject matter. It is a system set up to measure the quality of the product of the organization; in this case, the final product is patient care.

Yet, measuring quality of patient care is only one purpose that may be served by a quality management system. Purposes include

- obtaining accurate patient care feedback
- correcting care deficits
- motivating nursing staff to improve patient care
- verifying effectiveness of established nursing processes
- conducting nursing research relating structure, process, and outcome elements and seeking to identify effective nursing methods

Because the field is complex, at least two instrumental products may be measured as well as the primary subject matter of patient care, namely, the quality of nursing practice and the quality of management itself.

Also, three basic domains may be measured for any given subject matter: structure, process, and outcome. Although any domain may be measured for any product, traditions in nursing measurement have followed this practice: The

nursing organization usually is assessed on structure standards, nursing care activities usually are assessed on process standards, and patient status usually is assessed on outcome standards. For simplicity, these common linkages are used.

It is important to gather data from all three arenas when evaluating patient care because of the interlinkages among them. For example, the structures of the organization affect the type of nursing care that is offered, and the type of care affects the patient outcomes achieved.

A word about terminology: When the language used to describe a phenomenon changes, it usually signals a new approach to or perspective on the subject. Nowhere have the linguistic games been more in evidence than in quality management, including the "in" name for the whole endeavor at any given moment.

Originally, nursing used the name adopted from business: *quality control*. This was shortly replaced by a phrase more in keeping with nursing's softer touch, namely, *quality assurance*. Assuring the patient that he received quality care seemed more in keeping with the nursing ideology than did the harsher term *control*.

Later, a philosophy of continuous, ongoing improvement seeped into nursing. It was evident in such other changes as *coaching* instead of performance appraisal. After all, the employee could always do better, even the superstars. Quality circles were popular in this era. In terms of meeting standards, the attempt was always to move closer and closer to the ideal (e.g., fewer patient falls, fewer medication errors). Quality assurance entered the game and became *continuous quality improvement* (CQI).

Eventually, the CQI philosophy gave way to the notion of absolute standards with no exceptions tolerated: the zero errors mentality, the 100 percent conformity standard. CQI now sounded out of step and fell to the more neutral term *quality management*. Among quality control workers there has at times been a fetish to keep up with the changing language. However, by the time this book reaches the public, the language may have changed again. The reader's challenge will be to see what philosophy underlies any such change. For simplicity, the term *quality management* is used in this chapter.

The rest of this chapter attempts to give the nurse executive an understanding of the structure beneath the structure; in other words, it examines how a quality management system is constructed and applied.

SELECTING THE FORM OF STANDARD TO BE USED

The setting of standards is the first step of structuring a quality management system. As previously stated, in setting standards, one can choose to appraise from the perspectives of structure, process, or outcome and from the subject matters of organization, nursing, or patient.

Structure Standards

Until recently, if one looked at the standards used by most accrediting or standards-setting agencies in nursing, such as the American Nurses Association (ANA), the National League for Nursing (NLN), and the Joint Commission on Accreditation of Healthcare Organizations (JCAHO), it was apparent that they selected structure as the area of concern.

Although this pattern is changing—JCAHO, for example, has a decided commitment to a patient outcomes orientation—most standards written by these organizations still follow the structure format. Further, the JCAHO focus on outcomes has enabled it to move toward universal outcomes in which nursing and other services, including medicine, can be judged jointly by a single set of standards. For purposes of clarity, however, we limit our examples and discussion to illustrations more directly related to nursing.

The following standards (in documents, they may be stated as standards or questions) illustrate a structure format:

- A registered nurse is responsible for planning, evaluating, and supervising the nursing care of each patient.
- The nursing department provides ongoing retraining programs for all staff in cardiopulmonary resuscitation.
- Patient assessments are recorded within 24 hours of admission.

All these statements are directed toward assessing the structures by which nursing care is organized and managed, the arrangements by which nursing care is delivered. They examine the established frameworks for the patient care delivery system. Logically, accrediting bodies focus on structure because it is a single entity and stable, whereas nursing processes and patient outcomes are numerous and require an extensive sampling if one were to make judgments concerning them.

An accrediting body seldom has the time for such an extensive survey. For this reason, it tends to concentrate on structure, the only aspect of patient care that is singular and relatively stable. This is why, for example, so many accreditors will say things such as, "If it wasn't charted, it wasn't done." In essence, this means, if the act left no trace on the structure, it cannot be attributed.

Structure-based criteria identify necessary, but not sufficient, conditions for good quality care. It might be necessary for a registered nurse to plan patient care, but the fact that such care is planned by a registered nurse is no assurance that the planning is well done. Retraining in cardiopulmonary resuscitation may be necessary, but just because it is given does not mean the employee will apply it accurately when a need arises.

Criteria based on structure give conditions under which it is likely that good nursing will take place and that good patient outcomes will occur, but such criteria do not ensure that these goals will be achieved. Structure criteria address themselves to the way in which the subject matter is systematized; they evaluate the organizing frameworks.

The following statements illustrate structure standards for the organization, for nursing, and for the patient, respectively:

- *Organization:* There is a fail-safe system for removing outdated supplies from nursing units.
- *Nursing care:* The nursing process is applied in the derivation of patient care plans.
- *Patient*: The amputee has the capacity, motivation, and opportunity to learn ambulation.

Process Standards

Process standards provide a second perspective; they measure the actions taken by the subject matter. Typically applied to nursing care, process standards tell what the nurse will do and how—actual interactions between the nurse and the patient. The nursing process takes place within the providing structure; it is the action rather than the structure in which that action takes place that constitutes process. The primary difference between process and structure standards can be demonstrated by the conversion of a structure standard into a representative process standard.

- *Structure standard:* The nursing department provides ongoing retraining programs for all staff in cardiopulmonary resuscitation.
- *Related process standard:* The staff member demonstrates correct technique in providing cardiopulmonary resuscitation on the teaching mannequin.

The following illustrate process standards for the organization, for nursing, and for the patient, respectively:

- *Organization:* The nursing division reassigns staff on each shift according to the classification system data.
- *Nursing care:* The nurse turns the unconscious patient every 2 hours.
- *Patient:* The diabetic patient accurately tests his urine for sugar and acetone.

Outcome Standards

The outcome standard takes yet another perspective; it measures the result rather than the providing structure or the process used. The difference between a process standard and an outcome standard can best be illustrated by conversion of a process standard to an outcome criterion:

- *Process standard:* Nurse applies dressings with appropriate sterile technique.
- *Related outcome standard:* Patient does not develop a wound infection.

Patient outcome standards represent the ultimate goals of nursing measurement, for if the patient outcome is unsatisfactory, it matters little what nursing processes were used or what organizational arrangement (structure) supported that therapy. Nevertheless, outcome alone is not sufficient as a sole criterion. Outcome represents effectiveness. Ultimately, in nursing management, one must look for efficiency as well as effectiveness. This means that one also must look for the least costly ways of achieving the desired outcome.

The following illustrate outcome standards for the organization, for nursing, and for the patient, respectively:

- *Organization:* Absenteeism is reduced 50 percent.
- *Nursing care:* Every Nurse Clinician III can read and accurately interpret an EKG strip.

- *Patient:* Normal peristalsis is returned by the second postoperative day.

Patient outcome standards can be difficult to isolate from a nursing perspective. Ideally, one would like to be able to determine how much of the patient's health outcome is due to nursing, how much is due to medicine, and how much to other factors. Typically, the patient's health outcome is the result of multiple interacting factors of which nursing only is one. This is one of the reasons that new JCAHO regulations focus on combined service outcomes rather than isolating elements according to each profession.

Even when the effects of the nursing component cannot be isolated, its significance still can be assessed by changes in statistical outcomes that correspond with specific, identified nursing processes. To use outcome standards to assess nursing, given these conditions, means that one accepts the following assumptions: (1) There are some health outcomes primarily attributable to nursing, (2) there are some health outcomes partially attributable to nursing, and (3) regulation of nursing actions can produce statistically improved health outcomes for patients in these categories.

The statistical concept is important here, for no single outcome can be ensured. For example, suppose it is determined that nursing makes a critical difference in the number of surgical wound infections. This does not mean that nurses are responsible for all wound infections. Nor does it mean that the infection of any given patient can be attributed to nursing. The patient might acquire an infection from a variety of sources: the physician's poor technique during surgery, the intern's technique in changing the dressing, ineffective sterilization of dressings, the patient's own interference with the dressing, or nursing technique. Using a better nursing technique should produce a statistical change in the number of wound infections but not an elimination of all infections.

In addition to the problem of multiple causation of health effects, there is a difficulty in establishing desired patient outcome standards that have significance for multiple patients. At one extreme, if patient outcome standards must be developed singly for each patient, then there is no generalized standard against which the nurse may measure her patient's outcome.

With individualized standards, there is no constant measure against which to compare end results for various patients receiving different nursing managements. Some individualization of patient outcomes is done in the nursing care plan document. Even here, however, judgments are based on norms modified to take into account individual patient motivation, capacity, and opportunity.

At the other extreme, some institutions have tried to solve the standards problem by identifying universal standards applicable to all patients. Such a universal standard might read, "Each patient is returned to the optimal physiologic health possible within the constraints of his disease process." Although worthy as goals, such statements are meaningless as operational criteria against which to measure and compare outcomes.

The most useful solution to the outcome standards problem is the middle road, the classification of patients into groups that logically may be expected to have similar desired outcomes. For example, one can easily set a standard that all obstetric patients learn appropriate techniques for feeding and handling the newborn infant. Similarly, one might set a standard that all amputees suffering loss of one leg learn the procedures of safe crutch walking. For all patients with surgical incisions, one might set a standard of first-intention wound healing.

Common standards can be developed for patients grouped by similar diseases and conditions or by similar incapacities. They can be identified for all juvenile diabetics (similar disease) or for all paraplegics (similar incapacities) regardless of the source of their disease process. A taxonomy for the selection of patient groups for quality measures is shown in Table 27–1.

RELATIONSHIPS AMONG THE THREE TYPES OF STANDARDS

The relationship among the three perspectives of evaluation—structure, process, and out-

Table 27–1 Taxonomy for Selection of Patient Groups for Quality Management

Grouping Criterion	Examples
Disease	All new diabetic patients
	Cardiac patients
Like treatment	Preoperative patients
	All patients on renal dialysis
Like needs	Patients with immobility
	Patients with decreased vision
Geographic criterion	All patients in the outpatient clinic
	All patients on this unit
Life stage	All geriatric patients
	All teenagers
Illness stage	All patients needing intensive care
	All self-care patients

come—is self-evident. Failure in meeting an outcome standard may indicate a need for a change in the nursing process; failure in meeting a nursing process standard may indicate a need for changing organizational structure. For example, if several patients develop postoperative infections, a negative outcome, it may be that the staff needs to examine the process of caring for wounds. If nurses are lax in techniques of dressing wounds, it may be that the nursing structure creates pressures causing shortcuts in the proper process. Thus, results of assessments from one of the three perspectives may have implications for another perspective. The following evaluations of a cardiac resuscitation illustrate that all three perspectives can be used to describe the same event:

- *Outcome evaluation:* Patient survived, suffered no irreversible brain damage, and received no physical trauma such as cracked ribs. Patient understands what happened to him and has worked through his reaction to the event.

- *Process evaluation:* Appropriate verification of the state of cardiac arrest was made. Patient was placed on a hard surface. Air passages were checked for obstruction. Cardiac massage and resuscitation were begun immediately.

- *Structure evaluation:* Cardiac board and mechanical respirator were ready at hand in the treatment room. Respirator was equipped and ready for immediate use. Cardiac resuscitation team arrived within 3 minutes. Prearranged standing orders permitted them to provide defibrillation and medication at once.

CONSTRUCTING STANDARDS

After the subject matter to be measured and the type of standard (structure, process, or outcome) have been selected, the next step in quality management is construction of the relevant standards. Because outcome standards are the most difficult to compose, they are reviewed in detail.

The first problem in setting outcome standards is to reach consensus on the meaning of a standard. Two contrasting definitions are frequently used in nursing literature: (1) A standard is a criterion of excellence or attainment, and (2) a standard is a baseline against which to measure the event or behavior. In the first concept, a standard is written in terms of the optimally desired outcome; in the second concept, the lowest acceptable level of outcome is described. Although there is no right or wrong definition of a standard, it is essential that a group know what sort of standards they are composing.

It is important to set realistic goals in realistic time frames for the achievement of standards. Standards set for specified time periods represent the nursing prognoses for the given patient base. One problem in constructing outcome standards is that health outcomes change over time. For certain impairments, there are stages of illness; for others, there is a gradual progression from the initial illness to the final outcome. The setting of standards requires that one determine when outcomes will be measured.

To deal only with final outcome criteria begs the question. Even if a patient ultimately reaches the desired final outcomes, one cannot claim good nursing process if he suffered unnecessarily, had unnecessary side effects, and took longer to achieve the final outcomes than would have been the case with more expert nursing.

Some conditions virtually set their own critical measurement points. For example, most nurses would agree that postpartum patients should be assessed at the completion of the delivery phase and at the time of discharge. Other conditions may require arbitrary setting of times for outcome assessments.

It has been suggested that measurement take place at the end of a certain phase of illness rather than at a given time. The problem here is that the criteria for assessment may be identical to the criteria that mark the end of the given phase of illness. When this is the case, evaluation becomes a tautology: The patient is not out of the phase until he meets the criteria; therefore, he will always meet the criteria if he is measured at the end of the phase. This is one of the big problems in the evaluation of quality management for psychiatric patients.

In formulating outcome standards, it is helpful to classify them on three different axes: (1) attainment or avoidance option, (2) performance or state-of-being option, and (3) absolute or relative option. Consideration of these axes can help in planning adequate and uniform measurement tools.

On the first axis, an outcome standard is either *a state to be attained* or a *state to be avoided*. The standard "maintains normal urinary output" gives a desired attainment, whereas the standard "does not develop a bladder infection" represents an avoidance standard. Some authors of standards prefer to deal strictly with attainment standards; others use both types. Avoidance standards can be converted into attainment standards (e.g., the avoidance standard given above can be converted into "maintains bladder's normal microbial status," an attainment standard).

The second axis for outcome standards indicates whether the outcome is *something the patient does* or a *state he exhibits*. For example, the standard "walks on crutches with a four-point gait" is a performance standard. "Maintains intact skin surfaces," however, is a state-of-being standard. Note that when a desired outcome is a performance (process), then there is a conformity of a patient process objective with a patient outcome objective.

When using performance, it is necessary to differentiate between standards that indicate an *ability to perform* and those that require the *performance itself* rather than the ability. Ability to demonstrate full range of motion of the shoulder joint is adequate measurement of shoulder mobility. The patient's ability to administer insulin accurately, however, may not be an adequate measure if he ignores some doses. Here, the action itself rather than the ability might be measured.

The last axis determines whether the standard is *absolute* or *relative*. The standard "all skin surfaces remain intact" is absolute. In contrast, a relative standard may show progression (e.g., "The patient, following a cardiovascular accident, increases his ability to depress a hard rubber ball with the weakened hand"). This standard is relative because it is measured in relation to the patient's past performance rather than in relation to an absolute measurement of strength. Such a standard could be quantified—the percentage of strength increase per week could be given—but this would not change the fact that the percentage increase would be relative to the patient's past status.

Every outcome standard can be classified along these three axes: attainment or avoidance, performance or state of being, and absolute or relative status. In classifying the standards of a given measurement tool, one finds the biases of the tool's author. Many such tools have a disproportionate number of performance standards, with an inadequate number of state-of-being standards.

One basic problem in composing outcome standards is to know when one really has a patient standard rather than one directed to another agent. Probably the easiest way to judge whether a standard is a patient standard is to apply two rules: When the understood or stated subject of the standard is the nurse, the organization, the patient's family, an event, or anything other than the patient himself or some aspect of his being, it is not a patient standard. When the statement says what someone other than the patient does (e.g., "Patient is turned frequently"), the standard is not a patient standard.

Another problem in composing standards is deciding how specific they should be. The specificity of standard statements is closely related to the scope of content covered in the evaluation tool as well as the nature of that content. For example, if the evaluation tool is measuring all alcoholic patients in the stage of delirium tremens, it is possible to state the desired outcomes with great detail. Similarly, if the subject matter lends itself to easily quantifiable measures (e.g., blood pressure), then standards can be concrete and specific.

For performance standards, the format for behavioral objectives can be used. In contrast, state-of-being standards cannot be stated with action verbs, but they can be given equal specificity and concrete description.

As the scope of content of the evaluation tool broadens, the nature of the standard must change. Suppose one were to try to write outcome standards for obstetric patients who are being discharged. One could easily produce a list of 200 to 300 standards; clearly, this is unwieldy and impractical. For situations such as this, the evaluator reduces standards to a manageable number of critical indicators.

There are several different ways to form standards for a given objective. One may divide the subject matter into its component parts, forming one or more standards for each component. Not every subject matter lends itself to this treatment. Another alternative is to select indices of the whole. In this case, standards are addressed to critical points rather than to the totality of components. For example, feeding, diapering, and handling might be critical points in the physical aspects of mothering a newborn infant. Although these are not the only elements in care of the newborn, they would be sufficiently significant indices when it is not practical to measure all potential aspects.

A third alternative forms standards by the use of illustrations rather than indices or components. This method is used when the objective is a principle that has many different instantiations. By using examples rather than components or indices, the reader is taught to recognize an instantiation of the principle, even if it differs somewhat from those of the multiple illustrations. Consider a standard such as, "Patient shows positive response to staff interaction." Because there are many diverse ways in which a patient could show a positive response and it is not possible to identify each potential behavior, a list of illustrative responses can alert the evaluator to look for certain kinds of response.

Standards should be few enough in number not to overwhelm the evaluator and should be worded to encourage similar interpretations by different evaluators. Behavioral objectives are appropriate for some cases but will not suffice when differences in performance are allowable or when states of being rather than performances are the subject matter of inquiry.

Frequently, a standard is accompanied by the statement of a rationale. Unfortunately, so-called rationales often turn out to be explanations of the standard. Appropriately used, a rationale is a justification, not an explanation; it should tell why the preceding statement is important enough to be chosen as a standard and should not merely restate or explain the standard.

FORMATS FOR QUALITY MANAGEMENT TOOLS

Once the standards have been determined, a general format for the tool itself must be prepared. A rule to follow is to keep the format simple, easy to use, and easy to interpret. Some common formats are shown in Figure 27–1.

Format 1 is the least likely to produce different opinions among raters, but it requires each standard be defined precisely. Format 2 has the disadvantage of eliciting greater variation in raters' responses. Format 3 has the same disadvantage but may be useful for quantifying answers. Quantification has the advantage of promoting competition among nursing units or of permitting the nursing unit to surpass its previous grade. When using numerical ratings, one should not exceed the number of differentiations that can be made accurately; it is unlikely,

1. Standards	Met	Unmet	Not observed	Comments
Long-range goals written on Kardex				

2. Standards	Excellent	Good	Fair	Poor	Not applicable

3. Standards	1	2	3	4	5

4. Standards	Above Average	Average	Below Average

5. Standards category	First descriptive statement	Second descriptive statement	Third descriptive statement
Patient teaching	Patient has received no teaching	Patient has received some teaching but does not adequately understand material	Patient has received thorough teaching and understands what was taught

6. Standards	Frequently	Infrequently	Never

Figure 27–1 Formats for Quality Management Tools

for example, that an evaluator can actually differentiate among ten levels.

Format 4 has the advantage of stability, for as the average improves in an institution, the form is still applicable. Format 5 is the most difficult to construct but permits identification of specific levels of nursing care. Notice that in this particular example, two elements rather than one are combined in the standard: teaching and learning.

Often attempts to combine two or more elements fail. One can identify options that are not given in the illustrated format (e.g., "Patient receives poor teaching but learns anyway" or "Patient has received thorough teaching but adamantly refuses to learn"). It is suggested that each standard deal with a single element as it varies over the continuum of gradations.

Format 6 is used when the quality of the standard is not as important as the frequency with which it is carried out. Percentages of time may be substituted for descriptive terms using indicators such as frequently, occasionally, or seldom. When descriptions rather than numbers are used, the results can still be converted to scores so that data can be interfaced with other information in the nursing management system.

SOURCES OF EVIDENCE

Once the standards and format for the quality assessment tool have been determined, the next step is to identify the sources of evidence. Primary and secondary sources are usually combined, but when possible, primary sources are preferable. (Often, secondary sources are substituted because of the cost of obtaining primary data.) A primary source gives the rater direct knowledge concerning the standard.

For example, if a standard states, "Patient receives adequate oral hygiene," the rater goes to the source, the patient, to observe whether this standard is fulfilled. For the standard, "Emergency equipment is complete and ready for use," the observer again goes directly to the source, evaluating the equipment first-hand.

Not all standards lend themselves to immediate observation. "Promotion of independence" might require a careful evaluation of the patient over a period of time. Some standards combine primary and secondary sources: "Adequate hydration is maintained" might combine direct observation of the skin turgor with secondary observation of the intake and output records.

The patient's chart is such a frequent secondary source that evaluation of nursing via the chart often is either included in the quality check or developed separately as a nursing chart audit. But a chart is not an entirely reliable secondary source, for it is possible that nurses write things they do not do—or do things they do not write. Nevertheless, the chart is a popular secondary source because of easy access to it and because it is relatively easy to evaluate.

Another source of evidence is the patient's response to (satisfaction or dissatisfaction with) his nursing care. It is important that a group forming a quality management system determine ahead how relevant patient satisfaction is as evidence of professional care. Wording of questions to patients is quite important. Some questions can be worded to give more reliable responses: "Did the nurse discuss your surgery with you the day before the operation?" Others cannot be given similar weight: "Are you generally pleased with your nursing care?" The following sources are the most frequently used in quality management checks: charts, rounds, records, nursing care plans, interviews of patients, interviews of nurses, and interviews of other health personnel or of the patient's family.

It is important that methods of evaluation be specified for each standard. If five evaluators were told to rate blind patients in a rehabilitation unit according to the standard "Ambulates safely in known territory," it is conceivable that without further direction the evaluators might use five different methods to rate a patient:

1. noting the patient's performance on the standard as recorded in his chart
2. asking several nurses about the patient's ambulation
3. asking the patient about his ambulation
4. observing the patient for several days as he ambulates on the unit and grounds

5. giving the patient a specific test, such as telling him "Go to the solarium and get X"

Clearly, some of these evaluation methods are better than others, but the point is that uses of evidence must be identified if standards are to be judged equitably. The selection of methods often is a compromise between the ideal and the economic in time or effort.

SURVEILLANCE AND FEEDBACK SYSTEMS

Once the standards have been completed for a project, consideration is given to setting up the surveillance system.

It is important that the measurement form be used in a systematic way. One needs to determine who will evaluate what at what times. Answers to these questions must be based on the institution's needs, but the following guidelines have proved useful:

1. Schedule evaluation visits at periodic, unannounced intervals. The unexpected visit is more likely to reflect the normal quality of nursing care.
2. Not all patients of a given class need be evaluated; a sampling technique is adequate in most cases.
3. Patient sampling may be performed at random, or patients may be selected on the basis of which ones require challenging nursing care.
4. Persons should serve on the evaluation team long enough to become thoroughly familiar with the evaluation process.
5. If evaluation team members split the work, each member should grade the same portion of the checklist on all units evaluated.
6. When a surveillance system monitors several quality measurement projects, the evaluations of a given subject matter should be recycled according to need.

The final component of quality management is that of corrective action. A quality management system is useless if proper and immediate feedback is not offered to the nursing units involved. It is more productive, however, to have the staff view quality management as a challenge than as a threat. Supervisors and head nurses can be counseled to see the program as a diagnostic tool more easily if they have an integral part in it.

The feedback from process and outcome standards differs. Process standards immediately identify the deviant nursing process, the practice that fails to conform. That is not the case with outcome standards. Outcome standards tell what is going wrong in the patient's progress, but they do not tell what is wrong in the nursing process or how to correct it.

Outcome standards serve as starting points for research into nursing process because they do not assume that traditional nursing measures are the proper solutions to patient outcome problems. The research design for determining the cause of an undesirable patient outcome requires use of the scientific method, formulation of hypotheses, identification of possible variables, and systematic manipulation of variables until the cause of the undesirable outcome is identified and a corrective solution is found.

When the same subject matter is subjected to both outcome and process standards, it may be possible to establish correlations between them. Figure 27–2 illustrates a tool in which outcome and process have been systematically correlated.

In this tool, the nursing processes deduced to have impact on each desired patient outcome have been systematically correlated. Yet, it has been determined that the anticipated relations have not always occurred. Some interesting conclusions can be drawn from data such as those collected in Figure 27–2. In this illustration, the processes that were assumed to be critical to Patient Outcome A were not all essential because the patient goal was achieved even though Nursing Process 3 was not met. Processes 1 and 2 alone seem to be adequate for achievement of the goal. (However, these data do not guarantee that processes 1 and 2 are actually required for

QUALITY CONTROL TOOL SUMMARY SHEET

STANDARDS	MET	NOT MET
Patient Outcome Standard A	✗	
Related Nursing Process Standard 1	✗	
Related Nursing Process Standard 2	✗	
Related Nursing Process Standard 3		✗
Patient Outcome Standard B	✗	
Related Nursing Process Standard 1	✗	
Related Nursing Process Standard 2	✗	
Related Nursing Process Standard 3	✗	
Related Nursing Process Standard 4	✗	
Patient Outcome Standard C		✗
Related Nursing Process Standard 1	✗	
Related Nursing Process Standard 2		✗
Related Nursing Process Standard 3	✗	
Related Nursing Process Standard 4	✗	

Figure 27–2 Quality Measurement Relating Outcome and Process

goal achievement, which could have been due to variables not identified in this tool.)

Patient Outcome B is achieved when all the identified nursing processes are supplied. Here, again, it can be assumed that these processes are sufficient to achieve the outcome, although it cannot be asserted that all are necessary or that any particular one is necessary. Patient Outcome C appears to have identified a nursing process that is associated with the outcome: Even when all the other nursing processes required were provided, the desired patient outcome was not reached in the absence of Nursing Process 2. Process 2, therefore, appears to be necessary for goal achievement. Although such conclusions only can be tentative because unidentified variables may enter the situation in each case, it is likely that such correlated quality measurement will lead to identification of valuable hypotheses for nursing research. Obviously, the link between quality management and research is direct.

If research is to be done, all nurses caring for involved patients must follow prescribed care protocols; inconsistent care (use of different methods) proscribes correlating care and outcome. Today's care maps provide for such continuity.

COMPARISON OF QUALITY MANAGEMENT AND TASK ANALYSIS SYSTEMS

Task analysis is the second assessment technique presently used in nursing. The task analysis method of measuring reveals the influence of systems analysis on nursing; it measures only the nursing process. With this technique, systems analysts, using time studies, establish time norms for the most common nursing tasks. These norms are specific for the institution under investigation.

Such studies are of practical value in establishing criteria for distribution of staff or of patients. Time studies usually reveal that certain tasks are significant in determining patient nursing care hours and that other tasks are inconsequential. Drug distribution, for example, seldom affects patient care hours, whereas presence of a Levine tube usually is related directly to increased nursing hours.

Quality management and task analysis are useful tools for the nurse administrator, provided their purposes are not confused with each other. Quality management identifies instances when particular nursing teams are more productive of good care than are similar teams in similar circumstances. It may recognize appropriate nursing models for study and imitation. Although the task analysis method indicates failures of a nursing team to carry the expected number of tasks, it has no means of identifying group excellence in care. Table 27–2 compares some of the critical differences in purpose between the two systems.

Nursing measurement systems are the necessary basis for evaluation, research, and change in nursing practice. They enable the profession to compare nursing from one institution to another. Quality management systems and task analysis systems are the beginning of a real data base for nursing.

ADMINISTRATIVE ASPECTS

Because it takes evaluation expertise to construct and refine measurement tools, quality assurance often is placed in the hands of a specialized department or at least in the hands of a testing and evaluation expert. Sometimes, the quality assurance function is combined in a department with the nursing research function because both require knowledge of tool construction and research practices. In other instances, the quality function is linked with risk management because both are monitoring projects.

However the expertise is supplied, quality management must be done. To have tools revised by the experts does not imply that others are eliminated from the process of quality assurance. Often, the clinicians are the best source for establishing criteria.

When evaluation expertise is not available, an institution may elect to use tools created elsewhere and marketed for nursing groups. Others may make this choice if it is assessed to be the best way to achieve productivity in quality assurance.

When multi-institution corporations contain many nursing divisions, it is usually preferable that these divisions use the same tools to measure quality control. In this way, it is possible to collect comparable data and to explore for effects from institutional variables on the quality of care.

Because quality is a goal for every aspect of an institution's performance, sometimes nursing quality management is not separated out but administered under an institutional department of quality management. The best institutional arrangements may vary from organization to organization. As accreditors move in the direction of combining all elements of care and evaluation, it is likely that more institutions will move in this direction as well, making the quality management administrative unit institutionwide rather than distributed over various divisions.

SUMMARY

Creation of a quality management system, although oversimplified, can be summarized in the following steps:

- Have a purpose.
- Decide what areas to evaluate.
- Identify standards.
- Select a format and construct the tool.
- Set up a surveillance system.
- Set up a feedback system.
- Develop a system for change.

Table 27–2 Comparison of Task Analysis and Quality Management Systems

Points of Comparison	Task Analysis System	Quality Management System
Aim of the system	Fairly distribute nursing tasks	Evaluate the quality of care
Basic criterion	What is being done	What *ought* to be done
Concept of nursing	Nursing is a series of specific tasks	Different theories can be used
Deviations from the norm	Instances when a team completes more or less than the norm	Instances of exceptional nursing, both good and bad
Perspective	What happens in the delivery system	What happens to the patient

SUGGESTED READINGS

Al-Assaf, A.F., and J.A. Schmele. 1993. *The textbook of total quality in healthcare.* New York: National League for Nursing.

Ammentorp, W. 1991. *Quality assurance for long-term care providers.* Newbury Park, Calif.: Sage Publications.

Anderson, M.A., and L.B. Helms. 1994. Quality improvement in discharge planning: An evaluation of factors in communication between health care providers. *Journal of Nursing Care Quality* 8, no.2:62–72.

Bechtel, G., et al. 1993. A continuous quality improvement approach to medication administration. *Journal of Nursing Care Quality* 7, no.3:28–34.

Blackburn, R., and B. Rosen. 1993. Total quality and human resources management: Lessons learned from Baldrige award-winning companies. *Academy of Management Executive* 7, no.3:29–66.

Bulau, J.M. 1989. *Quality assurance policies and procedures for home health care.* Gaithersburg, Md.: Aspen Publishers, Inc.

Dineman, J., ed. 1992. *Continuous quality improvement in nursing.* Washington, D.C.: American Nurses Association.

Ernst, D.F. 1994. Total quality management in the hospital setting. *Journal of Nursing Care Quality* 8, no.2:1–8.

Fielding, J., et al. 1990. Exploratory project for development of nursing outcome criteria in long term care. *The Journal of the New York State Nurses Association* 21, no.3:19–23.

Green, E., and J. Katz. 1993. Practice guidelines: A standard whose time has come. *Journal of Nursing Care Quality* 8, no.1: 23–32.

Jacobs, R. 1993. TQM—More than a dying fad? *Fortune* 128, no.9:66–68, 72.

Jones, K.R. 1991. Maintaining quality in a changing environment. *Nursing Economics* 9, no.3:159–170.

Keenan, M.J., et al. 1993. Polarity management for quality care: Self-direction and manager direction. *Nursing Administration Quarterly* 18, no.1:23–29.

Krishnan, R., et al. 1993. In search of quality improvement: Problems of design and implementation. *Academy of Management Executive* 7, no.4:7–20.

Masters, M.L., and R.J. Masters. 1993. Building total quality management into nursing management. *Nursing Economics* 11, no.5:274–278.

Mitty, E.L., ed. 1994. *Mechanisms of quality in long-term care: Education.* New York: National League for Nursing.

Smith, P., et al. 1994. Planning for patient care redesign: Success through continuous quality improvement. *Journal of Nursing Care Quality* 8, no.2:73–80.

Strickland, O.L., and C.F. Waltz. 1988. *Measurement of nursing outcomes—Measuring nursing performance: Practice education and research.* Vol. 2. New York: Springer Publishing Co., Inc.

Waltz, C.F., and O.L. Strickland. 1988. *Measurement of nursing outcomes—Measuring client outcomes.* Vol. 1. New York: Springer Publishing Co., Inc.

White, L. 1993. Quality improvement consumer influence on perioperative services. *AORN Journal* 58, no.1:96–101.

Woodyard, L.W., and J.E. Sheetz. 1994. Critical pathway patient outcomes: The missing standard. *Journal of Nursing Care Quality* 8, no.2:51–57.

28

Performance Appraisal System

The performance appraisal system is part of an important feedback loop to provide the nurse executive with information about how well the organization is doing. With a well-articulated program, a performance appraisal system is an efficient means of gauging success. The performance appraisal system not only provides information about individual staff members but, in the aggregate, provides information about the accomplishment of objectives.

The performance appraisal system works best when there are clearly articulated goals and organizational expectations. A good performance appraisal system samples the range of outcomes to make sure that these goals have been met. In a well-expounded nursing program, the philosophy of care, the culture, the kinds of relationships that are expected, the values by which the organization lives, the organizational structure, and the standards by which outcomes of care are measured will be in place and guide the appraisals.

For example, if the nursing program were built around Orem's self-care theory, certain expectations would be different than if the program was built around Martha Roger's work. Nursing theories such as Orem's self-care come alive if the appraisal system supports the goals, appraising the staff on their ability to achieve them. The performance appraisal system becomes a continual benchmark for the nurse executive in determining just where the organization stands in aggregate performance.

The performance appraisal system is one of the main control systems of the nursing division, regulating individual employee behaviors by measuring them against and modifying them according to specified job standards. For the performance appraisal system to be effective, the nurse executive must consider all its elements: (1) input—the employee's behavior on hire or before evaluation; (2) thruput—those structures designed to modify and/or direct his behavior; (3) output—the employee's behavior after exposure to the thruput; and (4) feedback and control—the performance appraisal and the subsequent employee coaching and counseling.

This chapter reviews the performance appraisal system, the formats used for recording performance, the techniques of interview, and discipline elements in appraisal. Whether the nurse executive is using these elements to appraise those directly beneath her in the organization chart or whether she is guiding development of the comprehensive performance appraisal system, the knowledge will be essential.

THE STAFF BEHAVIOR SYSTEM

The term *performance appraisal system* is used here although appraisal is only part of the cybernetic system to regulate staff behavior. To look at the totality, a systems approach is used. First, one establishes goals. What does the nurse executive expect from the system, and in what way does performance appraisal contribute to those goals? Almost any nurse executive would be delighted if her staff behavior system accomplished the objectives of making satisfactory workers better, ridding the system of unsatisfactory workers, and improving the distribution of merit pay.

When performance appraisal is seen as an isolated entity, a form to be filled out once a year for employees with seniority, and more frequently for those who are new to the institution, these three objectives are not addressed. An appraisal system rightfully is more than a form: It tells who will do what, with whom, in what manner, when, and for what purpose.

Making Satisfactory Workers Better

Making satisfactory workers better is a good place to start. Satisfactory workers include everyone from employees who are just meeting baseline performance standards to those employees who give an exceptional level of performance. The objective of making all these workers better is optimistic, for it assumes that everyone can improve continuously year by year.

There is both truth and fiction in this assumption. Theoretically, it is always possible to conceive of one more ability a good employee might acquire even though he may already be excellent. However, managers talk about persons who are working at their maximum capacity. The real question is not whether the assumption of continuous improvement is true or false but whether it is an assumption effective for improving the work of most or even many workers.

This assumption has one important virtue: It treats everyone alike. If everyone is expected to set goals and work toward improvement, no one can say that it is unreasonable to expect it of him. The assumption of ongoing improvement becomes the underpinning for a complete system in which workers expect their faults and

deficiencies to be a focus of attention. It is expected that improvement of faults or acquisition of new capabilities will be goals for all employees.

If the goal of making satisfactory workers better is to serve as a goal, what components must the appraisal system contain? The following are logical components:

- The employee and his immediate supervisor must know what behaviors are expected of the employee. (*Goals*)
- The employee and his supervisor must know what behaviors the employee exhibits. (*Feedback*)
- The employee and his supervisor must be able to see where the employee's behavior fails to meet the requisite behavior pattern. (*Assessment and evaluation*)
- The employee and his supervisor must explore ways to change the employee's behavior. (*Adjustment*)
- The employee and his supervisor must agree on a plan for altered behavior. (*Adjustment*)
- The employee must put the plan into action. (*Adjustment*)
- The employee's changed behaviors must be compared with the original behaviors. (*Feedback*)

In a system designed to make satisfactory workers perform better, performance appraisal is a means rather than an end. Appraising the performance is only part of a cybernetic loop that also includes an adjustment component. For this purpose, the system uses a coaching process of employee counseling much like that used in training athletes: careful study of the employee's present behaviors and purposeful, practiced change in behavior to improve performance.

What are the responsibilities of the nurse executive, the evaluating supervisor, and the employee? First, the nurse executive sees to it that adequate job descriptions exist that identify desired behaviors. She must also see that adequate orientation to the requirements of each job is provided to all nurse managers and their employees. This is particularly important in an era when many new positions are being created. Each employee must be made aware of the goals for one in his position.

The nurse executive has responsibility for seeing that her nurse managers consistently use the coaching process. Coaching requires greater skills than does the typical appraisal process. One way for the nurse executive to teach the coaching process is through her own use of it with the employees she evaluates. Also, managerial training in the process is essential.

What are the responsibilities of an evaluating supervisor? They are knowledge of the job requirements for each employee under her direction and initiation of upward mobility for workers if warranted by improved performance. If promotion is not possible, given licensure and certification laws, and the employee has met all required job behaviors, then the supervisor is responsible for helping the employee determine appropriate new behavioral goals to enhance performance of the given job.

A supervisor must accept responsibility for developing skill in assessing and interviewing. Each supervisor must create the opportunity for close observation of each employee immediately under her direction; she must know the performance patterns of each employee she is to evaluate. No supervisor should have to manage more persons than she can observe and assess. When coaching is not based on accurate assessment, it should not be used. If a nurse executive expects coaching to be performed, then she must plan for a reasonable span of control for each manager. Coaching should be performed by the manager who is most familiar with the worker's behavior, the employee's immediate supervisor by whatever title.

Most employees enjoy coaching-based evaluation. Usually, it is rewarding to the employee to see himself continuously acquiring new skills and abilities. Some employees, however, resent this approach. When a competent employee is unwilling to put more effort into improvement on the job, he may see the coaching process as an unwarranted intrusion. In this case, the supervisor may need to use a different approach.

As a general rule, however, the coaching process is a singularly effective means of making satisfactory workers better. In the coaching process, performance appraisal is an essential step, but only one step. Performance appraisal is subordinated to the setting of behavioral standards and the planned alteration of work behaviors to meet those standards.

Dismissal of Unsatisfactory Workers

How would a performance appraisal system be designed to get rid of unsatisfactory workers? The coaching process is a good start, for it documents and compares required and exhibited behaviors. Also, it offers the worker an opportunity to change his behavior by setting specific behavioral goals with target dates and review periods. The coaching process alone, however, is only part of a dismissal system.

It is important not to overlook the legal, contractual, or quasilegal considerations involved in dismissing an employee. The employer has no right to be capricious and arbitrary in firing an employee, and in today's economy, a dismissed employee may seek legal counsel.

When a dismissal case goes to grievance or arbitration, the nurse executive must be certain to avoid the most common sources of failure:

- when the charges on which the dismissal rests are not proved
- when the charge is not sufficient to warrant the severity of the punishment (i.e., dismissal)
- when the cause of the firing is unrelated to job performance
- when the proper disciplinary procedures were not followed

One way to avoid these errors is to abdicate supervisory responsibility and tolerate the poor employee. One hears supervisors claim, "It is not possible to get rid of a poor employee here." In most cases, this is another way of saying that the supervisor is not willing to go to the trouble of getting rid of a poor employee.

Sometimes, a supervisor perceives lack of support by the nurse executive when, in fact, she has placed the nurse executive in a position in which the only reasonable action is to rescind a dismissal. No nurse executive is going to let a losing case go to grievance or arbitration. What is really needed between supervisor and nurse executive is a tacit agreement that the supervisor will do her homework on a firing. When the supervisor has followed appropriate channels and procedures, the nurse executive must support her managerial right to make the dismissal decision.

Failing to Prove Charges

One dismissal error occurs when a supervisor fails to prove the charges on which the decision rests. Proof for a firing need not be as explicit as proof in a court of law, but there must be a preponderance of evidence supporting the supervisor's position.

The first question concerns the facts of the case. What really happened? Most firings are the result of cumulative poor performances rather than the result of a single dramatic error. This means that the supervisor must be able to prove past as well as present poor behavior; there must be documented proof of past behaviors.

In addition to proof of facts, there may be questions of interpretation. The wise supervisor will have elicited the interpretations of all parties involved so that she may be able, if required, to substantiate her own interpretation and to refute those interpretations that label the offending behavior as acceptable.

The supervisor bases her case on the employee's actions and their consequences, not on the employee's intentions. One can be certain that a malicious intention will have become a benign one by the time the employee explains it to a third party. The supervisor should not focus on an employee's intentions but stick to the behavior and its consequences.

For discipline to be implemented, the supervisor must document her judgments and actions and those of her employees. Each supervisor must be held accountable for accurately, objectively, and consistently documenting poor performance.

Mismatch between Charge and Punishment

Another error occurs when the charge is not judged sufficient to warrant dismissal. It is hardly a new principle that the punishment should fit the crime. Errors occur when the supervisor does the firing in anger without weighing the punishment and the crime, or more commonly, when the employee's provoking behavior was simply the last straw. If previous poor behaviors have not been documented adequately in the disciplinary record, the single last straw is not likely to stand on its own.

It is particularly frustrating when one looks back at the problem employee's record and finds that he always was rated as average or above average. Such appraisals inevitably cause a hearing officer or arbitrator to reverse a dismissal decision that appears to rest on a single incident.

The nurse executive should make herself familiar with the performance-rating habits of each supervisor. If a supervisor routinely inflates evaluations, she should challenge the supervisor or reeducate her.

Firings Unrelated to Job Performance

Sometimes an inexperienced supervisor dismisses an employee seen as troublesome because of holding a high union role or fires an employee whose private lifestyle is considered offensive. Obviously, there is no way a nurse executive can support such dismissals. However, the opposite condition does not hold: These employees should not be protected if they actually are failing at the work. If the supervisor has good evidence of the employee's failings, she will be able to refute a claim that the firing was not performance-related.

Failure to Use Disciplinary Procedures

Another error in dismissal cases occurs when proper disciplinary procedures are not followed. Discipline and dismissal policies must be written policies. When a disciplinary system is not formalized, an arbitrator usually will accept the following series of actions as reasonable. The series can be used as a protocol for a formal policy:

- *verbal warning:* anecdotal notes to be kept by the supervisor
- *written notice:* on a standard form, with a copy to the employee
- *suspension* (usually two days to two weeks): this should not be given at the time of the offense, but later, so that the employee has time to submit a grievance over the suspension if he desires to do so
- *dismissal*

Failure to follow the appropriate disciplinary procedure as published and practiced in the institution or failure to follow a reasonable course of action as outlined above will leave the executive or arbitrator no choice but to rescind a dismissal. A word about suspension: Some employees tend to regard a suspension as a welcome vacation rather than a discipline. The supervisor must make clear the function of suspension as a step toward dismissal.

The disciplinary sequence may be bypassed in exceptional cases; some behaviors warrant immediate dismissal. These include instances in which the employee's behavior presents a clear danger to patients and other employees, involves illegal acts, or presents a case of insubordination.

Employment is a quasicontract in which the employee agrees to perform assigned tasks that fall within the scope of his job description. In return, the employing agency agrees to give him remuneration. The employing agency retains the right to select those assigned tasks; after all, that is what the agency is paying for. Provided these acts fall reasonably within the scope of the job description, the employee has no right to refuse to do them. Refusal constitutes a breaking of the contract between the two parties. Thus, insubordination, the refusal to carry out a legitimate assignment, is a case of self-firing. The employee breaks the contract and has no right to expect further benefit from the employing agency.

The most common case of insubordination in nursing occurs when an employee refuses assignment to a floor other than his regular one. If the assignment is substantially the same, as when an employee is moved from one medical-surgical floor to another medical-surgical floor, the employee has no right to refuse the assignment except for contract agreements. Nor can the supervisor afford to yield management prerogative because an employee refuses to accept a legitimate assignment. Many employees are unaware that a refusal of this sort constitutes grounds for dismissal. He should be informed of the nature and seriousness of his proposed refusal.

Cases tried under the Labor Management Relations Act have established that an employer has a fundamental right to assign employees to positions which he deems, in the exercise of his managerial discretion, to be most expedient. The supervisor cannot let patient needs take a back seat to employee preferences or perceived rights. The employer has the right to move personnel. From the employee's narrow perception, movement to another floor may appear unfair, but the supervisor cannot let such special interests work to the detriment of the organization.

Nor do employees have the right to change their work performance in rebellion to placement changes. Employees have the right to strike, but they have no right to continue working on their own terms while rejecting the standards desired by their employer. The supervisor must maintain control of assignments and demand that standards be met.

When disciplinary policies are not followed closely, one is certain to lose disputed cases of dismissal. Also, if common practice in an institution is to be more lenient than the written policy, then a nurse executive may lose a dismissal case that follows the official policy. Common practice is the standard to which the supervisor and nurse executive will be held if a case is contested.

Suppose, for example, the nurse executive wishes to implement a discipline policy strictly, when past supervisory policy has been lax. She first must notify every employee of the intention to enforce the policy. This must be performed in a way that ensures calling the change to everyone's attention. A notice on an overloaded and ignored communal bulletin board will not suffice in any subsequent grievance or arbitration case.

Consistency is also required in applying performance appraisal. Supervisors cannot differ in degree of strictness and laxity. If a disciplinarian fires an employee who fails to measure up to her standards, the employee will be retained if an arbitrator finds that other supervisors would not have fired him. What rules in any hearing is general practice, and if general practice is a low standard of work, the supervisor who is trying to improve standards alone will lose every time.

It is the obligation of the nurse executive to see that a uniform high standard of practice is enforced. She cannot afford to keep inefficient supervisors; their inaction ties the hands of the effective supervisors.

Another problem with uniformity of practice is the fact that no arbitrator will uphold a disciplinary action against an employee for a fault he shares with the supervisor. For example, if a supervisor is chronically late for work, she cannot discipline an employee for tardiness. The supervisor is supposed to be a role model, and her own record must be good before she can criticize a subordinate.

Unfortunately, one of the most common employee performance failures today relates to employee use of drugs. Because drug dependency has become frequent, it is important that an institution have a standing policy concerning how to deal with this situation. In creating such a policy, several different circumstances must be considered:

- Does the employee's behavior (use of a drug or drugs) decrease his ability to do a job or does it just do damage to the employee himself? Obviously, decreased ability to reason endangers patients.
- Does the employee's drug use involve illegal theft of institutional drugs? The nurse executive needs legal advice concerning how this is to be handled in her state. Legal requirements should be stated in the policy.
- If the employee holds a professional license, what are the mechanisms that must be used in reporting the problem to the licensing authority?

- What mechanisms, if any, are locally available for rehabilitation? What evidence of rehabilitation is acceptable for returning the employee to his position?
- What right does the employee have to refuse rehabilitation? If rehabilitation is rejected, how does this affect his vulnerability to dismissal?
- Which drug-related offenses call for immediate dismissal? Which call for rehabilitation and opportunity to return to work?

Creation of a policy for drug-dependent employees is not a simple matter. Note the difference between these cases:

- Employee A is known to staff to be a drug offender. However, when under the influence of drugs, the employee calls in ill. He has never reported to duty under the influence of the drug. However, he has disrupted the unit work by his frequent sick calls and the fact that one cannot count on his presence on assigned days.
- Employee B has been caught giving patients half-doses of ordered narcotics, while administering remainders to herself. Her judgment concerning nursing care has not seemed to be diminished by her use of drugs, but her patients have received inadequate analgesia.
- Employee C was found sniffing various anesthetic gases in the obstetrics department. She was discovered by a nurses' aide, disoriented and confused when she was the only nurse on duty in the labor and delivery suite.

Obviously, any standing policy should give definitive answers for handling these cases and others that can be envisioned. The policy must also deal carefully with the rights of the institution and of the individual. For example, does the institution have the right to inspect the arms of a nurse who chronically wears long sleeves and is suspected of mainlining drugs? Any rights asserted by the institution should be made known to prospective employees on hire. Even here, one walks a fine line between employer rights and the personal rights of the employee as a citizen.

The nurse executive will want to consult the institution's lawyers in devising a policy for the drug-impaired employee. The problem has become so widespread that many texts are available to the executive on this problem as well as its policy implications.

What, then, are the requirements of a performance appraisal system that works to get rid of unsatisfactory workers? The nurse executive needs a disciplinary policy that is clear and unambiguous, effectively communicated, and uniformly and consistently applied. When such a policy and its implementation are combined with accurate assessment of employee behaviors and coaching toward required behavioral change, then the performance appraisal system will accomplish the objective of eliminating unsatisfactory work.

Improving the Distribution of Merit Pay

To talk about merit pay, it first must be differentiated from a yearly increment, a cost of living raise, or any other salary adjustment based on a principle other than merit. To call a yearly increment a merit raise does not make it so. Arbitration cases have ruled in favor of employees when supervisors have tried to withhold yearly raises on the grounds that the employee does not merit it. If it is practice for every employee to receive a yearly raise, then it is not a merit raise.

A merit raise is financial compensation for performance above and beyond expectations. It may take the form of a one-time-only bonus or it may be in the form of an addition to the hourly, weekly, or monthly earning rate of the employee. When a merit raise takes the latter form, the nurse executive must realize that even a minimal merit award can be a substantial financial increment, for it will be paid every subsequent year in which the worker is employed by the institution by virtue of its incorporation into the base pay rate.

A merit raise also tends to increase other increments. When the yearly increment or the Christmas bonus or any other award is calculated as a percentage of the base salary, the merit raise will also increase these awards. In other words, merit raises are serious business and should not be handed out without careful consideration.

Because a merit increase is a reward for service above and beyond that expected or required on the job, the first requirement is a system that identifies employees who do exceed the expected job behaviors. Once again, the careful appraisal, which is part of the coaching process, can provide the answer. It is important that merit raises be tied to specific, identified job behaviors and accomplishments. Otherwise, they tend to become popularity awards. Most unions are suspicious of variable merit raises for just this reason.

Merit awards should require documented proof of superior performance just as discipline requires documented proof of performance below the standards. Identification of employee behaviors that exceed behavioral standards will not solve all the problems of merit pay. The nurse executive still must weigh the nature of each outstanding performance and the concrete accomplishments that can be attributed to that performance. She also must determine how to distribute merit pay among outstanding employees in all job classifications. Performance appraisal of job-related behaviors will provide a logical and defensible basis for making fund distribution decisions.

APPRAISING PERFORMANCE

In appraising performance of a subordinate, it is important to use as many sources of evidence as possible. Selected sources should be easy to use, valid, reliable, and objective.

First, one must ask what performance is to be identified? Is it the performance the employee evidences at *this* time? Or the performance norm that he has demonstrated over the past 6 months or year? Obviously, the data may differ. Both time frames have advantages and disadvantages. Although an evaluation of present performance is more contemporary, there are some employees who are lax 9 months out of 12, only giving performance of quality around the time of evaluation.

However, a normative judgment over a sustained period of time does not give recognition for real learning and improvement that is ongoing. An employee who has worked sincerely to improve performance may be discouraged when his rating is a gradation between past poor performance and present good performance that he has worked hard to achieve.

Most performance appraisal systems are designed to report normative behavior over a span of time. This perspective will be used here; it requires systematic appraisal throughout the performance period. Indeed, this is a major managerial responsibility: to collect sample behavior data over time, not to try to remember performance patterns once an evaluation deadline occurs.

The effective manager will provide informal feedback on performance when performance data are being collected. This continuous feedback with recommendations for improvement is a major managerial responsibility. Feedback and correction should be ongoing, spontaneous, and to the point. There should be no delay, no waiting for an official evaluation date.

To provide feedback, one must gather evaluative data on performance. There are two basic approaches to evaluation. In one, the manager selects a particular class of employees—all staff nurses or all staff development instructors, for example—and evaluates them on a selected day or week on a key job function from their job description. Observing a number of employees on the same dimension makes for better comparison. It enables one to eliminate false shading that often occurs because of personality and character differences. In the second approach, the manager tries to evaluate a single employee on all key functions of her job on a given evaluation day or week. There also is some merit to this, in that the employee may manifest behavior relevant to several key functions simultaneously.

There are many sources of evidence, but direct observation is always the best. Direct observation may be complemented by peer evaluation and employee self-evaluation if the manager so

chooses, but the manager should keep in mind the weaknesses and limitations of these two methods.

Usually when peer evaluation is applied, it is used at the staff nurse level. Peer evaluation may place some employees of this level under stress. If a worker knows that his raises depend on the judgments offered by his peers, then he is aware that those peers are looking carefully at his own evaluations of them. It is not unusual for an employee who has received a low rating to take revenge on peers whom he surmises have marked him negatively—even if the reports are kept confidential. The danger is greatest in situations in which the worker must rely on his fellow workers for assistance at the job. In these circumstances, an employee may perceive that it is not to his advantage to mark fellow workers poorly, whatever their actual performance.

These limitations considered, peer evaluation still offers some benefits. It cannot be entered into lightly, however, and it is unrealistic to think that peers can be involved with evaluation without extensive training. Responsibility cannot be delegated until the person who is taking over the task performs it at an acceptable level of accuracy—that is, the quality of the judgment is as sharp as it was before delegation.

A peer review system requires an organized program; it will take some time to implement. In some settings, it is reserved for only the most competent of nurses. It is the feeling of many that not all nurses should be involved in peer review. New nurses and nurses who have not achieved the expert level do not have the competence and the coaching abilities to do a good job. In many settings, only advanced nurses are involved in peer review. In some settings, nurses ranked at the top rung of the clinical ladder or the top level of the differentiated practice model are required to demonstrate the ability to do peer review.

Theoretically, very good evaluations and coaching can come from expert nurses. This input aids the nurse manager, who only sees a small picture of the staff nurses' performance. Peers who work side by side are more cognizant of strengths and weaknesses of peers and can suggest modalities for improvement easier than can a nurse manager who only sees the staff nurse infrequently by comparison.

This does not imply that the nurse manager lacks important things to say about the performance of the staff nurse. It does imply, however, that the broader view from the eyes of the peer group provide additional information and gives the staff nurse an opportunity to learn from peer experts.

Rather than being applied to judging a peer nurse's performance, sometimes the phrase *peer evaluation* is applied to the process of evaluating the care given to a selected patient (by one or many nurses). This task clearly falls within the obligation of the professional staff. This is not a managerial task but a professional one and is an appropriate task for peers.

Self-appraisal also is a limited tool for performance evaluation. The good performer typically is astute and recognizes his limitations, but the not-so-good performer may lack the insight to see his faults. Ironically, the better worker may be harder on himself in evaluation than is the less competent worker. If the manager allows these judgments to become part of the final evaluation judgment, then the system may penalize the most capable.

Some managers rely on nurses' basic honesty and willingness to reveal faults as a substitute for managerial observation. After the employee recognizes one of his own revealed faults carrying heavy weight in the final appraisal, he will soon cease helping his supervisor to downgrade his performance. When self-rating is used, it must be tempered with other measures.

Anecdotal notes help one to evaluate employees at all levels in the organization. Memory cannot be relied on: What seems clear today will have faded if the supervisor tries to recall it 6 months to 1 year later. Two types of observations occur in anecdotes: routine behavior samples and critical incidents.

The routine samples are behaviors noted when the manager goes out to check on behaviors related to key job functions as part of the routine collection of performance data. Here, the attempt is not to get anything unusual but to record the average behavior, be it good, bad, exciting, or mundane. It is important to collect enough samples to be able to assert that they represent the average, typical behavior.

A critical incident, however, is a single observed event that is so good or bad that it reflects on the total performance of the employee. For example, if the executive observes a supervisor refusing to listen to an employee's side of a problem, this single incident tells much about the supervisor's way of functioning. Similarly, if a nurse were observed to react to a subtle patient problem in a resourceful manner, the effect is the same in that a single event reveals sensitivities and abilities, or insensitivities and inabilities, as the case may be.

In collecting observations, it is important that a manager preserve actual descriptions of the behavior exhibited rather than just judgments about that behavior. Later that manager may have to substantiate her judgments if an employee contests the evaluation or action subsequent to the evaluation.

Secondary sources of evidence of performance may be used to supplement judgments drawn from direct observation. For evaluating the staff nurse, his nursing care plans may be excellent secondary sources. Although it is possible that a nurse may derive excellent care plans without following through on them, it is more likely that the care he gives is good if he is able to specify it in care plans than if he is not able to do so. Other documents such as incident reports and illness and tardiness records may be taken into account in deriving a performance appraisal.

Professional activities (speaking, writing) also may be considered in the case of professional nurses. Participation in institutional, divisional, or departmental committees may be considered—especially if the nurse has made significant contributions to such committees. In evaluating a manager, the superordinate manager will also consider the manager's reports and her attainment of objectives set for her department or unit.

When an institution has an effective clinical ladder, the ladder must be tied to the appraisal system in a meaningful way. Both a good clinical ladder program and a performance appraisal system attempt to rate nurse behaviors. Ideally, the nurse will be rated as to how he performs on the step of the ladder where he is placed. A performance appraisal might indicate the misplacement of a nurse, and a supervisor might well use the performance rating to initiate reclassification of an employee.

Placing Judgments on Data

When placing judgments on performance data, the nurse manager should be careful to avoid such common errors of judgment as the following:

- *Halo effect:* The individual whose performance in several known areas is good is assumed to be able to perform well in other, unknown areas. Sometimes this error is termed *trait carryover.*
- *Recency effect:* Recent issues weigh heavier with the rater than do events that occurred earlier in the evaluation period.
- *Problem distortion*: One poor performance weighs heavier with the rater than do 20 good performances that went unnoticed because they created no problems.
- *Sunflower effect:* The rater may grade all her employees too high because of a feeling that she has a great team.
- *Central tendency:* The evaluator may tend to mark everyone as average, especially if she is unsure of the real performance on a particular criterion.
- *Rater temperament effect:* Different raters may have differences in the strictness or leniency with which they rate employees.
- *Guessing error:* Some raters guess rather than record that particular observations were not made.

Feasible versus Ideal Observation

Although the manager must set aside time for evaluation, there is never enough time to do all the evaluation that one might choose. Because the manager cannot evaluate everything, it is important that she evaluate the key functions of an employee's job. Also, it is important that the employee be evaluated in any domain in which he previously was found to be deficient. Specific assignments can be devised to test improvement in such areas.

PERFORMANCE APPRAISAL FORMATS

Many formats are used for performance appraisal, including essay, ranking systems, rating scales, and checklists. Each format has advantages and disadvantages and may be adapted for different purposes.

Essay

Essay has the advantage of being free-form, allowing the rater to respond in ways that capture the unique performance of the employee. The disadvantage of essay is that it makes it difficult to compare performance across groups of workers.

Free-form essay can be improved if the rater uses a common list of critical topics to be addressed for every worker in a given classification. In this way, the subject matter corresponds from evaluation to evaluation, but the rater still is free to individualize comments on different subjects. The key job functions as reflected in the job description should be identified. Consistent use of the same categories also will enable the employee to compare his performance at any one time against his past performance.

When essay is used, the manager must be clear and definite in her description of the employee's behavior. She cannot let the meaning be lost in polite phrasing. Look, for example, at the following essay, taken from an actual performance report:

> Miss M conducts herself in a professional manner. She is an active member of the ANA. Her attendance is very good, and she remains flexible about time changes in her schedule.

She is knowledgeable about hospital policies.

Her rapport with nonprofessionals continues to improve. We established, together, the following goals: (1) become proficient in the role of primary nurse, (2) become accountable for documentation on progress notes and care plans, and (3) follow through on goals set for assigned patients.

Ironically, the supervisor and the employee came away from the conference at which this essay was discussed with radically different notions of the nurse's performance. The staff nurse reported to colleagues that the supervisor had no complaints about her performance.

The supervisor was astonished to hear this because, as she reported, one could infer many faults in the practice from the nature of the goals set. Because the goals set would not be needed in the face of good nursing practice, she had anticipated that the nurse would understand that the report was negative. Indeed, when the supervisor later produced this document at a grievance hearing, she lost the case because her warning to the employee was too disguised to be taken as a warning.

An essay is poor if it (1) is noncommittal, (2) addresses insignificant topics, (3) alludes to faults in a way that is indirect, or (4) speaks through omission rather than by explicit statement.

Ranking Systems

Ranking systems compare employees to each other by placing them in order according to their performances on the given categories. Often, the ranking of employees on specific job dimensions will help the manager to overcome prejudices and biases that may be related to personal factors.

A ranking system alone does not make a statement concerning the overall quality of the group or of any individual in the group being ranked. It merely reveals how the employees compare with one another. Ranking is a useful technique for considering candidates for promotion or for distributing merit pay fairly.

Summary judgments may be made about ranked candidates by scoring each dimension on which candidates are ranked according to its overall importance. This factor may be multiplied by the candidate's rank, as in Table 28–1.

In Table 28–1, three nurses are being compared and ranked on dimensions of the nursing process and the recording accompanying that process. Weights have been assigned to each component and have been multiplied by the rank of the nurse in each instance. Notice that the nurse who ranked highest was given a 3, not a 1, so that the mathematics could be calculated per highest score. In this instance, Nurse A's score is considerably higher than her two colleagues' scores.

Rating Scales

A rating scale allows the evaluator to make a choice from among a quantitative or qualitative range of options for every criterion being assessed. Such options may include, for example,

- Excellent—Good—Fair—Poor
- Above Average—Average—Below Average

Table 28–1 Ranking System—Quantified

Key Functions	Weight	Rank A	B	C	Item Score for Nurse A	B	C
1. Assesses patient needs	3×	3	2	1	9	6	3
2. Sets appropriate goals	2×	3	1	2	6	2	4
3. Formulates good nursing care plans	3×	2	3	1	6	9	3
4. Implements care plan successfully	3×	2	1	3	6	3	9
5. Evaluates and modifies plan	2×	3	2	1	6	4	2
6. Documents care	1×	1	3	2	1	3	2
Total Score:					34	27	23

- Yes—No
- Always—Frequently—Occasionally—Seldom—Never
- 1—2—3—4—5
- 0–25%—26–50%—51–75%—76–100%

Sometimes, the same range of options is given for each criterion, with an attempt to describe further the meaning of each option. In other cases, the options vary for different criteria; one criterion might be answered in terms of frequency, whereas another might be answered in terms of quality or degree of excellence. In more sophisticated rating scales, the options may be descriptive statements, as in Figure 28–1.

Most rating scales force the rater to select one or another of the given options. Some scales are constructed on a continuum so that the rater may use more discretion. A continuum may allow the rater to make more subtle differentiations among candidates who rank close to each other. The continuum, however, is subject to the same problem as is a scale with too many options. It becomes difficult to justify the degrees of differentiation that such scales offer.

The checklist is an alternative format for an evaluation system wherein each standard is checked either as met or not met. Checklists also may be given numerical values, either by a simple count of yes and no items or by weighting items as in a rating scale.

Whatever format is used, anecdotal notes and critical incident reports are used in determining the placement of the employee on each item. Some managers elect to have the employee fill out a similar tool and then negotiate a final judgment between the two reports, comparing that of the employee with that of the manager. The employee is likely to have an advantage, for by marking himself highly, he is in a position to negotiate his evaluation upward.

Whatever reporting method is used—essay, ranking, rating, or checklist—the format should provide room for supporting evidence for the judgments made. Clear, concrete illustrations should be given of the behaviors that led to the judgments. These become particularly important when coaching employees to improve or when an employee submits a grievance over the grade assigned him or over subsequent action based on the grade. The more concrete the illustrations of behavior, the better.

The format also should provide a place to record when and where the evaluation conference took place at which the report was shared with the employee. Most forms have a place for the employee to sign, indicating that he has seen the report. Sometimes, if he disagrees with the judgment, an employee may refuse to sign the report. When this occurs, the manager may stress that the signature only indicates that the report was seen by the employee, not that it was accepted. If the employee still refuses to sign, the manager will do well to have a witness sign that the conference did, in fact, take place.

Tool Deficiencies

Performance appraisal tools may suffer from many deficiencies. When the nurse manager is forced to use a poor tool, say one prescribed for institutionwide use by a personnel department, her job is made more difficult. Many a nurse executive has created her own tools just to overcome the defects in such a universal form. Even when use of such a form is required, there is no reason the nursing division cannot supplement evaluation with tools that provide meaningful records of employee behavior.

The problem with a universal tool used for all employees is one of validity. A single tool cannot possibly evaluate every employee based on

STANDARD	CRITERIA			
Supervisor's use of research	No apparent use or knowledge of recent research	Applies research findings on her units	Makes her units available to researchers	Devises and implements nursing research on units

Figure 28–1 Descriptive Rating Scale Sample

his job description. And if an employee is not evaluated on performance of the job he was hired to do, then the evaluation is invalid. The universal tool, because it cannot address performance, usually addresses personality traits and/or broad generalities of more or less importance in various jobs. Items typically include appearance, loyalty to the institution, quantity of work, quality of work, cooperativeness with others, professional manner, tardiness or absenteeism, and manner of dealing with patients or the public. Indeed, these few aspects are the only ones shared by personnel. Such a form is incapable of capturing the essence of each job and cannot accurately evaluate job performance. Each job classification should have a separate performance appraisal tool, one adapted to the key functions of the particular job.

The performance appraisal tool is invalid—fails to measure what it purports to measure—if the items of which it is comprised are poorly chosen. For example, if more items reflect incidentals and fewer items reflect the main responsibilities of the job, the tool will give a false measurement. Similarly, if weighting of items does not reflect their actual significance in the job performance, then the tool will be invalid. The rating scale or checklist is made representative by either balancing the original selection of items or by weighting items to create a balance that reflects the job requirements. The essay is balanced by identification of specific categories to be addressed.

Some tools err by failing to identify the acceptable level of performance. If a rating scale uses a range of 1 to 5, the evaluator and the employee need to know what number represents baseline acceptable performance. Is it 2, 3, or 4? If one uses such terms as excellent, good, fair, and poor, the same question arises. Is "fair" baseline performance? Or is "good" the acceptable level? For a checklist, it is assumed that each item itself is a baseline element and that a positive score is required as evidence of acceptable performance. In an essay, the evaluator must identify whether the performance in each instance is at an acceptable level.

Not only must one be able to interpret each item as it relates to baseline acceptable perform-

ance, but one must be able to place a summary judgment on the total performance as indicated in the tool. And one must be able to arrive at a final judgment that considers all the criteria and their marks. When each item in a ranking scale has a score, these scores may be added together and divided by the number of items to derive a total score. Where weighting is used, additional mathematics is required, but the score still is a mathematical derivation, not a judgment.

When descriptive scales are used, one must equate terms with values. Supposing, however, that "fair" is taken to be baseline acceptable performance, there are still questions to be answered. How many items may fall below the acceptable level before discipline or dismissal occur? On how many performance appraisals will substandard performance be tolerated? Are there certain critical items that must be at an acceptable level, while there may be some room for deviation on other less critical items? These same questions apply also to checklist items.

Simply put, the decision rules for how to interpret a summary score must be determined before the evaluation process begins. For essay, it is more difficult to draw a summary conclusion from the previous materials, but it must be done. Otherwise, the essay is not really an evaluative tool; it must place a summary judgment on the employee's performance as it relates to the job standards.

Appraisal tools also may suffer from deficits in reliability. When standards are poorly operationalized or when grading criteria are poorly described, different raters may use the tools in different ways. Precision is needed in both elements: constructing standards open to a single interpretation and describing judgments, be they numerical or verbal, so that they cannot be misinterpreted.

Criteria for an Evaluation Tool

A good evaluation tool meets the following requirements:

- *Utility:* The tool actually is useful in promoting change in employee behavior.

- *Simplicity:* It is easy to use, not requiring complicated procedures.
- *Validity:* It reflects the key job requirements.
- *Rating:* It defines minimal acceptable levels of performance.
- *Event-oriented:* Real behaviors, not employee traits, comprise the items.
- *Differentiation:* The tool allows one to differentiate among performances of various employees, without requiring an impossible degree of differentiation on the part of the evaluator.
- *Appropriate weighting:* The tool balances categories on the basis of their importance.

Although all these criteria are important, it is necessary to review the criteria concerning behaviors in detail. This is to avoid performance appraisal forms that deal with personal traits rather than work behavior. One should not pass judgment on the character of the individual being evaluated but on his work. This is not to say that some positive "traits" may not be required (e.g., a pleasant customer-oriented attitude toward patients). But these items can usually be described in behavioral terms with a little effort.

Use of trait categories places the evaluator at a disadvantage, for trait language represents a summary opinion derived from the observation of multiple behaviors. If the employee disagrees with the judgment of the evaluator, his typical response is to ask for examples that form the basis of the judgment. If the evaluator is unable to recall specific incidents, she looks inept. If the evaluator is able to identify events, there is still no guarantee that she and the employee will place the same interpretation on those events. In trait language, there is no way to resolve different interpretations of the same behavior. The solution to this problem is to revise evaluation systems to use event language rather than trait language.

In wording, the behavior (event) statements should be explicit so that they will have the same meaning for all raters. Each statement should identify the expected level of performance in precise behavioral terms. Both the job

description and the evaluation tool, if well constructed, will reveal the most critical elements of a position.

THE APPRAISAL INTERVIEW

There are many different aspects of the appraisal interview. This chapter looks at the context in which the interview takes place, the content of the interview, and the interview process.

Who, When, and Where

The ideal evaluator is the manager to whom the employee reports because this manager has first-hand knowledge of the employee's performance. This rating system also helps reinforce the appropriate lines of authority. If a supervisor evaluates the employees who work under a head nurse, for example, this undermines the head nurse's authority.

Another issue is the question of how often to evaluate personnel. The more often evaluation can be performed, the less stressful the situation becomes, and the more evaluation takes on the nature of guidance rather than of judgment. Yearly evaluations, for example, are too far apart to have vital impact on behavior patterns, yet the very rarity of the event causes high anxiety levels in both employees and supervisors.

One need not and should not wait for an official evaluation time, such as the employee's anniversary date, if the employee's performance is problematic. Evaluation should take place whenever an employee's performance warrants it. If an employee's performance is stable and good, the official evaluation times may be adequate. When an employee has been evaluated as unsatisfactory, it is legitimate to increase the frequency of evaluation; otherwise, it would take years to get rid of an unsatisfactory worker. The repeat evaluations should be scheduled at intervals long enough to allow the employee time to develop new desired behaviors.

The setting for the performance appraisal interview should be quiet and private. If an office is used, a secretary or switchboard operator should be notified to hold telephone calls. Not only should care be given to selecting the physical setting, but the psychological setting should also be prepared. The employee should be notified in advance so that he may plan for the conference. He may be asked to come prepared to discuss his performance, its strengths and weaknesses, his performance problems, and any needs for supervisory help in relation to performance.

The psychological tone is carried over into the conference itself, with the supervisor making it evident that the conference is serious and formal business by telling the employee, "We are meeting here today to review your performance for the past 6 months and to see how it might be improved." The conference neither begins nor ends as if it were a social occasion.

Content of the Interview

Evaluation interviews differ in content, depending on their purpose. The interview discussed here is the one aiming at improving employee performance. Such an interview is future-oriented and change-oriented and does not focus on placing blame but on correction. A prerequisite for such an interview is that the employee be acquainted with the desired work behaviors. A good way to accomplish this is to begin by reviewing the employee's job description to locate and explore differences in interpretation and attitude concerning the job.

Another useful technique for discovering different job interpretations is for the manager and the employee each to prepare for the interview by listing and ranking the key functions of the employee's job as they see them. Comparing and discussing differences between key function lists, as well as comparing them with the job description, will help the manager and the employee reach consensus. Differences in both content and priorities will help the employee see what functions the manager views as most important. Seeing the employee's list will help the manager understand the employee's work behavior.

Another prerequisite for a productive evaluation interview is to help the employee learn in what way his own behaviors fail to match those desired. In the average employee appraisal, judgment of the employee's behavior is the real focus of the interview process. The employee sits passively while the manager tells him what things he did right and what things he did wrong. In this context, hearing what he did right merely sugarcoats hearing what he did wrong. The right-versus-wrong mechanism forces the evaluation process into a trial-like judgment in which the employee simply hopes that the good will outweigh the bad. This type of evaluation will not change employee behavior, because his interest is focused on the judgment, on how well his performance balances out. The most he can do is accept or reject the judgment.

The employee needs to be oriented to the nature and the purpose of the interview. He needs to know beforehand that the purpose of the interview is to improve his job performance, not to congratulate him on his successes, although that may occur incidentally for the good performer. Given the purpose of improving performance, the best employee and the least effective one will experience similar interviews: Both will be structured around probing for ways to improve performance.

If the employee is capable of objective self-evaluation, his performance deficiencies may be identified in a mutual interaction between manager and employee. One of the ironies of the system is that the better the employee, the more likely he will be able to identify his deficiencies; the less capable the employee, the less likely he will be to see his defects. The capable employee usually knows what performance areas can be improved; he already measures himself against internalized standards.

The less capable employee may need assistance in identifying his deficiencies; in other instances, he may know them. When an employee is not objective, it is up to the manager to specify the behavioral deficiencies.

It is not prudent to go into all the employee's deficiencies if he has many. The weight of such a judgment is heavy and often nonmotivating. It is better to focus only on those that most urgently need changing, because it is unlikely that an employee will be able to work on more than one or two behavioral changes at a time.

With the employee whose performance is satisfactory, the manager may find it productive to let him select the behaviors he will try to improve. With another employee, the manager may have to specify which particular behaviors are major impairments in the employee's work. An exceptionally poor employee may have more than one or two behaviors that must be changed immediately if he is to be retained in his position.

Although it is unlikely that the individual will be able to make so many behavioral changes at once, at least the interview documents that the need for the changes has been communicated to the employee. In most cases, this will be documentation toward an eventual dismissal. In some rare cases, where the employee actually has the capability, he may show extensive improvement in many areas of practice after such an interview.

Like any other system, change-oriented employee evaluation must be used with judgment. The system works best with two types of employees: self-motivated achievers who enjoy working toward a goal and workers who clearly need guidance and direction from an authority figure. It is always possible, however, that a very good employee is not interested in making any further adaptations in his performance. In this case, the manager will be wise to alter the evaluation system if she wants to retain the employee. When an employee has, in effect, announced that he will go this far for the job and no farther, then the manager should accept that stand and decide whether to keep the employee on that basis.

In identifying behaviors to be changed, it is important that the manager not be overzealous in trying to inflict some ideal employee image on each worker. It is unrealistic to expect exactly the same behaviors from all employees. The manager who aims for this will rob herself of many of the best talents of her staff. For example, one nurse may approach his work with zest and enthusiasm and another may approach his work with cautious, steady planning. Both of these contrasting behaviors may be valuable contributions to the total work group. The manager should focus on developing the talents and abilities inherent in the employee's makeup. If the manager and the employee together identify the behaviors to be improved, these individual considerations will be taken into account.

A third prerequisite for the productive employee interview is for the manager to see that the employee learns how to change his behavior toward the desired pattern. Pinpointing an undesirable behavior and directing the employee to change it simply will not work. But together the employee and the manager can identify the new behaviors the employee will be expected to exhibit. These behaviors must be determined, action by action. For example, to say that the nurse will now distribute his medications on time does not help. It does not tell him how to modify the behaviors that now cause him always to be late.

A time limit should be set by which the employee is expected to have practiced and habituated the new behavior. However, some behaviors cannot be allowed to develop gradually, but these are in the minority. Usually, the employee can be given a grace period during which he can concentrate on effecting the behavioral change.

The last prerequisite of the successful employee interview is motivation, namely, that the employee leave the conference determined to change his behavior. If the process of evaluation is seen as assistive and not judgmental, a positive mind-set is more likely to occur.

Among the false conceptions about motivation, none is more wrong than the idea it can be supplied from the outside. Motivation is an internal principle; it is not possible for a manager to supply it. Threats of punishment or promises of rewards do not motivate, they manipulate. Some individuals can inspire others in such a way that they become motivated, but the manager need not rely on charisma.

When inspiration fails, the manager can require that certain behaviors be shown as conditions of holding a job, getting a raise, or getting a promotion. One way or the other, the employee will leave the interview with the knowledge that he must change his behavior. And he has an exact idea of what to do. After setting time limits for the behavioral change, the manager sets in advance one or more follow-up conferences to check on the progress.

The evaluation interview designed to improve deficient employee performance is only one kind of appraisal interview. For some employees, the manager will build on strengths rather than correct weaknesses. This is one way a successful employee sincerely can be commended. When a manager helps an employee develop incipient talents, this is the best form of employee recognition.

Processes of the Interview

There are at least four managerial objectives for the interview: (1) to convey information, (2) to foster actual behavioral change, (3) to keep the interview situation comfortable and as free of tension as possible, and (4) to maintain control of the situation. These goals are facilitated if the manager goes into the interview with clear purposes in mind. She should know in detail what kinds of change she wishes to bring about in the employee and how she will suggest those changes be implemented.

Preparing

It helps if the supervisor has some strategies for the interview prepared in advance. By thinking ahead into the interview situation and anticipating the employee's responses, the manager can prepare her own tactics for dealing with the anticipated responses. When criticism of performance is necessary, defense mechanisms are likely to be invoked: withdrawal, denial, excuses, or challenge and confrontation. She must get beyond these immediate responses if the employee's behavior is to be improved.

Keeping Control

To keep control during the process of the interview, the supervisor must be both an involved participant and a disinterested removed judge of the process that is going on. She must watch for power shifts between herself and the employee.

Sometimes, she can allow the employee to take control of the interview but not if such control threatens the purpose of the conference. The manager can reassert control when required if she has clearly asserted her prerogatives at the start.

Content of the Interview

The content of the interview should not be allowed to drift from the established purpose. If the employee is a facile conversationalist, the supervisor may find that she must bring the conversation back as often as required.

The manager should be sensitive to both the facts and the feelings that make up the interview. At one instant, she may find it appropriate to focus on the facts being discussed; at another time, it may be advantageous to discuss the employee's feelings.

Communicating

One major part of communicating involves listening to the other person. Listening to the employee means letting him do much of the talking, letting him finish sentences, not thinking ahead into one's response while he is still talking, and checking to see if the message he was trying to convey was actually received.

Listening alone is only half the job of communication; the rest involves mutuality. The manager can assure two-way communication by preparing a number of pivotal questions to ask the employee—questions that require thought and discussion, questions that cannot be answered by a "yes" or a "no." The key function comparison scheme mentioned earlier is another activity that creates two-way communication. To make the interview two-way, the employee should be advised to prepare for the evaluation just as adequately as does the manager. Another way to establish two-way communication is for the two individuals to discuss their mutual expectations of each other.

One of the best ways to maintain good communication during an evaluation interview is for the manager to avoid falling into common interview traps, such as

- conducting a one-way (telling) conversation
- interrupting the employee's thoughts, explanations, and questions
- criticizing the employee rather than the performance
- smoothing over real deficiencies and problems too fast
- failing to investigate facts before expressing opinions
- passing the buck by claiming that one's corrective measures originate higher up
- allowing the interview to fall into charge–countercharge cycles
- allowing the interview to fall into charge–denial cycles
- allowing the interview to fall into charge–excuse cycles
- allowing the interview to deteriorate into a social visit

During an interview, the manager continuously evaluates what is happening in the interaction, recognizing what she is doing as well as what the employee is doing.

Response Options

The greatest asset a manager can have is the knowledge that she need not stick to any particular response pattern. She can keep her options open. If she is to respond thoughtfully, however, she must take time to think before she speaks. She must actually listen to what the employee says and dare to take the time to think rather than rush into an unconsidered reaction.

For every statement made by an employee, there are many ways to respond. Unconsidered responses tend to be limited to one of two typical patterns. The first pattern is to respond with a judgment of the employee's statement. In an interview situation, this response creates a trial-like atmosphere. The second pattern is to react directly to the content of the employee's statement. There are many times when this is an appropriate response, but there are also times when other responses are better. To evaluate some response options, let us examine an interview that has fallen into the charge–excuse cycle:

> *Head Nurse:* ". . . also, you failed to give Mrs. Jones her passive exercise all last week."
> *Staff Nurse:* "You are thinking about last Thursday, and that day she was so upset she wouldn't let anyone touch her."
> *Head Nurse:* "I'm not thinking just of Thursday. You didn't exercise her weak side on Friday either. "
> *Staff Nurse:* "On Friday her doctor did that spinal tap and took all morning at it. No one could have gotten in there to exercise her."
> *Head Nurse:* "But nothing went on Friday afternoon, and you still didn't exercise her."
> *Staff Nurse:* "I was taught that patients were to lie flat and quiet after a spinal tap to prevent a headache."

This head nurse has fallen into a deadly trap, for the staff nurse can probably find an excuse for any charge the head nurse can think up. The head nurse has in each case responded to the content of the staff nurse's statement. As long as she continues this, she will neither break the cycle nor make her point.

To break off this unproductive cycle, the head nurse needs to recognize that such a pattern takes two to keep it going. As soon as one participant refuses to play, the cycle is interrupted. One simple solution is for the head nurse to admit that this line of conversation is unproductive and break it off, going to another topic.

A better option might be to answer the last response with a question or suggestion that directs the employee out of the cycle. "Why don't you review for me your plans for Mrs. Jones last week. Maybe we can explore what happened to them."

The head nurse also might switch from content-directed charges to exploration of feelings. She could direct a question to the staff nurse concerning her feelings about Mrs. Jones. Another choice would be for the head nurse to point out that Mrs. Jones' care is only part of a larger problem and then return to the bigger problem instead of haggling over one instance of behavior.

Another useful response option is for the head nurse to call the staff nurse's attention to the excuse pattern of her responses. They might then explore why this pattern dominates her explanations of her work. Many paths can be taken to restore the interview to a productive session. The critical factor is simply that the manager recognize the defective communications pattern and use a constructive response option.

Producing Attitudinal Change

Managers often use the evaluation interview to encourage changes in employee attitudes. It is impossible to change attitudes that are couched by the supervisor in trait language, such as "You are hostile," "You are racially prejudiced," "You are headstrong and impulsive." The logical way to achieve desired attitude change is to identify the behavior or behaviors that give evidence of the trait. To tell an employee that he is impulsive does not tell him how to change that trait, nor does it make him wish to change. It is possible, however, to identify past behaviors that demonstrated impulsiveness and impaired the work process. In this fashion, it is legitimate to require that an employee change a nonfunctional attitude.

Many authorities agree that the best way to change attitudes is to change behaviors first. Once an individual is routinely doing a particular act, he is likely to develop a positive attitude toward that act.

Final Accountability

The manager is obligated to make absolutely clear what she means in an interview. For example, if the session is a last warning before a potential dismissal, she must make certain that the employee understands the situation. Otherwise, some employees may interpret as casual conversation what the manager sees as serious. In all such disciplinary instances, the manager follows the conference with a letter to the employee summarizing the interview, the problems

discussed, and the goals set. Although disciplining an employee is never an easy task, use of an event-focused evaluation system makes the job less difficult.

When possible, the manager seeks agreement concerning deficiencies and goals. However, the interview cannot be reduced to a bargaining session. The manager may need to assert her authority when the employee is not in agreement; employee acceptance is desirable but not always possible. The manager should listen, but she has no need to negotiate. Ultimately, she will determine the significance of the situation, including the final judgment to be passed on the subordinate's behavior.

Ending the Interview

Managers often have difficulty knowing when and how to end an interview. Although there is no absolute rule for timing, almost any interview can be easily contained within an hour. If a manager tends to hold longer conferences, she is likely to be doing one of two things: either turning the interview into a social visit, or belaboring the same essential points. Both of these patterns are to be avoided.

A good way to end the interview and give it a sense of completion is for the manager to summarize the events of the interview. She can briefly identify the problems discussed, the agreements reached, the goals set, and the proposed behavioral changes. This summary gives the employee a final chance to compare her interpretation of the interview with the manager's interpretation. Any differences in understanding can be revealed and settled. Also, summarizing clearly announces to the employee that the interview is at an end. The summary includes a review of what happened in the interview, the agreements reached, and any direct orders from the manager.

SUMMARY

The performance appraisal system is a major control system of the nursing division. It provides an aggregate measure of staff performance for the nurse executive as well as providing guidance for individual employees. Many diverse purposes may be served by employee appraisal, including personnel decisions, quality improvement of patient care, and staff motivation.

Creating an effective performance appraisal system includes many steps, from creating a system with useful feedback to devising good job descriptions and personnel evaluation tools. The system and the judgments made within it may be correlated with many other systems from clinical ladder placement to promotions and dismissals to merit increments. Also, managers at every level will need to build skills in the processes of employee assessment and interview.

SUGGESTED READINGS

Bushardt, S., and A. Fowler. 1988. Performance evaluation alternatives. *Journal of Nursing Administration* 18, no. 10:40–44.

del Bueno, D.J. 1990. Evaluation: Myths, mystiques, and obsessions. *Journal of Nursing Administration* 20, no. 11:4–7.

Fosbinder, D., and H. Vos. 1989. Setting standards and evaluating nursing performance with a single tool. *Journal of Nursing Administration* 19, no.10:23–30.

Fralic, M.F. 1992. The nurse case manager: Focus, selection, preparation, and measurement. *Journal of Nursing Administration* 22, no.11:13–14, 46.

Haas, S. 1992. Coaching: Developing key players. *Journal of Nursing Administration* 22, no.6:54–58.

Heslin, K. 1991. The staff nurse employment interview: Predicting performance outcomes. *Canadian Journal of Nursing Administration* 4, no.4:30–36.

Kohn, A. 1993. Why incentive plans cannot work. *Harvard Business Review* 71, no.5:54–63.

MacKay, R., et al. 1990. Evaluating the competence of clinical nurses from beginning to advanced practitioner. *Canadian Journal of Nursing Administration* 3, no.3: 25–29.

Mann, L., et al. 1990. Peer review in performance appraisal. *Nursing Administration Quarterly* 14, no.4:9–14.

Tayler, C.M. 1992. Subordinate performance appraisal: What nurses really want in their managers. *Canadian Journal of Nursing Administration* 5, no.3:6–9.

29

Staff Development

Staff development is the term used here to refer to those educational functions that are handled in or through the institution to prepare its employees for better role fulfillment or for advancement to other positions. Sometimes called *inservice education,* such instruction is always judged by its efficacy in improving patient care. Employee benefits from education are of a secondary interest (although important). But enhancement of employee talents is justified economically only if it improves patient care.

LEARNING NEEDS

In the typical staff education department, two related needs are meshed: staff development and orientation. Although employee orientation includes some needs for education (or verification that education is at a satisfactory level), primarily it deals with informing, not educating.

Education and information are differentiated here by noting that education gives the learner transferable knowledge that could be applied in diverse settings (e.g., learning about a new clinical procedure, a new disease, a new drug therapy). Information, however, has more to do with the pragmatic ways and means of a given setting (e.g., where the procedure books are kept, how to page the physician on call, the system for reporting a fire). Information items are those bits of knowledge that help an employee function in this institution at this time. Education, in contrast, adds to one's professional/occupational knowledge and competencies.

Although most of staff development deals with education, orientation—in most cases—focuses on information giving. In neither case can it be assumed that knowledge inevitably translates into action. An employee may demonstrate a procedure in a laboratory examination only to fail to apply it correctly in a real patient situation on a unit. Similarly, he may ignore certain information if not motivated to apply it. Educating and informing cure ignorance; they do not ensure subsequent behavior.

When a staff development department is free to determine the learning needs of a nursing staff and how the needs are to be met, it faces a tremendous challenge. The complexities are several: (1) staff education has no curriculum set in stone. Indeed, the learning needs shift constantly, as patient care needs change and as staff changes; (2) the student population is not homogeneous; various levels of workers have different education needs; (3) education must always be at a high level (application, not mere knowledge); (4) the education function must interface with other functions, namely, practice and administration; and (5) the education function is always secondary in the organization, not taking place for its own sake. Because of these complexities, staff development is vulnerable to conflicts arising in the immediate press of care delivery as well as other pushes and pulls inherent in the organization.

ORGANIZATIONAL ARRANGEMENTS

Nursing staff development may be provided through various organizational arrangements from (1) total integration (with each patient care unit providing its own education and orientation), (2) to centralization in a separate nursing education department, (3) to centralization in an institutionwide department of education and orientation. Recent trends lean toward the latter conformation, especially as accreditation outcome criteria blend professions (and their patient outcomes) more frequently. In this case, the education department may be located in nursing, under personnel management, or elsewhere in the organization.

When education is decentralized to the nursing care unit level, costs may be exorbitant unless educators have secondary care provision duties on their units. However, if the knowledge and skills that must be taught for an employee to deliver care on that unit are unique, it may be that this system will be effective. As nursing *de facto* divides into more and more specialties, this situation grows common.

Another option that some institutions select is to decentralize education for the staff of some unique and insular units while still centralizing education for most of the staff. A blended solution may meet the needs of many organizations.

In most cases, staff development is provided by a department within the nursing division. Because this is still the norm, we will focus on this situation. Within a nursing department, the staff development function (education and orientation) may be insular or the function may be combined with other departmental functions such as quality management, risk management, research and development, affiliations management, or community liaison.

For clarity, the person heading a nursing staff development department is called a *director* for the rest of this chapter to differentiate her from the nurse executive. In most organizations, the education director reports directly to the nursing executive. She may be placed equally with nursing vice presidents (e.g., directors of major nursing divisions) or somewhat higher or lower. In any case, she is usually considered to be a major player in the core of nursing administrators.

Education as a Secondary Goal

One advantage in separating out a department of nursing education is that it gives more clout to education than might occur when it is handled by the same officers who provide for direct patient care. In decentralized models, managers often are tempted to sacrifice educational needs for more immediate care needs.

Even when education is provided centrally, each director of an educational program will have to devise her own strategies to prevent disruption of planned educational projects by pressing care needs for staff. When a director can give visible demonstration that her programs contribute to care outcomes, she is likely to build greater cooperation and support among other nurse managers.

LEARNING METHODS

In addition to charging the staff development department with responsibility for identifying employee needs for both education and information, the nurse executive must be concerned with how the education department goes about meeting those needs. This involves both teaching effectiveness and economy of methods used.

In today's resource-scarce environment, many directors of education have concentrated on efficiency and economy in the delivery system. Often, this has led to enhanced use of computer-assisted education programs and extensive audio-visual libraries, often providing learning materials to staff for use at the convenience of the learner. Use of such prepackaged learning modules makes education fit staff time instead of reversing the process, and it encourages the self-directed sort of learning that should be appropriate, at least at the professional level. Further, self-directed education supported by available educational packets makes it easier to deliver education on off-shifts.

Multi-institution corporations also are enhancing staff development by sharing personnel and learning packages. Often, the system is enhanced by television linkage among participating institutions. In these circumstances, there may be a single corporate nursing education director with education staff at multiple sites.

Once an education system has been put into place, including purchasing or creating of most necessary packages of learning, it may be possible to decrease the teaching staff, retaining enough staff for those learning elements requiring a faculty member present as well as providing faculty hours for evaluating and updating the learning system itself.

An environment in which the nurse seeks out materials for his own learning needs will not happen just because the appropriate learning tools and learning packages are available. The nurse executive and the director will have to foster this sort of self-learning accountability. If managers fail to allow and validate such learning time (which may involve the nurse leaving the patient care unit for a period of time), the whole system will fail.

MULTIPLE REQUESTS FOR SERVICES

Continuous advances in nursing and medical therapy create an environment in which nurses should be constantly seeking new information. The rate of obsolescence of knowledge and skills makes education a challenging race. The presses experienced by a staff development department will partly depend on other resources available to the institution. Is there a health library? A school of nursing? Or does the staff development department supplant such services?

In many settings, the demands placed on the staff development department will overextend its available resources despite technological efficiency. This requires a fine sense of prioritizing on the part of the director. Further, she needs clear operational policies concerning whether services of the department are limited to nursing division staff or extended to others. In many places, routine physician (or other) retraining requirements are placed within this department. Obviously, there are advantages to working cooperatively with the rest of the organization as long as clear guidelines have been established concerning who is accountable for what.

STAFF DEVELOPMENT DRIVEN BY QUALITY OUTCOME MEASURES

Gone are the days when staff development can provide the "nice to know" programs. In the resource-driven model, as resources become constricted, more cost benefit analysis must be performed on staff development programs to ensure acceptable outcomes. The staff development department must be concerned with preventing problems before they happen. Education and competency testing are built into the way care is delivered.

Problem solving is a major concern here. Once an educational problem has been discovered, this department must be concerned with understanding what the problem is, changing practices as rapidly as possible, and quickly helping the nursing staff to learn new behaviors in a short time.

The staff development programs must also continually assess areas of potential risk and go "looking for problems." Staff development educators must be in the patient care areas looking for practices that indicate a knowledge deficit. Are there breaks in sterile technique? Is it a management problem that reflects an information need (lack of compliance with policy) or lack of knowledge in correct technique?

Are there areas of potentially unsafe practice—such as staff failing to recognize when a patient develops symptoms of shock—and what is the plan to correct this? Are patient falls occurring because staff are unfamiliar with the falls prevention protocol? Are staff making mistakes because there is not adequate time available to make a thorough assessment? In the latter example, staff educators have to decide between problems based on lack of knowledge and problems related to managerial practices.

Few of these problems would have been recognized by a staff educator of the previous era, one who concerned herself with formal classes, seldom seeing a patient unit first-hand. One advantage of new teaching technologies is that staff educators can be freed up for this sort of educational troubleshooting on the patient care units.

The staff development department has as its customers the patients. It is charged with educating the staff to perform safe care. Therefore, the staff development staff must be intimately associated with patient care. Indeed, the director of the staff development department can take her marching orders directly from the results of the quality program and by anticipating future needs.

Not only must an education director be driven by quality management outcomes, but she must see that all education activities are themselves measured for effectiveness. The best measurements are those in which changes in staff behaviors can be identified and attributed to educational interventions.

Evaluation of every project may involve answering the following questions:

- Was an appropriate problem the basis of the educational project? Was the problem correctly defined and delimited?
- Was the problem properly analyzed? Were the causes correctly identified? Was a multisource problem wrongly diagnosed as a single-source problem? Were contributory causes considered in planning the educational project?
- Were the selected remedial staff behaviors appropriate to reach the desired client outcomes? Were the staff taught behaviors realistic for the environment?
- Were the best possible learning experiences selected to teach the desired staff behav-

iors? Were alternate learning experiences considered and tried?
- Were appropriate tools used to measure both change in staff behavior and change in client outcome?

POWER RELATIONSHIPS

Although the director of staff development has primarily a staff relationship within the nursing department, it is not unusual for disproportionate power to gather in the role. The reasons for this are obvious. First, in other than a university setting, the director may be one of the best educated members of the nursing staff.

Second, the department, if centralized, has knowledge of and input from all of the nursing departments and often from out-of-division departments as well. This, incidentally, is probably why the function of troubleshooting is so often laid at the door of the director; it fits her "wide-scope" orientation. Hence, a relatively small department gathers power by virtue of its extensive relationships and information-seeking function within the organization.

Power Plays over Control of Staff

Even though line managers want their staff educated, their primary drive is to supply patient care, and that may interrupt education on any given day if all control remains in the hands of the line managers. This means that the education director and the line managers need to come to some clear agreements from the start concerning who controls what portion of the staff's time.

Educational programs (those that are not packaged for self-study) can be very expensive if anticipated attendees do not appear. An education director does not want to put extensive faculty time into preparing educational programs that have few students or that must be repeated many times. And that situation is demotivating for the faculty.

Sometimes control of staff becomes the issue in orientation programs. In some locations, the new staff are assigned by the staff education department until "released" to the line management staff for regular service. Unfortunately, with shrinking resources, this pattern is not feasible everywhere. Because a poor orientation is a main cause of premature resignations, it is a pity if immediate care demands give a new employee too much work before he is prepared for it.

Whatever the circumstances, evaluation of a new employee is critical. In most places, this responsibility is shared between education and line management. Whoever is responsible, it is to everyone's advantage to eliminate unsatisfactory workers as early as possible. Many places still observe the custom of maintaining a probation period during which a new employee can be dismissed without much need to justify the action.

At one time, new employees might receive orientation to many units of the institution, but this practice has declined. It is more common for the clinical orientation to be limited to the two or three units where the employee is likely to be based or to float. Increasing specialization has made the comprehensive orientation impractical, not to mention expensive.

Further, the internship programs once available to new graduates or new employees also have been curtailed, again because of economics. Interestingly, there is a counter-demand at present from university educators that service settings bear the cost of ongoing collegiate staff education at various levels. It is a demand many settings cannot afford to meet, no matter how much they would like to make such a commitment.

ORGANIZATION OF THE STAFF DEVELOPMENT PROGRAM

The staff development program is the totality of activities planned and implemented by the education department; it consists of all departmental projects taken together. As we mentioned earlier, this may include other related functions such as quality management or research—or it may be limited to the more traditional education projects. Most typically, the program includes staff education, orientation, and in some places, nurses' aide and technician training. Education programs are designed for induction, remedial, maintenance, preparatory, or supplemental education. See Table 29–1 for examples.

These five basic types of education might be identified as "get up," "catch up," "stay up," "move up," and "move out," respectively. Analysis of the distribution of projects over these five basic purposes provides a useful assessment of departmental functions.

Another perspective on education looks at services from the perspective of the recipient. Exhibit 29–1 illustrates this point. Although services to patients are key to the success of the program, services to nursing administration are also important. Further, services to staff members may be important in areas of the nation where there is heavy competition for staff.

Predictably in today's environment, in which staff are more likely to be cut than expanded, services for nursing staff are being cut. Indeed, many institutions that once had open enrollment in upward mobility programs have eliminated them. Institutions no longer pay staff to get higher degrees and advanced certification if positions requiring those skills are not available within the institution.

Services to the community, however, have tended to increase for at least two reasons. First, a customer relations program may be very important in securing potential clients. Community groups have been quick to discover the bargaining power this gives them. Public relations can be greatly enhanced by offering community health education programs that meet neighborhood interests.

Also, other programs are offered to raise monies, and these may include programs for the public or for professional groups. Some staff development departments are expected to carry many of their own costs; selling education is one way they do it. Indeed, the education department often contains the entrepreneurs of the nursing staff.

ADMINISTRATIVE ISSUES

The director should keep careful records of her programs, their content, and participants.

Table 29–1 Taxonomy of Educational Purpose

Form	Sample Project
1. Induction Education	
a. New job	Technician training, nurses' aide training
b. New function	LPN medication course
c. Orientation	
i. New environment	New employee orientation
ii. New position	Promotion
2. Remedial Education	
a. Foundational supplement	Nurse internship
b. Reentry supplement	Refresher course
3. Maintenance Education	
a. Recurrent training	Cardiopulmonary resuscitation practice
b. Updating	Training in new technologies
4. Preparatory Education	
a. Upgrading clinical education	
i. Nurse technician programs	Coronary care course
ii. Nurse associate programs	Pediatric nurse associate
iii. Clinical nurse specialist	MA programs
b. Upgrading functional skills	
i. Educational skills	Methods-of-teaching course
ii. Management skills	Principles of case management
iii. Research skills	
5. Supplemental Education	
a. Education applicable to direct nursing practice	Psychology, sociology, biology
b. Education facilitative to nursing practice or function	Languages, economics, management theory

Exhibit 29–1 Scope of Educational Services

1. Services for Nursing Staff Members

Educational projects—workshops, courses, classes

Career educational counseling—academic, certificate, and continuing education information

Coordination and promotion of educational opportunities available outside of the home institution—conventions, seminars, workshops

Maintenance of personnel records on educational acquisitions of all employees

Maintenance and control of educational materials—library holdings, circulation of materials, selective distribution

Consultation and problem solving—as needed or requested for nursing care problems

2. Services for Nursing Administrative Staff

Advising and participating in formulation of policies, practices, and procedures

Troubleshooting—analysis of problem situations in the division, proposal of solutions

Nursing research—identification of areas of need, construction and implementation of proper research designs

Quality management systems design, monitoring, risk management

Staffing—placement of staff on the basis of individual competencies

Serving as a catalyst in design groups or committees

Preparation of grant proposals—initiating use of grants, helping others in preparations

Serving as an educational expert—assisting others with their own educational projects

3. Services for Patients

Preparing programs for patient education

Providing direct education to patients

Teaching staff members methods of patient education

Construction of valid patient questionnaires to identify needs for change

4. Services for Community

Educational programs on normal health needs

Education for special interest groups—family planning, diabetic education, emergency care education

Nursing vocational counseling—for high school groups and others

Managing relations with affiliating nursing, medical, or allied health students

Usually, a double system is required whereby participation and evaluation are also entered on the attendee's personnel record. The record-keeping function increases as many departments of staff development seek authority to grant continuing education units or, alternately, submit many of their programs for such credit. Also, many departments are getting into the business of offering courses that qualify participants to sit for various certification examinations. When a program relates to any sort of credential for participants, records must not only be exacting but kept over time. More and more employees are using their inservice education records as unofficial transcripts.

If an education program is to succeed, it must have the support of the nurse executive and nursing management. The support must be attitudinal as well as structural, with the work processes designed to reinforce educational projects.

When the staff development department is responsible for negotiating with academic programs over student placement, another opportunity presents itself. In today's market, many tradeoffs take place whereby, in exchange for student placement, an education department can call on academic faculty for various educational services. This is a great way to extend the educational resources of a department.

Also, in exchange for student services, faculty appointments are often extended to practicing nurses, frequently including qualified staff educators and directors. In such negotiations, no rules can be set; what matters is that each side believe that it has reached an appropriate reciprocity. Both sides should come out of a bargaining session feeling that they have made an equal trade of services and benefits.

SUMMARY

An effective staff development program calls for a balance of activities designed to meet the unique needs of the given organization. Staff education may be seen as the corrective component of a feedback systems loop, designed primarily to enhance patient outcomes but also to serve administrative or public relations needs.

The education director and her staff must be skilled educators, able to work with diverse education methods and willing to work intimately with the nursing staff on the patient care units. Economy in delivery of educational programs has become a must, influencing not only the functions and programs of a staff education department but also its methods. The staff development function, however organized, demands close work with the quality management program.

SUGGESTED READINGS

Ament, L.A. 1993. Competency assessment versus credentialing: Promoting professional nursing practice. *Journal of Nursing Staff Development* 9, no.3:155–157.

Aulback, R.K., et al. 1993. Collaborative critical care education: The educator link. *Journal of Nursing Staff Development* 9, no.2:63–67.

Brown-Steward, P. 1992. JCAHO: De-mystifying the staff development role. *Nursing Staff Development Insider* 1, no.1:1, 6–7.

Brunt, B. 1993. Outcome studies. *Journal of Nursing Staff Development* 9, no.2:96–97.

Cummings, C. 1993. Ethical issues in staff development. *Nursing Staff Development Insider* 2, no.2:6–7.

Finnick, M., et al. 1993. Staff development challenge: Assuring nurses competency in quality assessment and improvement. *Journal of Nursing Staff Development* 9, no.3:136–140.

Jambunathan, J. 1992. Planning a peer review program. *Journal of Nursing Staff Development* 8, no.5:235–239.

Ozcan, Y.A., and R.K. Shukia. 1993. The effect of a competency-based targeted staff development program on nursing productivity. *Journal of Nursing Staff Development* 9, no.2:78–84.

Rodriguez, L. 1993. Linking staff development to the organization's goals. *Nursing Staff Development Insider* 2, no.3:3.

Sheridan, D.R. 1993. The potential demise of staff development departments editorial. *Nursing Staff Development Insider* 2, no.3:1, 8.

Part VIII

Nurse Executive As Leader

This is an era when the nurse executive role has shifted from that of manager toward that of leader. In other words, the nurse executive can no longer be the person who simply tends to the operation, no matter how effectively. Today's nurse executive role requires operation by broader strokes, greater vision, and more setting of future goals and roles.

Today's nurse executive needs a wider view on the world of health, society, and the forces likely to have an effect on health care delivery now and in the future. His monitoring of the situation must be constant and thoughtful; his role is corporate, not limited to the nursing division. It is no longer a world in which nursing can operate in isolation. Close coordination with physicians, other professionals, and institutional administrators is a must.

The nurse manager role of prior years was easier: One learned the components of the role and their related processes and procedures. A good manager could be created with the proper education. Although benefiting from the right education, the leader cannot follow preset formulas. The astuteness of today's nurse executive is more important than the thoroughness of yesterday's nurse manager. In essence, the most valuable human traits and capacities required of a nurse executive are changing. Today's nurse executive must be clever, able to seize the moment, hopefully charismatic, and able to cast a vision others will want to follow.

30

Nurse Executives and Transitions

Nurse executives come to their roles from a variety of situations. Every situation brings a set of opportunities distinctly different from any other situation, and each must be handled uniquely. A nurse executive may find himself in a position in which his predecessor lost the job in a traumatic termination process. Or the previous nurse executive may have chosen not to swim the stormy waters in the wake of a merger or acquisition.

In some situations, the new nurse executive may be filling a freshly conceptualized position, created because the organization found itself in a crisis and needed a nurse executive to quickly turn around a situation threatening the organization's survival.

In some cases, there has been an extensive leadership change in the top level of the organization, and the nurse executive may be part of a new team brought in by a new chief executive officer. The job of a nurse executive is greatly influenced by such circumstances.

However, a nurse executive may find himself on the other end of a transition. He might find himself no longer suited to the position, or someone else in the organization may find him no longer suited. A nurse executive who has always experienced success in his role may find that his style is simply incompatible with that of a new chief executive officer or he may think

that he is unable to work under a new organization design.

Not all nurse executives are capable of or interested in working in a new organizational design. For example, a nurse executive losing line authority as an organization makes the transition from a departmental focus to a service line structure might find the transition traumatic and resign or be terminated because of resistance to the new plan.

THE CHALLENGES OF TRANSITION

Each of these situations and many others that might be described brings its own unique set of opportunities and problems for the nurse executive. Around these problems and opportunities, he must build a program and a career. Today, any nurse executive is likely to be faced with at least one main transition, maybe many—even if he remains in the same institution. Transitions are difficult for executives who remain in place and struggle to adapt to new circumstances. They are difficult for the nurse executive who is making an organizational move, too. This chapter focuses on the nurse executive moving to a new organization, but many comments apply equally to an executive changing jobs in the same location.

In many ways, this transition period can be simplistically likened to that of a family that loses one parent and takes on a step-parent. The organization must get used to a stranger who comes with a whole new set of values and expectations and who demands that the organization follow a new path. Some step-parents and some nurse executives handle this transition with grace and style, and the organization benefits from the experience of the transition. In other situations, the transition period is not handled well and the organization, at least temporarily, becomes embroiled in turmoil and nonproductive activities.

The transition into a new nurse executive position can be an extraordinarily stressful time for the nurse executive, whether he comes from an internal promotion within the organization or from an outside appointment. In many cases, being from outside the organization means coming from outside the immediate geographic area as well.

Not only is the nurse executive confronted with a new position and a new region of the country (with a different set of cultural beliefs and values) but he also is faced with the practical trauma of moving. And the stresses and strains of relocating occur simultaneously with the executive's challenge of establishing a new set of social relationships as well as work relationships. Commonly now, nurse executives relocate with families, magnifying the stresses of relocation.

ON MAKING THE RIGHT TRANSITION

Ideally, when faced with a leadership change, the organization will have thought through the issue of the transition and will have identified the kind of person and the particular characteristics he will need to fill the position. This means the involved officers have considered what sort of nurse executive is needed in the light of the long-term mission and their vision for the health care facility.

For example, when teaching and research are heavy commitments, the nurse executive will need doctoral preparation to hold his own in the power structure. Similarly, a need for tough competition within the managed care market may influence the characteristics the organization requires in its nurse leader.

Often today, an executive search firm is in charge of a search for a top nurse executive. Most of these businesses are dedicated to finding the right person for the right slot, but some are more interested in filling the position and moving on to the next assignment than worrying over whether the match of institution and executive has been a good one. Commonly, search firms that make themselves available to health care facilities provide an organizational assessment to the nurse executive candidates. Such a profile helps one determine if the fit between the nurse executive and the health care facility is right.

Much of the success of the nurse executive rests in the "job fit" between him, the chief executive officer, the staff, the physicians, and the community. It is not uncommon that nurse executives fail, not because of lack of expertise but because of the lack of "job fit" between the person and the position.

BEGINNING A NEW POSITION

The first few days of the new job are very important because the nurse executive is under intense scrutiny. The organization will be watching to see how he actualizes the role. This is a time for the executive to consciously think about the messages he wants to send throughout the organization. For example, if this is a situation in which a fast turnaround of operations is required, the message should convey that fast action and restructuring can be anticipated. This needs to be heard immediately so that the organization will know what to expect.

However, in some organizations, perhaps those in excellent condition except for an instability created by rapid turnover at the top or loss of revered leaders, the needed message may be that there will be no radical change and that the tradition of excellence will continue. The nurse executive is then placed in a position of proving in the first few weeks that he can do the job as well as his predecessor.

Whatever the circumstances, the last thing that the new executive should do in the initial stages is to criticize the former nurse executive. Regardless of the performance of his predecessor, there will be people who are loyal to this person—and people who are not. When the new nurse executive demonstrates respect for his predecessor, the staff will be assured that the new leader has character and sensitivity.

The process of taking on a position should be thought out and handled similarly to the way one handles project management. Endpoints must be conceptualized in terms of when the nurse executive will have the organization restructured and developed.

Stages of Adaptation to the Role

In *The Dynamics of Taking Charge,* Gabarro (1987) delineated several stages the new executive goes through in transit to the new job, determining these stages through interviews and field studies. They are as follows (pp. 10–38):

1. *Stage 1—Taking Hold.* In this stage, lasting 3 to 6 months, the new manager takes hold of the position and comes to understand the problems and opportunities it presents.
2. *Stage 2—Immersion.* Here, the manager becomes immersed in the running of the organization, learning how improvements can be made and how practices should be altered.
3. *Stage 3—Reshaping.* This is a phase in which the new person makes structural changes and reconceptualizes how the job and the work should be performed.
4. *Stage 4—Consolidation.* The manager evaluates the outcomes of the reshaping stage and makes changes and refinements to consolidate the new organization pattern.
5. *Stage 5—Refinement.* In this stage, no major organizational redesigns are made, but additional improvements are instituted based on new information.

With these stages as a guide, the new nurse executive can prospectively determine how to move through the process of learning the job, restructuring, and consolidating practices.

Many of the previous chapters of this book outlined what the nurse executive does and what needs to be performed by him. When these functions are broken into stages and processes, a prospective plan of action can be developed. It is common that the nurse executive does not think that he "owns" the job for at least $1\frac{1}{2}$ to 2 years.

Divisions of nursing are very complicated. Assessing the organization and developing a plan takes extensive thought and application of the skills of synthesis and analysis. It is crucial for the nurse executive to think his plans through at this early period of time, using all resources possible, such as the knowledge of organizational design, change theory, and knowledge of interpersonal relationships. If the stages of taking charge are successfully navigated, the tenure of the nurse executive is off to a good start.

Developing a Management Team

Beyond the stages that Gabarro delineated, there are other important processes for this phase of transition. One involves looking downward at one's own nursing management team. Beyond determining who the players will be—and their respective powers—the nurse executive must build the relationships between and among these people so that a fully functioning team evolves. Without this teamwork, the nurse executive's effectiveness will be limited. In *Making a Leadership Change,* Gilmore (1988) pointed out that the leader must determine the critical challenges, decide what roles will be needed to meet those challenges, and assess the present staff to ascertain which players can become a part of the new management team. After he makes these decisions, he builds the team.

Gilmore said that a useful way to assess the staff is to examine their performance where they work now, enhancing this judgment through observations of them at retreats (when their performance in formal activities as well as informal activities can be assessed). It is seldom the case that a new nurse executive will want to maintain the old nursing leadership intact—nor should he be expected to. If nothing else, there are usually some personnel changes incurred by a new organization chart. Indeed, before taking a new position, the nurse executive should be certain he will have the authority to build his own team.

An even worse mistake than taking a position where one cannot make changes in the nursing team is going into a situation and replacing everyone. Some executives try the tactic of importing their old team and superimposing it on the new facility. This high-handed replacement of all management staff is bound to have bad repercussions. Further, it costs one the opportunity of finding the good people among those already in place.

If one brings along too many people from one's former position, there is a real danger of forgetting that every institution is different. All too easily, the "old team" will try the old solutions, ignoring the realities of the new situation. Worse, the executive will get a reputation as a raider, decreasing his future career opportunities. The executive should leave the former place of employment in good shape, with an intact staff ready to carry on effectively until a new nurse executive is appointed.

Once his new team is established, the nurse executive must develop and communicate a new vision and program. The vision should appear to come from the entire management staff; if he has built wisely, that will be true. Once this group has a shared view of the values, purposes, and mission for the organization, the executive team will be an effective, efficient force in performing the work of the organization.

Good Working Relationships

Beyond one's own nursing management staff, other working relationships need to be fostered to develop one's role productively. Gabarro (1985) found that, by the end of the first year, the most important predictor of exec-

utive success was the quality of the working relationships that the new manager had established. When good working relationships were developed, the transition to the new position was successful.

When relationships were poor, the manager was failing to move successfully into the new position. The nurse executive needs to purposefully develop working relationships with other departments throughout the organization so that the goals of patient care can be met. This involves assessing other departments, their leaders, and their relationship to the division of nursing; it also involves defining shared outcomes, determining what needs to be done in the context of the relationship, and setting each relationship on a firm basis.

Sometimes, good working relationships can be established by simple dialogue and joint planning. In other cases, they are more complex and need more attention so a shared vision of patient care and mutual goal achievement can be accomplished. Nor can the nurse executive be parochial in this effort; the goals of the other leader and his department/division must be taken into account in making a relationship work.

Mechanisms such as liaison committees between the division of nursing and problematic departments can quickly solve many problems if people can be put together in face-to-face situations. Often, when other departments understand the strategic direction of the division of nursing and believe that they are a part of it, the right kind of relationships will develop.

The nurse executive must also be sensitive to the origins of interorganizational problems. Are they really problems arising among the divisions and departments, or are the problems created by competitive rivalries among corporate executives? It would be nice if everyone in health care were motivated simply by what is good for an institution's patients. Unfortunately, this is not always the case. Simply, the presence of a strong nurse executive with a large piece of the corporate pie may be enough to stir up corporate jealousies and confrontations. Each problem will be better handled if the nurse executive can fester out "where it is coming from."

Relations with One's Boss

In the early phase of transition, the nurse executive must establish an excellent working relationship with his boss. Each new nurse executive will have different role expectations both for himself and for his boss. Building a successful relationship with the boss means negotiating roles and developing a shared vision of how these roles should mesh and be operationalized. Some role preferences will be shared, some will be independent, and others will need much negotiation. At this stage, the nurse executive is well advised to manage this relationship with much thought as to strategy. Gilmore (1988) gave several suggestions important in this role negotiation with the boss.

1. Determine the strategic challenges and negotiate shared expectations for these challenges.
2. Thoughtfully analyze the style differences between the boss and oneself.
3. Understand from the boss's perspective, his picture of the world, and determine how the issues at hand need to be addressed based on this.
4. Analyze the boss's strengths and weaknesses and determine how they fit with one's own.
5. Regularly ask the boss for feedback and determine how one's position can better support what the boss needs.

When taking charge, the new nurse executive must be concerned about managing relationships with subordinates and with horizontal and upward relationships in the organization. When one can develop mutual expectations, mutual trust, and a commitment to working together for the good of the organization, a high-performing management team will ensue.

THE TRANSITION IN LEAVING A POSITION

In addition to the transition into a new job, the nurse executive must also face a transition out of a position. The transition of termination happens for a variety of reasons. Career opportunities can take the nurse executive away. Or a nurse executive may resign when he finds himself positioned poorly within a merger. Sometimes, the nurse executive will be asked to leave because of conflict with a new boss or a perception that he is performing poorly.

Transition, whether from dismissal or through resignation, evokes a grief process, with all the similar stages. Indeed, Barba and Selder (1995) equated loss of a high-placed nurse executive job with the emotional experiences faced by a patient who has suffered a major permanent physical injury. Selder's (1989) life transition theory is a good model for the process.

Jacoby (1986) stated that "the changing of the guard can be exciting and stimulating if positive attitudes prevail and the climate of friendship and mutual interest is sustained" (p. 205). But when one is personally involved, it is easy to be self-centered and think of one's own feelings first.

The most appropriate thing to do is to exit without causing harm to the organization and to the people who are left in the organization. The best thing a person can do in this situation is to plan carefully and introspectively to make an effective farewell. According to Maholick and Turner (1979), the plan must consider all the audiences affected, such as one's boss, those directly reporting to the person, people outside one's reporting relationship, and people outside the facility.

Depending on how this is handled, people can resign with style and grace or can do great harm to the organization and to themselves by not thinking through the best way to handle the transition.

Rituals

When the nurse executive makes a decision to take a new job, there are important rituals to mark his termination from the old position. Bon voyage parties and recognition ceremonies serve their functions well, providing a time for people to express their gratitude and to say good-bye. Such events formally and symbolically allow the executive to terminate from the old position and clear his head for the new one. If the executive does not psychologically leave the old position, he may mistakenly live out that position in the new one.

The executive most likely to fail is the one who arrives at a new position with a set of strategies and goals in hand—those that worked on the prior job. No two situations are the same; each requires a unique approach. The executive will need to distance himself from the old situation if he is to attack the new one effectively.

The worst thing an executive can do is to leave one position on Friday and begin another on the following Monday. And the demands of the new job are often so pressing that people will want the nurse executive to start as soon as possible. However, a "time-out period" between jobs is the best way to clear one's head and to think about how to conceptualize a new job.

SUMMARY

Transitions in the nurse executive role are really like reaching new plateaus. If the transition is planned well, the nurse executive can reach that new plateau and so can both the receiving and losing organizations. If the transition is not carefully planned, however, the endeavor becomes fraught with many slips and falls. Planning for the transition phase enables one to advance in the new position, moving forward on a consistent path. And it allows the old organization to appreciate one's contribution rather than resent one's departure.

Transitions for nurse executives are difficult because their roles are complex and because the institutions for which they work are full of ambiguities and contradictions. The nurse executive who anticipates the challenge of the transition process will manage it better than the executive who is unprepared.

REFERENCES

Barba, E.A., and F. Selder. 1995. Life transition theory: It works for the unemployed nurse executive as well as for patients. *Nursing Leadership Forum* 1, no.1:4–11.

Gabarro, J. 1985. When a new manager takes charge. *Harvard Business Review* 63, no.3:110–123.

Gabarro, J. 1987. *The dynamics of taking charge.* Boston: Harvard Business School Press.

Gilmore, T.M. 1988. *Making a leadership change.* San Francisco: Jossey-Bass, Inc.

Jacoby, E. 1986. The changing of the guard. *Journal of Professional Nursing* 2, no.4:205.

Maholick, L. and D. Turner. 1979. Termination: That difficult farewell. *American Journal of Psychotherapy* 33, no.4:583–591.

Selder, F. 1989. Life transition theory: The resolution of uncertainty. *Nursing and Health Care* 10, no.8:436–451.

SUGGESTED READINGS

Aulatta, K. 1985. *The art of corporate success.* New York: Penguin Books.

Beckhardt, R., and R.T. Harris. 1977. *Organizational transitions: Managing complex change.* Reading, Mass.: Addison-Wesley.

Bennis, W., and B. Nanus. 1985. *Leaders: The strategy for taking charge.* New York: Harper & Row.

Brown, B. 1983. What is business savvy? *Nursing Economics* 4, no.1:53.

Dooley, S.L., and J. Hauben. 1979. From staff nurse to head nurse: A trying transition. *Journal of Nursing Administration* 9, no.4:4–7.

Freund, C.M. 1985. The tenure of directors of nursing. *The Journal of Nursing Administration* 15, no.2:11–15.

Grove, A.S. 1983. *High output management.* New York: Random House.

Kelly, J.N. 1980. Management transitions for new appointed CEOs. *Sloan Management Review* 22, no.1:37–45.

Lebsack, C. 1986. Dealing with leadership changes. *Nursing Success Today* 3, no.12:32–36.

Levinson, H., and S. Rosenthal. 1984. *CEO: Corporate leadership in action.* New York: Basic Books, Inc.

McCaskey, M.B. 1982. *The executive challenge: Managing change and ambiguity.* Boston: Pittman.

Vancil, R.F. 1987. Corporate look at CEO succession. *Harvard Business Review* 65, no.2:107–117.

Zaluzinek, A. 1967. Management of disappointment. *Harvard Business Review* 45, no.6:59–70.

31

Nurse Executive As Builder of Teams

One of the most important measures of the success of the nurse executive is his ability to work with groups. Not only does he need to manage groups within the division but also groups outside the division. Most of the work of the nurse executive is performed through committees, task forces, or small informal meetings.

The nurse executive works in groups all the way from top management groups, to task forces, through work with staff nurses on the front lines. The effectiveness of these groups can be measured by the quality of their output, by the degree to which people work interdependently to get the job done effectively, and on how well the group contributes to the growth and personal well-being of team members (Hackman 1990).

Different teams vary on the degree to which they achieve these criteria. High-performing teams have learned to work well together, developing synergy. By synergy, we mean that they achieve more together than they would as separate individuals. Sometimes, it is difficult to develop high-performing groups and teams at the executive level. People come to the executive level because they are competitive and high achievers. At times, they have private agendas, sometimes in conflict with organizational goals. Rivalry for the executive's attention or competition for resources often makes for a corporate executive with a mind-set that makes teamwork difficult.

Katzenbach and Smith (1993) pointed out that the way to build a successful team at the top is to find real work that the executives can do together. This often is difficult for the executive team because of time constraints and because of a sense of individualism common to many members. However, these authors believe that, if collective work products and approaches can be identified, the executive team will develop the mutual accountability that is characteristic of good teams.

The nurse executive is well positioned to help develop this kind of mutual accountability at the executive level. It is not uncommon to find that the nurse executive is the most skilled in interpersonal relationships and group dynamics because of his clinical education.

Cross-functional groups are important mechanisms in compensating for the hierarchy in vertically designed organizations. Cross-division teams provide excellent means for re-engineering the work processes and getting the work of patient care performed more efficiently and at higher levels of quality. Basic to this concept of cross-divisional work teams is a move toward self-governed and self-managed teams. In the best of all possible worlds, highly synergized self-managed teams can work throughout the organization from the very top to the bottom.

BUILDING TEAMS AT THE PATIENT CARE LEVEL

Often the nurse executive desires to instill a democratic process of self-rule within the patient care units of his division. This will not happen without a lot of work and preparation. Knowledge of group work on the executive's part can facilitate the process of building such self-managing teams at the bedside on the unit level.

According to Dwyer (1987), the current interest in groups and teams had its roots in the Hawthorne studies (in which the group responded to manipulations of the work environment conditions), in Likert's analysis of participative group management, and in McGregor's work on developing managerial teams. Certainly, these are three of the hallmark works that have influenced nursing management.

Empowering of the work force is a goal of many effective nurse executives. Manz and Sims (1989) pointed out that the goal of a manager should not be to become a super-leader but to convert his control to the staff so they can internalize accountability and manage themselves. Manz and Sims believed that the manager should lead others to lead themselves. Thus, a self-governed team moves from empowering individuals to empowering the full team to work as a unit. Groups evolve from participative management through shared governance to self-directed and empowered teams that develop synergy and high productivity.

When this movement toward teamwork matures, a highly sophisticated group of nurses can, in fact, manage themselves without a nurse manager. Once their tasks are clear, self-managed teams can organize themselves to do the jobs and to evaluate themselves as well. Indeed, some prestigious nursing divisions already have such self-managed nursing units with highly synergized effective teams of staff members.

Most professional practice models advocate professionals managing themselves. Unlike health care (in which roles such as nurse manager, supervisor, and director prevail), not all professionals organize themselves in hierarchies. Lawyers, for example, organize themselves in partnerships with self-governed structures in which the partnership team manages the enterprise.

There is a basic conflict between traditional management science, geared to managing the blue collar technical worker, and the notion of managing white collar or professional workers. Some argue that the traditional model does not work well in nursing, that nurses leave nursing because they feel overmanaged. When they have the opportunity to realize full professional status in self-managed teams, attrition decreases. With experience and sophistication, master clinicians can take on the traditional work of managers: doing their own peer review, hiring their own staff, and performing strategic planning for their unit.

In these models, the nurse manager becomes a coach and facilitator, not a director and controller of practice. The manager merely sets the wheels in motion and watches as highly performing self-managed teams take over the management functions and produce excellent outcomes.

The move to shared governance and other employee empowerment models behooves everyone, the nurse executive, the management team, and staff, to become experts in managing groups and in understanding group dynamics. The task is made easier because groups are predictable. They go through definite stages of forming and finally synergizing.

Much of what the nurse executive does is achieved through the process of bringing diverse groups of people together to complete tasks. This is successful when they share the commitment and are mutually accountable for specific activities. Larson and LaFlastel (1989) pointed out that there are four necessary features for effective team structures:

- clear rules and accountabilities
- an effective communication system
- methods for monitoring individual performance and providing feedback
- emphasis on fact-based judgment

These authors also admit the necessity for having a "clear, elevating goal, a results-driven structure, and competent team members," as well as a unified commitment. Also, Hackman (1990) noted that there are five mistakes that leaders of groups often make (pp. 493–504):

- managing members as individuals rather than as a team
- failing to balance managerial and team authority appropriately as the team evolves
- assembling people to accomplish a task, then failing to provide members with enough structure
- skimping on organizational support for the team
- assuming that people automatically have confidence to work well as a team

Shared governance models work best if true teamwork and a sense of synergy develop in the task forces and committee structures that get the work of the organization done. The nurse executive is challenged to provide the educational support necessary for shared governance structures, allowing the staff to take on more accountability over time. As staff nurses lead shared governance teams, they also must have the opportunity to learn how groups work.

SUMMARY

Highly synergized productive work teams have been shown to be much more effective in terms of cost and quality of outcomes than over-managed structures. Furthermore, when professionals are not accorded full professional status, productivity suffers. Autonomous and highly effective work groups are a great vehicle for facilitating and achieving the goals of management.

The resource-driven model challenges the nurse executive to get the work done with better methods, with controlled costs, and better outcomes. As the world of business has proved, self-managed teams can achieve more than can a few individuals functioning alone at the top. Nursing organizations can feel proud that shared governance structures of this kind have been in place in nursing for many years. The challenge for the nurse executive is to become an expert in developing teams so that the organization can be successful in these models.

REFERENCES

Dwyer, W. 1987. *Teambuilding: Issues and alternatives*. 2nd ed. Reading, Mass.: Addison-Wesley Publishing Co.

Hackman, J.R. 1990. *Groups that work (and those that don't)*. San Francisco: Jossey-Bass.

Katzenbach, J.R., and D.K. Smith. 1993. *The wisdom of teams*. Boston: Harvard Business School Press.

Larson, C.E., and F.M. LaFlastel. 1989. *Teamwork*. Newberry Park, London: Sage Publications.

Manz, C., and H. Sims. 1989. *Super leadership*. Englewood Cliffs, N.J.: Prentice Hall.

SUGGESTED READINGS

Benjamin, G. 1989. Effective staff functioning in dealing with executive teams. *Nursing Administration Quarterly* 13, no.2:55–58.

Brown, M. 1989. Building and promoting the executive team. *Nursing Administration Quarterly* 13, no.2:vii–viii.

Craig, M. 1989. Reflections of the executive team. *Nursing Administration Quarterly* 13, no.2:61–62.

Davis, P. 1992. Unit-based shared governance: Nurturing the vision. *Journal of Nursing Administration* 22, no.12:46–50.

Farley, M., and M. Stonger. 1989. The nurse executive and interdisciplinary teams. *Nursing Administration Quarterly* 13, no.2:24–30.

Mills, J., and M. Oie. 1992. Autonomous staff selection teams. *Journal of Nursing Administration* 22, no. 12:57–63.

Robinson, J. 1989. Creating the foundation for an effective executive team. *Nursing Administration Quarterly* 13, no.2:44–51.

Sands, J., and B. Garabedian. 1991. The product-line management team. *Nursing Administration Quarterly* 15, no.2:45–48.

Taft, S., et al. 1992. Strengthening hospital nursing, Part III. *Journal of Nursing Administration* 22, no.7–8:41–50.

Thyen, M., et al. 1993. Organizational empowerment through self-governed teams. *Journal of Nursing Administration* 23, no.1:24–26.

Tonges, M. 1989. Redesigning hospital nursing practice: The professionally advanced care team. *Journal of Nursing Administration* 19, no.9:19–22.

Tonges, M. 1989. The executive team: Part II. *Nursing Administration Quarterly* 13, no.3:vii–viii, 1–74.

32

Strategic Planning and Marketing

Strategic planning and marketing are discussed here as if they were separate functions, when, in fact, they often intertwine. Marketing concerns are an inherent part of most strategic planning, and strategic planning, in turn, is an integral part of successful marketing. Strategic planning and marketing arise from a similar view of the world: Both reflect a bottom-line, product-oriented mentality. Both are sensitive to the environment and respond to sudden changes within it. They are concerned with positioning an organization in the environment to be competitive and to take advantage of business-enhancing opportunities that arise.

STRATEGIC PLANNING

Strategic planning, briefly addressed in Chapters 2 and 3, is an approach applied in determining the goals, objectives, and activities of an organization (or a component within that organization) and moves swiftly to take advantage of environmental changes; it is designed to provide for quick response in a changing world.

One way to understand this concept is to compare it with management by objective (MBO). MBO is a more static process wherein one sets goals and organizes to deliver on them. As discussed in Chapter 2, in MBO the goals come first. How goals are determined is not specified, but tradition (e.g., what a nursing service division typically does) or some ethical stance (e.g., what a nursing division should do in an institution of this sort) may be the source.

In MBO, the goals are set, the environment is assayed to determine the ways and means needed to achieve the goals, and finally the plan is put into effect. The length of the plan may be variable. Some institutions and some nursing divisions plan year by year; others have longer planning cycles. To create such a plan assumes that one has knowledge of the ways and means that will deliver on the selected goals. It also assumes that the world will continue to operate in much the same way for the totality of the planned time period.

The traditional MBO planning model has proved of limited value given the rapid shifts in the environment of today's health care organization. For example, the imposition of the diagnosis-related group (DRG) reimbursement model caused major upheavals in the long-term plans of many institutions. Now, the imposition of managed care and price dictated by insurers exerts a similar state of continuous upheaval and replanning.

Strategic planning has arisen as the favored alternate form of institutional planning, adopted when the more static forms fail to work. Historically, Mintzberg (1973) identified three different strategies for management:

- *planning model:* characterized by goal setting with systematic and detailed plans for achievement; reliance on rationality and scientific techniques; anticipatory decision making
- *adaptive model:* characterized by reactive and remedial decisions aimed at reducing conflict; ongoing negotiation and adjustment to the environment; incremental decision making
- *entrepreneurial model:* characterized by an active search for new opportunities; proactive leaps forward in the face of uncertainty dominated by a high-risk, high-gain mentality

If MBO epitomizes the planning model, then strategic planning can be seen as a modification of the adaptive model. Planning ahead is still the aim, but what gets planned depends on the situation. The following assumptions underlie strategic planning:

- Management is relational: The major environmental characteristics that have an effect on one's business must be recognized and taken into account in planning.
- The environment may change suddenly and unpredictably, and one must be prepared to change one's plans accordingly and rapidly.
- Methods and even goals are contingent on the environmental opportunities; they are not fixed.
- Constant surveillance of the environment, including one's competition, is necessary for rapid interpretation and response.

Strategic planning is a management process that evaluates markets and competition, identifying and taking into account the environmental circumstances that are likely to have an effect on the organization. It is a philosophy and method of opportunism, enabling the institution to select goals that accentuate its strengths and to select markets that will benefit from those strengths (benefiting both the client and the organization).

Strategic planning starts with an analysis of the organization. It is scrutinized for both strengths and weaknesses. Past mission statements are explored in the light of current organizational realities. The new missions considered are pragmatic: what will work to the organization's advantage in these times.

This perspective is then juxtaposed with an analysis of the potential customers (present or untapped future users of services). The market analysis assesses potential customers in the light of environmental factors, primarily economic ones. In most cases, the institution must compete for customers, and its marketability is viewed from this perspective.

Many definitions of strategic planning assume the financial bottom-line is a driving force in the institution's survival. Others may see the financial environment as just one environment among others to be assessed. For example, an analysis may include looking at technological, political, and industrial environments as well as the economic realities.

Major differences may be seen between the MBO planning model and strategic planning. First, strategic planning hones in on the main, but not all, environmental issues. It seeks to isolate trends that will endure and have impact. Strategic planning tends to act with a broad brush, whereas MBO uses a fine-lined pen. Strategic planning sets key thrusts for the future, without trying to compose a comprehensive plan for all possible future actions. It concentrates on the key organizational goals and actions. It is more focused yet less comprehensive than an MBO plan. Generally, a strategic plan is bolder and takes more risks.

Strategic planning also is more flexible. It involves devising alternate plans, not just a single plan. Commitment to a plan lasts just as long as the plan is effective. Constant monitoring and evaluation provide continuous feedback, allowing for quicker recognition of a plan gone awry and providing for fast changing of gears when required. There is less psychological investment in the plan and more in the outcome. When a plan fails, an alternate is quickly put in its place.

A failure of a strategic plan is regrettable, but a failure to recognize when a plan is not working is worse.

The greatest difference between an MBO planning model and strategic planning lies in the different ways in which goals arise. In the MBO model, all planning begins with the goals. In strategic planning, goals are selected contingent on the analysis of the environment and the potential customers, and decisions concerning what the institution is in the best situation to create and market.

Nursing Use of Strategic Planning

In taking a strategic approach to its planning, a nursing division uncovers many opportunities for contributing to the institution. Nursing is one of the chief services in a health care institution and, as such, provides and can create products and services that meet many consumer demands. Additional consumer demands can be created for products by skilled marketing techniques.

More important, a strategic planning approach allows the nurse executive to take a creative new perspective on the work of the division. Restructured nursing practice, a movement taking place across this nation, is a result of strategic planning. Namely, restructured practice was a response to a unique environmental constraint: constantly decreasing funding along with continuously increasing nursing salaries. The challenge presented by this circumstance was to find ways to deliver quality care within these constraints.

Building Revenue Streams

In some instances, strategic planning comes closer to Mintzberg's entrepreneurial strategy than to his adaptive model. In this resource-driven era, the nurse executive is challenged to develop new revenue streams, and to this end, many are developing, marketing, and selling new nursing products. Along with an entrepreneurial spirit, market survey techniques help the nurse executive determine what nursing products can be developed profitably.

Many nursing divisions have initiated for-profit services to enhance their divisional income. Rather than being entered on the general ledger, sometimes such income is set aside to maintain excellence in nursing, paying for staff to attend nursing seminars, and to support travel for nurses attending off-site conferences.

Customers of these entrepreneurial efforts may be patients, nurses, or other professionals. Nurse-run clinics are one example of patient services. Community information/education sessions are another source of income. One hospital in an air-polluted environment, for example, developed an ongoing series, "Living with Asthma," for the general public.

Many staff development departments are marketing their educational services (e.g., programs preparatory to various credentialing examinations, pharmacy courses) to nurses in their own and other institutions. Some nursing education departments become self-supporting or even generate revenue with a program designed to be customer-oriented.

Nor need traditional programs be the only possible products. If the facility has particular areas of excellence, nursing related to these specialties can be marketed to produce revenue. For example, an institution with a nationally known cardiovascular program might develop a consultation service or market a short nursing internship so that nurses (nationally and internationally) may come and visit for a fee.

Nonclinical specialties can be used in this way also. Often organizations with successful case management programs offer consultation services; some even market their case maps. If the organization is distinguished in shared governance, materials could be sold and/or consultation fees charged for learning about this program. Programs of this sort can involve people coming to the facility or experts going off-site to other institutions.

Internally developed/programmed learning texts, video tapes, or various manuals (patient education, case maps, nursing procedures) are all products that can be developed and marketed to generate revenue. With an entrepreneurial marketing orientation, the staff can develop many products that will sell and generate revenue.

Nor need products be limited to nurse clients. Some staff development programs, for example, are selling programs required for relicensure (e.g., child abuse education, infection control education) to practitioners from all professions. Projects that aim to sell a product or a service require a blending of strategic planning and marketing skill. A good idea, even a good product, is not enough without the right marketing approach.

Outside of traditional acute care, nurses are forming their own corporations and companies for various health care services. They market well-health programs to industry, alternate site care to ill and convalescent customers, as well as life enhancement and recovery programs to the growing health-conscious public. Strategic planning, with market assessment, opens new possibilities for nurses in old and new settings, established and new businesses. In many cases, nurses are competing successfully with physicians, providing similar services at cost-competitive prices.

Most nurse executives use strategic planning to analyze all their ongoing nursing practices and programs. The strategic planning model, based on an economic bottom-line perspective, is simply more compatible with today's fast changing challenges and opportunities than are older planning models.

MARKETING

Marketing in a narrow conceptualization is the successful selling of a product or service. At one time, the health care industry did not have to rely on marketing to attract clients. Marketing vision, at best, consisted of attracting eminent physicians to the staff. Today's health care environment is far more complex. Institutions compete for customers in all sorts of ways. Those that are less effective do not survive.

Nor can the nursing function be separated from the institution's overall marketing efforts. The fate of the nursing division is tied to the fate of the total institution. Marketing of her institution's and her division's services is one of the chief responsibilities of today's nurse executive.

Basics of Marketing

Many major institutions use the services of professionals for marketing; others have their own experts on staff. Nevertheless, the nurse executive can benefit from a basic understanding of the broad tactics and strategies used in marketing. This section gives a brief overview of these aspects.

Bond (1981) described marketing as a process that considers *product, promotion, price,* and *place.* The decisions reached concerning these elements comprise the marketing plan.

When one considers *product,* the questions asked are, What is our business? What is being sold? Most products are goods or services, but identifying one's product may not be simple. Is the nursing product a patient's recovery or his comfort during an illness and its associated therapy? The same product can be seen from many different perspectives. I am reminded of a time when my niece was selling toothbrushes to pay for a school trip. When I told her I did not need a toothbrush, her eye roamed to my finger. "Actually," she said, "I'm selling ring scrubbers." How one defines a product dictates how it will be marketed. My niece had applied the first rule: Address the customer's need.

Who is the customer? Why would he want the product? The same product may have different appeals to different customers. Recognizing this is the first step in segmenting the potential market. It is easier to market a product to a specific target group than to try for generalized appeal to a larger, more diverse audience. Effective marketing involves segmenting potential customers according to their interests. Then the product and its advertising are slanted toward the needs and preferences of the given segment.

Part of marketing involves determining how one's goods or services differ from those of the competition. Why, for example, would a patient select the nursing care in this hospital over the nursing care at the competing institution? What edge does one have over the competition? To what audience would this difference appeal?

Once the nature of the product (or service) has been determined, its target audiences selected, and the thrust of the message to be delivered decided upon, *promotion* can be addressed. There are many ways to promote a product. Advertising is the common one. Promotion through advertising is differentiated from promotion through public relations by the fact that the seller pays directly for advertising. Public relations, although often costly, result in "free" publicity because of voluntary media coverage.

Advertising involves selecting the best media to convey one's message. Media include but are not limited to radio, television, and print media (magazines, newspapers, and circulars). These are the traditional media; of course, one can get as creative as a budget allows—using everything from messages on blimps to sky writing.

Unlike advertising, promotional events and news stories involve public relations (i.e., they attempt to capture the interest of the media because they are newsworthy). A press release illustrates this sort of promotion. However, one does not achieve the desired publicity just by wanting it. Many press releases are ignored, and the press may elect not to show up at a promotional event. (They are more likely to show up if the issue addressed is critical and if food and cocktails are included.) To make one's product newsworthy takes careful planning and effort. Even using the right format for a press release can make the difference in whether it receives publicity.

Public relations campaigns often aim at increasing consumer knowledge or changing the public's behavior. Most people working in the media avoid covering any event that is a barely disguised form of advertising. To attract coverage, one usually has to address public concerns, with one's more self-serving message secondary. (We provided this unique health fair for the community. It proves we care—so use our facilities.) Also, "me, too" events have little appeal to the press. The *second* hospital to open a rehabilitation wing for blind leper poets can forget about coverage. Location can affect publicity. A

small town may be more desperate for news than a big city.

Even company logos, newsletters, and calling cards are forms of promotion. Packets of materials prepared for prospective employees or entering patients are good forms of promotion for a health care institution.

Price is the next factor in a marketing strategy. All products have associated costs, and most pricing strategies are a compromise between what it costs to produce the goods or services and what others are willing to pay for them. For many products, the fixed price per unit interacts with the volume sales. Lower prices mean more sales; higher prices, fewer sales.

Determining an optimal pricing strategy is a delicate matter. Often in health care, other players and values other than the profit motive enter the equation. For example, a clinic may wish to set its fees as low as possible if its aim is to serve a large segment of the local community. In major care institutions, the free market has less to do with pricing than does the insurance industry. Governmental constraints, third-party payers, and other factors may artificially set or limit prices for many health care products and services.

The final element for a market analysis, *place,* focuses on how the product gets to the consumer. The distribution system includes such elements as (1) the transport system (e.g., freight costs, speed of delivery, delivery reliability), (2) warehousing elements (e.g., storage costs, location of plants and markets, size of inventories), and (3) management of orders (e.g., lead time needed to fill orders, cost of processing orders, the cost of handling returns).

Until recently, the health care system was not really concerned with place factors. The health care consumer was expected to come to the service, whatever his inconvenience. In today's competitive market, however, things have changed; ambulatory services are taken to the consumer's home, services such as emergency care or surgicenters are located conveniently throughout the community. In a competitive environment, customer convenience is no longer overlooked, and place of service delivery is part of today's marketing.

Marketing in the Nursing Division

Within the acute care facility, the nurse executive is concerned with marketing on two levels: marketing the facility itself as a health care organization and marketing the division of nursing. Because most of health care is focused around what nurses do, the nurse executive is in a pivotal position to develop marketing programs about what the organization does best, (i.e., providing care to patients). The nurse executive who can market programs that make the institution look good is in a powerful position indeed.

Personalized marketing is what consumers are looking for. Hence, community service programs can be instrumental in indirect marketing of an institution. Programs such as "Ask-a-Nurse" (in which people can call a facility and have a nurse answer questions about health care) are very effective in positioning the organization as a patient-centered facility. Beth Israel Hospital in Boston, for example, has been very effective in marketing itself around a program of nursing excellence. The nurse executive is pivotal in designing and enhancing such marketing programs.

Community-based programs work to develop an image of nursing and an image of the facility. Such programs position the health care facility in the community. Also, association with the health care facility may bring recognition for and from the community. Recently, for example, one nursing division held a public relations event, unveiling a mural painted by teenagers from a nearby underprivileged neighborhood. The work-study program for teens gave press and pride to the community as well as establishing the caring concern of the nursing department.

Programs on television that highlight the work of nurses, in direct and indirect clinical care, or that feature volunteer work with constituencies in the community such as the homeless give a very positive message to the community. Nurse-managed health fairs also create positive press.

Innovative programs attract media attention: programs with interesting speakers, award programs for nurses, or "Walk a Mile" programs in which prominent citizens follow staff nurses for a day to see what nurses really do. However, as mentioned earlier, the ease or difficulty of obtaining publicity for such events partly depends on the location of the institution—and the number of other events competing for print and television news space.

Print media such as hospital publications and newsletters sent to patients and potential contributors are other tactics often used. These also can help create the kind of image desired. Smaller institutions may interact more intimately with their community, making image less of a problem, but every large institution is in the business of image marketing these days. When the nursing division contributes to positive image marketing, it increases its clout in corporate quarters.

In addition to formal marketing programs aimed at the public or some targeted segment of it, some nurse executives are very effective in marketing programs to managed care companies and in acquiring other necessary contracting. If the nurse executive is competent in marketing skills, she is invaluable to the organization for external marketing programs and for those external negotiations that demand a great deal of selling to the prospective buyer.

The nurse executive's role in fund raising cannot be underestimated. The nurse executive is well positioned to market the institution to potential donors. Prospective patrons often respond to personal interest stories about patients and nurses. The nurse executive can be very effective in presenting financial needs in a way that is highly personalized and touching for the potential donor. It is not unusual that a grateful patient's request to send candy to the unit can be reframed so that he will make a generous gift to a nursing scholarship fund instead. Nurse executives have been very successful in teaching staff nurses to informally present projects to potential donors.

In addition to marketing outside the institution, the nursing division can be marketed internally. Other departments throughout the facility do not automatically believe that nursing is wonderful and important to the institution. Marketing the division of nursing to other departments helps them buy into nursing's programs. An effective nurse executive tries to market the division of nursing as a collegial partner with other divisions rather than a competitor.

Within the division of nursing, the nurse executive continually markets nursing positively to nurses. Nurses do not always take as much pride in their profession as other professions do. To develop the staff's pride in the profession and pride in the nursing offered at one's facility can be a challenge. Internal programs that celebrate individual nurse's achievements or celebrate national events such as nurses' week contribute to building pride.

In addition to ceremonies, vehicles for this work include internal newsletters, adoption of slogans that define the mission of the division in two or three words, and personal visits by the nurse executive to various units to recognize achievements. The focus of this internal marketing is to differentiate this nursing program from others in the minds of the staff and to create the pride that nurses must have for a successful organization.

One of the great challenges for the nurse executive is to help the nursing staff market themselves to patients. As patients perceive nurses, so they perceive the facility. It is common that a nursing staff can give excellent care but that patients will perceive that the care is poor because the nurses have not done what patients perceive as important, namely, very personalized, individualized care.

If nurses appear rushed, unconcerned, uncaring, and inattentive, they are marketing themselves poorly to the patient. Many hospitals have used guest relations training in an effort to market the staff to the patients. But it really goes beyond customer relations. There has to be a deep concern on the part of every person on the staff, an understanding that they must market themselves to patients.

In a competitive environment, the key to success is for staff to develop a bond between themselves and their customers—patients and their families. Families cannot be forgotten in this equation. They are the ones who notice what is going on in the organization when the patient cannot. Families become the opinion makers.

The nurse executive has another consumer of services: the physician. A nurse executive who sets the nursing division in conflict with the physician staff does a disservice to the institution. Consistently, physicians choose an organization because of their perception of the nursing staff. They also leave based on their perception of the nursing staff. The nurse executive is charged with the responsibility of marketing the excellence of the nursing staff to physicians, through reports at various physician staff meetings, at other meetings where many members are physicians, and by handling complaints and resolving problems fairly and quickly.

The nurse executive is challenged to market new programs that may be controversial to physicians. Being sensitive to the needs and interests of the physician market will enable her to do this in a way that obtains their support. Nurses on individual units are also charged with marketing unit-based programs to physicians. Committees that involve physician–nurse collaboration are an excellent vehicle to help physicians understand how nurses create excellence and also provide a way to find out what physicians as customers want and need to facilitate their practice.

SUMMARY

A marketing strategy involves many steps, including determining how to posture the product, determining the target populations, deciding on objectives for the marketing campaign, setting a strategy for achieving the objectives, and evaluating and adjusting the strategy as needed. A marketing strategy involves a compromise between what can be afforded and the ideal marketing campaign that could be envisioned. It involves many choices, all of which can be made better with the help of a marketing expert. These choices include products, target audiences, prices, promotions strategies, media, timing, and anticipated audience response.

Marketing goes hand in glove with strategic planning, a system that allows the nurse executive to devise fluid plans, contingent on environmental changes. Strategic planning and marketing are two approaches that fit the health care environment of today. As long as competition and bottom-line economics are dominant features determining the fate of any health care institution, nurse executives do well to make these tactics work for them rather than against them.

The nurse executive must be involved in strategic planning and marketing, not only for the nursing division and its projects but also for the institution or corporation as a whole. The more effective the nurse executive is in applying these two techniques to her operations, the more power she will accumulate in the organization.

REFERENCES

Bond, R. 1981. Marketing disciplines for medical group practices. Paper presented at Florida Medical Group Management Association Annual Meeting, Clearwater Beach, Florida.

Mintzberg, H. 1973. Strategy-making in three modes. *California Management Review* 16, no.2:44–53.

SUGGESTED READINGS

Alward, R.R., and C. Camunas. 1990. Public relations. Part I, A skill for nurses. *Journal of Nursing Administration* 20, no. 10:28–34.

Alward, R.R., and C. Camunas. 1991. *The nurse's guide to marketing*. Albany, N.Y.: Delmar Publishers, Inc.

Andreoli, K., et al. 1988. Marketing strategies: Projecting an image of nursing that reflects achievement. *Nursing Administration Quarterly* 12, no.4:5–14.

Beaupre, B. 1988. An administrative marketing strategy: A different perspective on the nursing process. *Journal of Nursing Administration* 18, no.11:37–41.

Dienemann, J., and L. Wintz. 1992. Designing a marketing plan that works. *Journal of Nursing Administration* 22, no.1:23–38.

Farley, M.J., and J. Nyberg. 1990. Environment as a major element in nursing administration practice for theory development. *Nursing & Health Care* 11, no.10:532–535.

Ireson, C., and D. Weaver. 1992. Marketing nursing beyond the walls. *Journal of Nursing Administration* 22, no.1: 57–60.

Johnson, J., et al. 1988. Writing a winning business plan. *Journal of Nursing Administration* 18, no.10:15–19.

Pattan, J. 1991. Nurse recruitment: From selling to marketing. *Journal of Nursing Administration* 21, no.9:16–20.

Porter-O'Grady, T. 1988. Restructuring the nursing organization for a consumer-driven marketplace. *Nursing Administration Quarterly* 12, no.3:60–65.

33

Communications in Nursing Management

In this chapter, a general communications model is offered and its application in nursing executive management is considered, together with related topics of special interest to the nurse executive—institutional relationships, the successful management of meetings, and media appearances.

COMMUNICATION MODEL

An understanding of communication theory begins with an analysis of the functional unit of communication. The simple components of any single communicated interchange are shown in Figure 33–1.

The system consists of a sender with certain goals. He encodes those goals (translates them into symbols) to form a message. That message is transmitted via some medium (audiovisual-sensory input system) to the intended receiver. On its sensory intake, the receiver decodes the message (interprets the symbols) and responds to its perceived content. How he interprets the message and how he responds to the content he perceives are influenced by his goals in relation to the sender and in relation to the message's subject matter. When the response includes communication feedback to the sender, the receiver assumes the sender role and the communication cycle begins again.

Function of Communication

The sender always communicates for some purpose, to have some effect on the receiver.

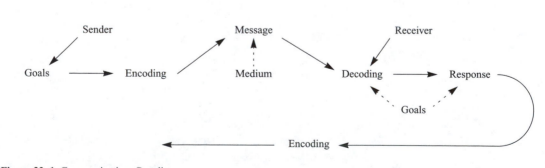

Figure 33–1 Communications Paradigm

Common purposes include to inform, to entertain, to inquire, to persuade, and to command. The goal may be to evoke a particular attitude or a particular behavior, verbal or actional.

The success of a communication is usually judged in terms of the goal–response relationship. Organizations usually define a good communication as one in which the goal of the sender was attained. This definition, however, has a limited perspective because it assumes that only the goals of the sender have importance. In truth, sender and receiver goals may mutually interact, each modifying the goals of the other. This consideration leads some authors to define a good communication as one in which both sender and receiver achieve ultimate goal satisfaction.

Structure of Communication

Communications can take place in two ways: by direct action and through symbols. A pat on the back and an opening of a door are examples of direct communication. Even such actions, however, are subject to misinterpretation. Most communication is of the symbolic type. Verbal communication is the most common form, words standing for meanings.

When symbolic communication is used, the degree of common understanding achieved between sender and receiver depends on whether they both interpret the words or other symbols in the same way. For example, telling the man in the street to do something *stat* would not produce the same effect as using that term with a nurse. However, the man in the street might pick up the meaning of stat from the speaker's direct communications, such as the urgency in the voice of the speaker or the apparent seriousness of the situation. The point is that some form of common understanding of the symbols used must be reached between sender and receiver if communication is to take place.

The act of putting meaning into a symbolic form is called *encoding,* and the act of extracting meaning from symbols is termed *decoding.* The degree of agreement between the message sent and the message received will depend on the degree to which the symbols have the same meaning for the two parties. In the model shown in Figure 33–1, arrows branch from the goals of the receiver toward both the decoding and the response, indicating that goals can affect not only the receiver's response but even his interpretation of what is being conveyed to him.

Methods of Communication

Methods for communication include talking, writing, showing, and all the various possible combinations for sensory input. These sensory messages can be delivered face to face or by the communications medium of choice. Media have their own particular effects on the message. Consider, for example, the delivery of the same message face to face or by letter, by film, or by slides. Effects such as closeness, distance, warmth, and coolness add overtones of meaning to the message.

These then are the primary components of a functional communications system: sender, goals, encoding, message, media, decoding, receiver, goals, and response. Both the parts and the relations of the parts are important in analyzing or constructing a communication.

NURSE EXECUTIVE AS SENDER AND RECEIVER OF COMMUNICATIONS

In the role of sender, the nurse executive's underlying personal, cultural, and professional biases direct her goals and her way of encoding messages. She must recognize that the receiver also has personal and cultural biases that color his decoding activity. When the nurse executive's biases are different from those of the receiver, she must allow for such differences.

She needs to encode in symbols that have the same meaning to the receiver as to herself. Failure to use clearly understood symbols is probably the most common sender problem in communication. Transcultural nursing has a message for the nurse executive when it comes to reaching common understandings—and the difficulties that may be incurred in reaching that goal.

Another sender problem is the general failure to communicate to all who need to know. For any communication instituting a change in policy, practice, or procedure, the nurse executive should carefully identify all individuals who need to receive the message. The executive needs to consider not only the face value of the message but the implications it may have, not only for her staff members but for other departments of the institution. Poor personnel relations are bound to follow if changes are instituted without proper communication.

Not all communication problems are sender problems; many are problems of message reception.

Selectivity

People tend to see or hear messages in which they are interested and to miss messages in which they are disinterested. This mechanism is called selective attention. Selective perception is another factor; with this phenomenon, the receiver selects those parts of the message that conform with his desires or expectations. Such picking and choosing can cause either incomplete or distorted interpretation of the message.

Anticipation of Content

Some persons assume that they have grasped the essence of a message before really hearing it out or reading it carefully. These persons tend to tune out the message because they think they already know what is being communicated.

Thinking Ahead into the Sender Role

Some persons become so enamored of their upcoming response to the message that they are mentally formulating their answer rather than really digesting the message. Persons who think ahead into the sender role often are guilty of interrupting the speaker and responding to incomplete messages.

Receiving Skills

Receiving skills are seldom given sufficient attention. Conscientious effort should be made to apply such basic listening techniques as the following:

- Give the speaker your full attention; try to hear what he is saying, not what you expect him to say.
- Do not interrupt or begin to formulate your answer mentally until he has finished his statement.
- Listen for both facts and feelings. What has the speaker said, and how does he feel about it?
- Tell the speaker what you think he has said; see if that is really what he meant. Use questions to clarify meanings.
- Suspend judgment until the speaker finishes talking.

Reading skills follow similar patterns:

- Read for what the author says, not what you expect him to say.
- Periodically summarize in your own words what the author is saying and doing. What structures is he building? Where is he leading?

The nurse executive must be a sensitive message receiver because of the nature of her job. At times, messages to her may be distorted due to the attempts of her staff or others to please. Her receptivity to messages must be such that staff do not feel inhibited when delivering unfavorable reports. Other messages may be designed to irritate. For all messages, it is important to differentiate between the message and the overtones. Each may require a response, but neither element should cloud the other.

MESSAGE CONTENT

Receptivity of the message is greatly affected by the media selected. In a face-to-face communication, confusion is resolved by immediate feedback and interaction among the individuals involved. The nurse executive, however, does much of her communication in written form when such immediate corrective feedback is not possible.

Clarity

Before publication, messages should be carefully checked for clarity of meaning, accuracy of content, and completeness of detail. The nurse executive who has problems with written communication may find it useful to have her messages read by a disinterested party who can suggest needed revisions. A good executive secretary can perform this function. Lacking a reader, the executive can usually evaluate her own messages if she lets the document get "cold" and rereads it before sending it out.

Tone

Half of the art of management is knowing what to communicate and when. Unfortunately, there is no set of rules to follow for making those decisions. At the outer limits, the executive might ask if the communication is necessary (or desirable) and whether it has the potential for coming back to haunt her one day.

Sometimes, tone is more important than content. A memo written in anger is almost always a mistake. If possible, the executive should wait and write the memo later. If she must respond immediately, she must be very certain that her anger does not show in writing. If there is an issue involved, she should let the facts of the case speak for themselves rather than letting the anger carry the message. Anger never does anything but let another person know one is out of control (or, in some cases, that he got the response he wanted). The underlying tone of any communication should convey the sense of a reasonable person. This is particularly important should a communication later get sent up the chain of command (by writer or receiver).

The tone and message also should reflect the appropriate organizational relationship. For messages going down the chain, it is important to differentiate between an order and a suggestion, and there should be no penalties for suggestions not followed. Sometimes, other managers use an inappropriate tone or wording in power moves against the nurse executive. For example, a vice president (he happened to be a physician) couched all his memos to the nursing vice president as orders despite the fact that their positions were equal on the organization chart.

She elected a soft approach to the problem instead of a direct confrontation. Every time she responded to one of these memos, she would start by saying, "I have considered your suggestion, and . . ." She would then go on to tell him her decision, praising his notion if it were valuable, explaining why it was rejected if rejected. This approach ultimately did more to establish a collegial relationship than would have any number of lectures on the subject.

COMMUNICATION FORMS

Any nurse executive finds that a great percentage of her time is spent in communications of one sort or another. Communication forms are identified in Table 33–1. This taxonomy has two axes; the first one runs from the one-to-one relationship through the one-to-many. Discretion is required in selecting options on this axis. A common error is communicating content that should be reserved for the one-to-one relationship in the one-to-many situation. Discipline of an employee in front of his peers, for example, is seldom an appropriate form. Nor is it appropriate to waste the time of a group of persons to discuss issues pertinent to only one or a few members.

Another defect exists when the nurse executive chronically communicates to some of her immediate staff to the exclusion of others. The nurse executive must be extremely careful not to penalize some staff members by accidental withholding of necessary information. Some executives use a weekly newsletter for top administrative staff to avert such accidental omissions.

Table 33–1 Forms of Communication

| Sender–Audience Relationship | Science | Communication Mode | |
		Face-to-Face	Mediated
One-to-one	Interpersonal relations	Conversation	Correspondence, E-mail, voice mail
One-to-small group	Small group dynamics	Meetings, task forces	Films, tapes, slides
One-to-many	Rhetoric	Speech making	Mass media: radio, television, E-mail

The one-to-small-group situation is a communication form that is most useful when the communication affects the group as a whole rather than as individuals. This provides for clarification, feedback, and reinforcement immediately within the group that will have to function with the same understanding of the message.

The second axis of the communications taxonomy has two poles, face-to-face and mediated communications. A mediated communication is any form presented through some device such as films, slides, or tapes. It is possible to combine mediated presentations with face-to-face communication (e.g., showing a movie and then having a group discussion of its content).

Here again, selection depends on the goals of the communicator. Person-to-person communication has advantages such as forcing the receiver's attention to the issue, providing immediate feedback and clarification, and allowing the message to be adapted to a specific audience. Mediated forms also have their advantages; the message can be given to different groups with no alteration in the tone or meaning. Appealing to more than one sense (combining visual and audio) also is more vivid than mere speech. The mediated form allows a complex idea to be edited and tested until the presentation has optimal clarity. The mediated communication has the effect of formalizing and recording a decision. Mediated forms can be retrieved for future reference to the subject.

Some communications are most effective when combining the two processes: face-to-face communication followed by written repetition. When communications require specific actions on the part of the recipient, it is effective to follow the personal communication with a written reiteration. It is also possible that several alternative modes may be viable for any one communication. A policy change may be announced at a mass staff meeting, published in a general memo, or discussed with small groups (one unit at a time).

Selection of the proper mode of communication can be very important in effective leadership. Factors to be considered in selecting a mode of communication include the message content and the anticipated audience response. An additional Christmas bonus may easily be announced in a printed memo; anticipated layoffs announced in this manner would not only be insensitive but would represent the worst of strategies. Some questions to consider in selecting the communication mode are the following:

- Is the message easy to understand? Does it need a mechanism for feedback? Is the feedback need immediate or will delayed response be adequate?

- Who is the audience? Will the message reach all who need to know?

- What is the audience's anticipated response? What is the intensity of the issue? Will it cause a change in routine practices?

- What need is there for formal documenting of the message? Is the content proper for a policy statement, procedure statement, memo, or other form?

- What are the abilities of the nurse administrator? With which mode of communication is she most comfortable and most adept?

Directional Flow

Another factor to consider when discussing communications in an organization is directional flow. Communications are necessarily influenced by the hierarchical structure of an organization. Communication lines between the nurse executive and all relevant persons in or closely associated with the organization can be visualized as in Figure 33–2.

It is easier for the nurse executive to control outgoing communications than incoming ones. If the nurse executive learns to express herself clearly, to control the tone of messages sent, and to consider who needs to know for all communications, her outgoing messages have likelihood of success.

There are, however, many ways in which she can foster good incoming communications. For example, many nurse executives use the mechanism of required reports to gain information from subordinate managers and nursing division committees. In some instances, minutes of meetings will suffice; sometimes, informal reports are satisfactory. If the incoming information is not what she needs, the nurse executive may create a reporting format that addresses the vital topics.

INSTITUTIONAL RELATIONSHIPS

The effect of group membership is another factor that has an impact on organizational communication. Many of the nurse executive's communications are directed toward groups rather than toward individuals. Even when a communication is directed to an individual, he still reacts on the basis of his group memberships.

Symbolic interactionists have always asserted that all things derive their meanings out of social interaction. Human beings act toward things on the basis of the meanings those things have for them, and those meanings are social products. For Blumer (1969), for example, even a physical object is a symbol and a social creation; its meaning comes from the society, not from the object itself.

This concept has implications for the nurse administrator because work groups are also social groups. Responses to communication will reflect the group as well as the individual. If a group places a certain meaning on a communication, there is pressure on individual members

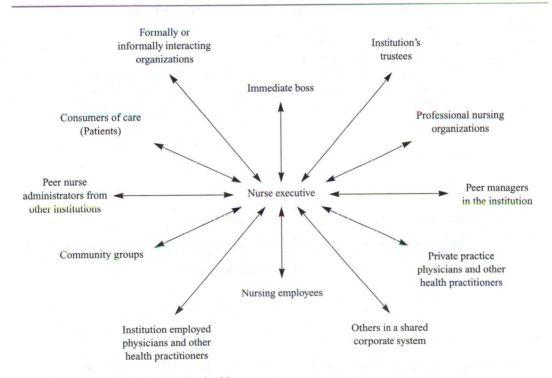

Figure 33–2 Communication Lines in Nursing Management

to conform to the group interpretation. In many instances it is more productive for the executive to deal directly with group feelings and reactions than to focus on the members as individuals.

An interesting traditional means of communicating with groups is the administrative nursing rounds when the nurse executive visits selected patient care units, views and evaluates the care of selected patients, and talks at random to staff members. This is not really a serious attempt to evaluate care; only gross deficiencies would be picked up in this manner. Instead, the important purpose is that of providing a two-way exchange with staff members.

The mere periodic presence of the nurse executive on the working unit decreases the employee's perceived distance between himself and the executive. Employees are more apt to identify with the executive's goals when she is personally known. Her physical presence can act to increase discipline or enhance motivation because the employees think that the executive really cares about what is going on. The executive's presence is a symbolic means of communicating her leadership.

Sometimes, joint rounds are made with several executives accompanying the nurse executive, ideally including the chief executive officer. The presence of these two executives together on the clinical units gives a powerful message of administrative unity and corporate concern.

Figure 33–2 indicates the major communication links that the nurse executive addresses in her role performance. These communication links require constant attention. In general, the more communication links that the nurse executive is able to build, the greater her power and her ability to get things done. The executive's network of communications will extend her information power; when she knows the values, interests, and modes of operation of these groups and individuals, she is better prepared for negotiations with them. Networking is an important component of the executive role.

GROUPS IN MEETINGS

The nurse executive typically finds herself directing many types of meetings. The abilities needed for this function vary, depending on the type of meeting. For example, for a major formal meeting of a large group or assembly, it is essential that the nurse executive know the procedures to be followed. Large groups can function only when detailed procedures exist; there simply is not time for all to participate, and consensus may be very difficult to reach.

Usually, this means that the nurse executive must know parliamentary procedure. Indeed, she should become expert in parliamentary procedure if she is to succeed in situations of this sort. The executive's personal input in presiding over large groups is minimal compared with the leadership she can offer in small groups, but such a meeting can be destroyed by a leader who is unsure who has the floor, what motions can be made, or how to use her prerogatives as chairman.

Sometimes, a nurse executive will address a large group on an informal basis. For example, she may set up periodic staff meetings to keep people abreast of a major institutional project that is underway. Here, a different set of skills is required: not parliamentary procedure but the ability to address and respond to a public.

Managing Committees

Much communication of the nursing division is done through committee work. Chapter 11 addresses the structure of committees; the material given here deals mostly with processes necessary to make committees work. The director needs two sorts of skills for effective committee work. She needs to be able to create and structure committees that will achieve their objectives, as well as to run committee meetings successfully. These skills are even more important on those corporate committees for which she has been assigned leadership.

The term *committee* is used here as a general term to describe a relatively stable group that meets periodically for an identified purpose or purposes, has official status and sanction of the nursing organization or the corporation, and has some established mechanism for maintaining and selecting members as well as for recommending or implementing its group decisions.

Corporate committees usually are formed by the chief executive officer or by the corporate top management team. The nurse executive should expect to do her share of heading and working on such committees. If her leadership is never requested, she should discuss the oversight with her boss. Obviously, her good work as a team member should make her leadership abilities self-evident. In forming committees of the nursing division, the nurse executive first examines the objectives and functions of her division to decide which objectives and functions can be best met through committees and which can be best handled by other means.

Committee structures are preferable for two kinds of situations: those requiring multiple input for goal attainment and those in which diverse representation facilitates implementation of proposed activities. Multiple input is required when the combined knowledge of various specialists is needed for completing the committee charge. Still other committees simply need multiple input for brainstorming and for reaching the most satisfactory solution. Diverse representation on a committee also may help in project implementation, lending legitimacy to projects and encouraging acceptance of solutions because of the democratic appeal.

Still, committees have their limitations, and many projects are better assigned to a single individual. Projects that require complex research and planning are better given to a single individual who can become familiar with and sensitive to each aspect of the project and its effect on other aspects of the project.

Nor should a committee be used to supplant the authority and responsibility of line managers. Committees are not designed to handle most day-to-day decisions. Indeed, the splintered responsibility in a committee makes it easy to avoid such decision making. Committees are better able to handle the larger issues, such as major policy changes or long-term divisional plans.

In designing committee structure, the nurse executive determines what goals and functions best can be handled by committees, decides what committees will exist, and examines the relationship of the committees to each other.

Some questions the executive may use as guidelines in evaluating committee structure and function are the following:

- Are there adequate committee structures to enable the division to reach its goals? Are there any obvious omissions?
- Does each committee fill a vital need that is not within the scope of any other committee?
- Does each committee have a clear reason for existing?
- Are the purposes of the nursing committees consistent with the avowed divisional definition of and philosophy of nursing?
- Is the total number of committees logical for the size of the nursing division and the thrust of its objectives?

Committee Power

One consideration in forming a committee is its degree of power. A group needs to be given enough authority to fulfill its objective. For example, a committee should not have to rely on persuasion if its directive is to produce action. Even intracommittee factors may be important. Does the committee, for example, have the power to delegate assignments to members?

Another power issue is the committee's ability to implement its decisions. The executive may give a committee power to recommend or power to decide. Committee members must clearly understand their powers in each case.

There are two main forms of decision making by committee: majority rule and consensus. The executive may deal only with consensus decisions or be content with majority decisions. Once more, it is important that committee members be given a clear directive.

Committee Membership

The committee should be viewed primarily as a means of getting work done, not as a means of meeting status needs, a popularity contest, or an exercise in democratic process. There is no use appointing a member to a committee if one can predict him to be noncontributive to the committee's objectives. One should appoint persons most likely to do a good job. However, the executive must be cautious against using the same reliable people on all committees. Design groups are often more creative and productive than committees based on organizational position because they tend to have the right membership.

In selecting committee members, the executive also must consider who needs to know in the implementation phase. One often sees such catastrophic events as a group of higher-level employees planning a change for a lower-level group without any representation from the latter. Representatives should usually be included from the group that is to implement any proposed change. There will be times, however, when confidentiality at a selected management level is needed, particularly in early planning stages for major divisional changes. Then, the executive must use discretion in determining appropriate committee membership.

To avoid a misuse of human resources, a committee should consist of the smallest number of persons who can meet the committee's objectives. Committee membership can be controlled on large projects by creating a small stable force for the total work, giving them the option to call in others as needed at various stages of the project development.

Committee Feedback Mechanisms

If the committee project is a long one that is expected ultimately to bring about a change in nursing practice, it may be wise to publish periodic status reports to the nursing groups that will be involved in the change. These reports will serve to create interest in the project as well as to prevent the resentment that arises when a plan suddenly materializes full blown and ready to be implemented.

Periodic status reports are useful for the nurse executive because they let her know the direction, rate of progress, and general productivity of the committee. Also, preparing periodic status reports forces committee members to return their attention to the original goals and to evaluate progress toward those goals.

In addition to creating communication channels from committees, channels to committees should exist whereby organization members who think that they have something to offer can submit ideas and suggestions. Creating input channels helps to build general acceptance for committee recommendations and decisions.

Committee Productivity

The nurse executive is responsible for making optimal use of staff time. Nowhere is there more danger of unproductive use of time than in committee work. When, for example, ten head nurses sit around a table for 2 hours and accomplish nothing, the cost in salaries is tremendous. Chronically unproductive committees must be closely examined.

Often a committee is unproductive because it does not really need to exist (e.g., when its objectives are either not attainable or not important at the particular time). When the objectives are judged valid but the committee is still unproductive, it is trying to do the job with the wrong people. A committee leader without appropriate skills also may be the problem. Another possibility is an incompatible mix of members, incompatible in regard to the objectives of the committee, not necessarily incompatible in their interpersonal relations with one another.

Because a design group is a single-purpose entity, it is easier to hold this group's feet to the fire. The nurse executive can give a task force time deadlines from the start. Communication here is easily managed: it deals with a single task.

Committee Functions

Committee functions may include any number of processes: problem solving, researching, standard setting, designing, implementing, monitoring, or evaluating. Communications used to complete the tasks include expressing, informing, recommending, arguing, clarifying, taking sides, compromising, harmonizing, encouraging, summarizing, consensus taking, voting, reasoning, and socializing, to name a few. Analyzing committee processes along these dimensions may be useful. Suppose, for example, a committee socializes at the expense of other pertinent processes. In another committee, a norm of excessive arguing may require intervention on the part of the leader.

COMMITTEE LEADERSHIP SKILLS

Basic Rules

There are a few basic rules that will help the nurse executive run committee meetings. Some of these rules concern preparation for the meetings; others direct the leader's activity during the meeting. Preparation rules are simple and self-explanatory (see Exhibit 33–1).

Leadership functions

During a meeting the leader has two functions: structuring the business to be done and directing and controlling members' behavior. It is not always so easy to tell where one leaves off and the other begins in an actual meeting.

Structuring the Business To Be Done

In structuring the business, the leader should plan to start each topic with an orientation, including a brief review of past actions and decisions on the topic (if the topic is not new) and a clear statement of what is to be accomplished with regard to that topic. Once the objectives are stated, the leader usually turns the action over to the committee members. She prepares a lead-in question or suggestion for this purpose.

Exhibit 33–1 Preparation Rules for Committee Meetings

Preparation of the physical environment

1. Comfort should be ensured by
   a. adequate ventilation, light, and heating
   b. comfortable seating
   c. good visual arrangements
   d. adequate space for the writing or reference materials of each participant
2. Convenience for participants can be ensured by
   a. supplying paper, pencils, name cards, if indicated
   b. minimizing interruptions
      i. informing the telephone operator of who is in the meeting and who will take messages
      ii. marking all entry doors to signify what meeting is in progress
   c. preparing and checking out all necessary audiovisual aids
   d. supplying agendas and documents to be discussed (do not assume that everyone will remember to bring her original copy)

Preparation of participants

1. Distribute detailed agendas long enough in advance for necessary preparation or research.
2. Distribute for advance preparation any documents to be approved or analyzed.
3. Indicate any materials that the participant should bring to the meeting.

Leader preparation

1. Prepare an agenda that clearly indicates the purpose and content of the meeting.
2. Review the status of all agenda topics to date.
3. Gather all necessary background information and supportive data on agenda topics.
4. Determine who needs to be invited as resource persons based on agenda topics.
5. Prepare a list of critical questions that can stimulate committee interaction on agenda topics.
6. Prepare such handouts or audiovisual presentations as will facilitate committee understanding of topics.
7. Prepare a strategy or strategies for handling the meeting.

The primary duty of the leader during the meeting is to keep the committee to its task, reminding the group of its objectives when the conversation strays. The periodic use of short summaries of committee progress also helps, but the leader must be cautious not to rush groups into premature decision making. At the meeting's termination, the leader summarizes what has occurred, identifying the decisions reached and the responsibilities accepted.

Not all meetings reach their intended goals, so the leader must recognize when a group is stalemated and can go no further toward task completion. This may happen when not enough information was available for drawing of conclusions or when there is no agreement among factions with equal power and equal conviction concerning alternate plans. This will be evidenced in the recycling of the same arguments by their various advocates. (Sometimes this can be avoided by an agreement that any single position can only be presented once.)

Whatever the cause of a stalemate, it calls for termination of the meeting, possibly with a plan to meet again when further information is available. Or the power for decision making may be removed from a committee that obviously will not reach agreement. Sometimes, a nurse executive who hopes for a consensus must be satisfied with a majority vote. When no new arguments are being offered, it is time to close the discussion, vote, or dismiss the committee. Alternately, in a multipurpose committee meeting, one may move on to the next item.

The structuring of the business to be done varies with the type of communication desired from the meeting. Some meetings aim at information transmittal, the simplest form being when the leader merely wishes to inform the group of something—a one-way communication. Essentially, the meeting remains in the control of the leader.

In contrast with this tell meeting, the sell meeting is one in which the leader is anxious not only to inform but to convince the group of the worth of her particular idea. When persuasion is the intent, the meeting should be allowed to develop into a three-way interaction. After the leader explains her idea to the group, she al-

lows them to pose questions and give reactions. Also, she allows time for the members to discuss the proposal with each other.

A third type of information transmittal meeting is the one in which the leader wants information from group members concerning a particular topic. In this case, there is a one-way flow of information from each member to the leader.

Meetings not intended for information transmittal are usually focused on decision reaching. Brainstorming is the simplest form, because the communication flow is one-way, from each member to the leader. In the brainstorming session, judgment of ideas is suspended; the purpose is to collect as wide a variety of tentative solutions as possible in a short time.

The advice-seeking meeting is the next level of decision reaching. In this meeting, the leader wants to gather the opinions and judgments of committee members on an issue. Often, this involves extensive interaction among committee members, and it is likely that the leader will find these interactions a useful part of the advice giving.

The highest level of decision reaching is that in which the members are asked to work together to arrive at a single best solution to the problem. This problem-solving meeting involves three-way interactions between and among leader and group members.

One of the most important leadership activities in structuring the committee's business is to make clear to committee members the purpose of the meeting. When the leader fails to do this, people act on the supposition that problem solving is required. When a committee expends the time to reach a decision, members are resentful if their solution is ignored.

Directing and Controlling Human Behavior

The leader's second function during meetings is the directing and controlling of human behavior. Here, the leader has two objectives: She wants to maintain a position of control while still encouraging active interchange among members.

Part of directing behavior is done by the leader in setting the tone of the meeting. At the start of the meeting, the leader sets the stage for free interaction by seeing that members are acquainted. Introductions include enough information about each member to let the others know what talents and knowledge he brings to the group. Until the members get to know each other, the leader facilitates interaction by directing questions to appropriate individuals.

When the leader is dealing with a familiar committee group, she has a different set of problems, namely, the reaction patterns of individual members and anticipated interactions among members. For the counterproductive reactions that can be predicted, the leader can have compensating strategies ready should those behaviors appear.

The leader both maintains control and promotes interaction by suppressing overactive members and drawing out timid or reticent ones. The leader also uses restatement and redirection. For example, she rephrases a contribution from a member and uses it as a pivot for changing the direction of the conversation. This is particularly important when a committee has overworked one section of the problem and should be moving on.

The functions of the leader during the committee meeting can be summarized: (1) focusing the issue, (2) refocusing when conversation strays, (3) changing the focus when an issue has been covered adequately, and (4) recapping the status of each issue, the decisions made, and the commitments for action.

Immediately after running a meeting the leader should ask herself: Did I meet my objectives for the meeting (i.e., did I really get the business done)? Did I facilitate appropriate interactions among members and divert unproductive interactions?

Committee Participation

In addition to responsibility for committee leadership, the nurse executive often serves on corporate committees. In this capacity, she may be a member more often than a leader of a group. Obviously, she cannot be less prepared

for meetings when she is a member rather than for those when she assumes leadership. One's participation in corporate meetings often sets the tone for how others regard the nurse executive and the nursing division.

The nurse executive always seeks access to the policy-making and influential committees of the organization. Sometimes, she may settle originally for a lesser status on a given committee (e.g., accepting presence and participation but no voting rights). Half a loaf can be the first step in a more comprehensive plan. Personal networking with the institutional and corporate-level officials is often an essential first step to one's inclusion in decision-making bodies.

EFFECTIVE MEDIA COMMUNICATIONS

To promote the visibility of her organization and her division, the nurse executive must be adept at the use of mass communication. Most institutions have a public relations department or employ a communications firm for this purpose. Often they are more than willing to help if called on. With or without expert help, the nurse executive will want to develop her own skills in professional writing and in making public appearances. The executive should keep her eyes open for events that can be used for publicity. If she is opening a new unit for patient care, trying some new mode of care delivery, or entertaining important international guests—whatever the potentially newsworthy event, she should optimize on opportunities for public visibility.

Any publication of the executive or a staff member in a refereed professional journal, whether or not its purpose is public relations, will reflect positively on her institution. Some executives also become skilled in writing letters published in the opinion/editorial pages of local newspapers. The nurse executive also should learn to address large crowds (or unseen crowds via television or radio). There are courses available on public speaking, and improvement comes with practice. A few brief rules may help the novice:

- Be conscious of your voice characteristics; listen to tapes of your presentations to cultivate a pleasant speaking voice.

- Do not read papers to an audience; learn instead to speak from notes. Be conscious of your effect on a crowd; speak as if you were enthusiastic about and committed to the ideas you are presenting.

- Plan your presentation to suit the audience. Do not present, for example, a professional paper to a lay audience; fit the level of complexity of the subject matter to the average audience member and his level of understanding about the subject.

- Develop a sense of timing, neither rushing nor belaboring a point. Learn to pace yourself so that the material covered fits the time allotted.

Interviews are more tricky than speeches. Much of the control is in the hands of the interviewer. The executive may try to obtain agreement ahead as to what will be covered. She can then plan answers in advance for those questions. Nevertheless, she should anticipate confrontational questions as well, preparing to address any pressing matters that the interviewer may have heard.

During the interview, the executive need not answer a question exactly as it has been phrased. If a question needs to be recast to be fair, she should do that. Some reporters will pose questions devised to put the interviewee in a bad light however they respond. Even though the executive may not wish to be tricked into answering the wrong question, she must be careful to answer fair questions even if they are tough ones. When there are problems, she will do better to be forthright, not to look as if she is trying to hedge.

If an interview is for written publication or delayed broadcast, a copy can be edited for any errors in fact. Most reporters will not change the slant of their article or interview to please the executive, but at least she will know what to expect. Nor should she hesitate to request the opportunity of a rejoinder if a reporter has really misinterpreted things. Finally, an executive

should never assume that any part of a discussion with a reporter will be off the record.

SUMMARY

The nurse executive should be a master of communication techniques—delivering communications, selecting the right forums, presenting messages in the right fashion. This includes communications within the institution and outside of it.

Like it or not, the executive is the representative of her institution, even if speaking as a private citizen. Effective communications grease the wheels of an organization and help the executive achieve her goals. The role of today's executive is more visible than ever before. She cannot expect to be effective without communication expertise.

REFERENCE

Blumer, H. 1969. *Symbolic interactionism: perspective and method.* Englewood Cliffs, N.J.: Prentice Hall.

SUGGESTED READINGS

Baillie, V.K., et al. 1989. *Effective nursing leadership: A practical guide.* Gaithersburg, Md.: Aspen Publishers, Inc.

Barnum, B. 1995. *Writing for publication: A primer for nurses.* New York: Springer Publishing Co., Inc.

Clampitt, P.G. 1991. *Communicating for managerial effectiveness.* London: Sage Publications, Inc.

Fondiller, S.H. 1992. *The writer's workbook.* New York: National League for Nursing.

Glendon, K., and D. Ulrich. 1992. Using cooperative decision-making strategies in nursing practice. *Nursing Administration Quarterly* 17, no.1:69–73.

Jones-Schenk, J., and P. Hartley. 1993. Organizing for communication and integration. *Journal of Nursing Administration* 23, no.10:30–33.

Long, L. 1992. *Understanding/responding: A communication manual for nurses.* 2nd ed. Boston: Jones and Bartlett.

McKay, L. 1993. Overcoming resistance to change. *Canadian Journal of Nursing Administration* 6, no.1:6–9.

McNeese-Smith, D. 1993. How effective are your leadership skills? *Journal of Nursing Administration* 23, no.2:9–10.

Northouse, P.G., and I.L. Northouse. 1992. *Health communication: Strategies for health professionals.* 2nd ed. Norwalk, Conn.: Appleton & Lange.

Orchard, M.L.H., and G.N. Swenson. 1993. Enhancing professional communication: A formal computerized nurse-to-nurse system. *Nursing Administration Quarterly* 18, no.1:66–79.

Smith, S. 1992. *Communications in nursing: Communicating assertively and responsibly in nursing—A guidebook.* 2nd ed. St. Louis: C.V. Mosby Co.

34

Role of the Nurse Executive

In examining the nurse executive role in management, we look at the historical classic literature as well as the more modern approaches. The historical frameworks are important because they have set the categories in which people think about management.

The classic management literature reflects a basic division between a focus on the people in the work setting and on tasks. Some researchers and authors approach management through identifying and examining tasks; others view management by observing those involved in the work process. Even authors who take a broad view of management tend to do it by including both tasks and people in their models rather than by developing models with other categories.

PEOPLE ELEMENT IN MANAGEMENT

The management literature that looks primarily at people in preference to tasks takes many different perspectives, but primarily it focuses on the leader, the followers, or the interaction between them. Within those choices, there are further differentiations.

A Look at the Manager

In examining the manager, it is possible to look at his traits (personality factors) or his leadership styles (modes of approaching the leadership task). We might differentiate between these two approaches by saying that one asks who the manager is whereas the other asks how he operates.

Trait Orientation

Early management studies often tried to capture the constellation of personality traits that made for a leader. Supposedly, if one could recognize the traits and identify who possessed them, then one could put the born leaders in managerial positions.

Notice that this goal marks the difference between management and leadership. Managers are persons who hold positions in which they are responsible for other workers and goal achievement; leaders are persons who, for one reason or another, have a followership. There may be people in managerial positions with little or no leadership ability; conversely, there may be leaders holding no formal positions in places of business. The early literature sometimes blurred the terms *manager* and *leader*. The studies that sought to identify leadership traits often were disappointing because they generally revealed leaders to have many and diverse personality traits.

Although looking at who the leader is (rather than what he does) has been out of style for de-

310

cades, this approach is coming back strong in transformational leadership—a new concept that looks at both who the leader is and his style of leadership. We will examine this trend later in the chapter.

Leader's Style

The Ohio State University studies improved on these studies by switching from inherent traits to leader behaviors (Korman 1973). The leader of a group, whatever his personal makeup, was found to be the person who (1) defined the roles of self and others in relation to goal achievement, (2) structured and interpreted the situation to the group, and (3) showed respect and consideration for the ideas of other group members.

Of the studies that concentrated on style rather than personality traits, perhaps the best known is one that classified managers according to their tendencies to be autocratic, democratic, or laissez faire (Stogdill 1974). Although the study calls these three tendencies leadership styles rather than managerial styles, the term *leadership style* is a misnomer because one may have a laissez faire manager but a laissez faire leader, by definition, is not a leader.

A more useful set of managerial styles was one that discriminated among idiocratic, democratic, technocratic, and bureaucratic tendencies (Nelson 1957). An idiocratic supervisor was one who related to his staff as individuals, in a one-to-one manner. In contrast, a democratic supervisor related to his staff as a group. In both of these categories (idiocratic or democratic), the relationship to people, not to task, was dominant.

The other two categories relate to task. The technocratic supervisor perceived himself as the super technician. In the case of nursing, this might be a supervisor who serves primarily as a clinical consultant or an expert manager. The bureaucratic supervisor was one who perceived his job as enforcing the rules, namely, the policies and procedures of the institution.

Both of these classification schemes (democratic, authoritarian, and laissez faire, or idiocratic, democratic, technocratic, and bureau-

cratic) may be useful for a bit of self-analysis. One may then go the next step beyond identifying instinctive styles to deciding which styles should be selected (i.e., fostering learned behaviors in which a preferred style is purposefully applied).

When a manager is advised to make his style fit the unique circumstances, the approach is contextual—a more sophisticated approach than an either/or choice. The situational approach to management is called contingency management. For example, in evaluating and improving performance of staff members, an idiocratic approach might work best for the nurse executive. His staff might have highly discrete functions requiring this one-on-one individual approach. In contrast, for directing the general work of the nursing division, he might meet with top management staff as a body, using the democratic style. When there is a need for shared information, this system is more efficient.

Alternatively, when meeting with a group of subordinate managers working with budget variance, he might adopt a technocratic style, especially if he thinks some of the managers need education in the techniques of determining and interpreting budget variances. Finally, if the nurse executive were administering some aspect of a labor contract, he might adopt a bureaucratic style, knowing the dangers of deviating from its contractual language.

Ideally, then, the nurse executive becomes aware of his own instinctive style of management, learns other styles that are not instinctive, and determines when to apply each style, making sure the style fits the situation.

An important work that borders on the style-oriented approach is that of McGregor (1960). He defined two different managerial beliefs about workers, each of which encourages a different style of treating workers. McGregor's theory X describes a manager with these beliefs about workers:

- People dislike and avoid work if possible.
- Direction, coercion, and control are needed to obtain performance from workers.
- People inevitably try to avoid responsibility.

- Personal goals inherently conflict with company goals.
- It is not reasonable to have high expectations of people.

The manager with a theory Y perspective holds contrary beliefs about workers:

- Work is natural, and people generally enjoy it.
- People are capable of self-direction and self-control.
- People seek and enjoy responsibility.
- Personal goals can be achieved through company goals.
- It is reasonable to have high expectations for people.

A manager who holds McGregor's theory X philosophy will be likely to be a task master; he will focus on high control of workers, and his attention will be riveted on task completion. The manager who holds to theory Y, in contrast, is likely to be people-oriented. He will focus on providing an environment where human potential will develop and be productive. (Here again, one can see a task orientation versus a people orientation.)

Sometimes, an additional category is amended to X and Y: theory Z (Ouchi 1981). Theory Z is based on a philosophy of bottom-up management dominant in the Japanese culture. Unlike the pattern originated in the United States (where managerial orders tend to flow downward from the top to lower levels), the Japanese reverse this direction. New ideas and methods are developed at lower levels and then sold to ever higher levels of management. In this cultural pattern, executive management ratifies and enacts decisions made at lower levels (those that stand the tests of coming up through the managerial ranks). This pattern has spread in the United States as Japanese firms have established businesses here using a theory Z approach.

Theory Z often is accompanied by a cultural pattern in which workers are perceived as lifetime employees. Whether theory Z is actually a different belief system about workers from the-

ory Y might be debated. In this country, it is popular to implement certain aspects of theory Z, typically one hears about quality circles. In this notion, workers from the same group (e.g., a unit of staff nurses) get together to evaluate and try to improve the work processes.

Seldom, however, is this model applied with consistency in American-run companies, least of all health care. The nurse executive is almost never perceived as a mere enactor of policy decisions made at the lower levels. It is hard to imagine that such an executive could survive in today's competitive health care environment.

Workers

Some of the people-oriented management literature focuses on the worker rather than on the manager. Sometimes, workers are analyzed as individuals; more often, they are treated as a group. When the workers are analyzed as a group, two approaches are found: one looks at how they are organized and the other looks at the group psychology. The first approach can be seen in nursing in participative management and self-governance. At Johns Hopkins, for example, many units have firmly established administrative vehicles for self-governance.

Another organization model that looks at worker groups recommends management of a nursing organization by committees. Although management by committee has been successful in some academic settings, it is difficult to apply to nursing administration, which calls for many rapid decisions. Team nursing was another organization approach arising out of a worker orientation.

Historically, psychological approaches to work groups have included such fads as transactional analysis and sensitivity training. Group dynamics also has been applied in studies of the work group.

Sometimes, workers are viewed as individuals instead of as members of groups. The job enrichment movement, the clinical ladder, and the coaching notion of management take this position. Assertiveness training, when it was popular, also looked to changing behavior on the individual level.

Some of the best-known work on the individual employee was the series of studies originated by Herzberg and associates (1957). They studied work motivation and discovered that the aspects of a work situation that caused job satisfaction or dissatisfaction are not opposites but separate items. Satisfying factors in a job related to work tasks, whereas dissatisfactions related to the job environment. Poor salaries, short lunch periods, or cramped office space—Herzberg et al. called these hygiene factors—could create dissatisfaction. Good salaries, long lunch periods, and spacious offices, however, do not provide contentment. What gave people satisfaction were factors such as ability to manifest talent, a sense of having turned out a good piece of work, or recognition for work achievement—Herzberg's motivation factors. The findings of Herzberg et al. have been the basis for many subsequent studies, including some that arrived at contradictory conclusions.

TASK ELEMENT AS IT RELATES TO MANAGEMENT

Classical studies that looked at tasks did so from two different perspectives: either they looked at workers' tasks or at the tasks of managers.

Workers' Tasks

Many studies of the tasks of workers have focused on time and motion. In health care, for example, institutions have studied nursing activities to find out how long various procedures normally take. These norms have been used as a basis for patient classification systems and for calculating staffing needs.

These studies are undergoing renewed popularity in today's cost-conscious environment where time is money. Norms of all sorts (nursing and other) are being collected for benchmarking (i.e., setting norms against which to gauge one's subsequent improvement). Benchmarking usually begins with a systems analysis approach to defining all the tasks of an organization and describing them in quantitative measures. It is not surprising that this approach is occurring simultaneously with restructured practice—a reorganization that takes the same task-distribution focus.

Managers' Tasks

Managers' tasks have been discussed in two different ways in the management literature: in terms of the skills required to complete the tasks and in terms of the specific tasks themselves.

Managers' Skills

In a schema that still makes sense, Katz (1974) identified three managerial skills: the technical, the human, and the conceptual. He broke with the task-versus-people dichotomy by adding the conceptual skill necessary to see an enterprise as a whole and to relate it appropriately to its environment.

Managers' Activities

There have been many approaches to identifying the tasks of the manager. In some proposals, the managerial tasks are seen as occurring simultaneously; in others, the managerial acts are seen as following an invariant sequence. Among definitions of management following the former pattern is the old standby, POSDCORB, an acronym standing for Planning, Organizing, Staffing, Directing, Coordinating (or Communicating), Rating (or Reporting), and Budgeting. This classic can be traced back to its first publication in 1937 (Gulick), yet the scheme is still used by many managers today.

The sequential models include management by objectives (MBO), which sequences activities starting with goal definition; the management cycle—planning, organizing, directing, and controlling; or the systems model, which is the equivalent of the management cycle—problem definition, systems design, programming, operating, feedback, and evaluation. Variations of these models have been explored by many authors.

COMBINING AN ORIENTATION TO PEOPLE AND TASKS

Some authors combined the task and the people side of management. Blake and Mouton (1968) evolved a management grid that measured both a manager's concern for production and for people involved in production. They found no contradiction in a manager having high scores simultaneously on the two variables.

Other authors looked at combined people and tasks elements as they related to the work context, as did Fiedler (1964). Although Fiedler took an either-or approach to the task-versus-people orientation, his orientation was not an instinctive perception or a personal preference as in McGregor; instead, it was a selected strategy. The manager selected either the task orientation or the human orientation on the basis of three variables rated high to low:

- how well the leader was accepted by the group
- how structured was the group's task
- how strong was the leader's formal position power

When these variables fell to either extreme, Fiedler suggested a task-controlling style be elected; when the variables fell within a middle range, he suggested a permissive human relations approach.

ROLE THEORY AND THE NURSE EXECUTIVE

Role theory breaks down the division between people and task orientations because the concept of role involves a set of expectations concerning how a person will enact a given societal position. Both the person and the acts are included in the concept of role.

There are at least two opposing views of how a person interacts with his roles. The first views the role much like a stage role—as something to be put on at appropriate times and taken off at others. In this conception, the role and the person are separate; the person plays or enacts a role and then leaves it off when he moves, temporarily, out of that particular role. The person is separate from the roles he plays.

In contrast, an existential philosophy might claim that the person is nothing more or less than the roles he dons. This perception is captured in Sartre's old tale of the person looking for the essence of the onion by removing layer after layer—only to finish with nothing left.

Whether the person is separate from or part of his roles, a role has both a psychological and a sociologic component. The person is highly involved with the roles he plays, and he plays them in the light of (or conscious of) social expectations for the roles.

There are two kinds of roles: ascribed (those for which one has no choice [e.g., white female]) and achieved (e.g., nurse executive, artist). One may argue that some roles bridge these categories. For example, a person may have elected motherhood but may not have realized that it would cast her in the role of "Laurie's mother" for all the small fry of the neighborhood.

We are concerned here with an achieved role—that of nurse executive. This is a peculiar type of achieved social role, a highly prescribed occupational position. A role of this sort adds another dimension to the psychological and sociologic elements, forming

- *the sociologic component:* what others in the society expect from a person in this position
- *the rationalized:* the specifics of job function and responsibility as detailed in the job description
- *the personal/psychological:* how the role incumbent chooses to enact this job based on his unique being

Much of the nursing literature encourages role making instead of role taking for the nurse executive in keeping with the executive's need for an active stance. The nurse executive decides in advance what sort of role he wishes to play as administrator, then constructs his behaviors to convey that notion to others—role forming versus role norming.

It is possible to change most roles because they have elasticity: leeway in the social component, the job description fulfillment, and in the personal component. The nurse executive can use this elasticity to create the role image he desires. It is easier for a nurse executive to make a role when beginning a new position than after he has held a position for some time because staff come to expect a given pattern of behavior from him. Suppose that a new nurse executive wishes to play the executive role in a more powerful way than his predecessor. Then he will deliberately act so that others see him from the start as decisive and in control.

Role Models

Observing executives at work, Mintzberg (1975) identified ten major roles executives play. These might be viewed as subroles within the executive role. Mintzberg's roles include:

1. *figurehead:* functioning as symbolic formal head of the division, filling ceremonial functions
2. *leader:* directing subordinates to goal achievement, motivating and working with staff
3. *liaison:* building a communications network; establishing contacts outside the vertical chain of command
4. *monitor:* scanning the environment for information pertinent to the job; keeping abreast of changes in the power structure or the organization direction
5. *disseminator:* sharing and distributing information with staff; determining what goes to whom, when, where, why
6. *spokesperson:* speaking for the division, addressing key external and internal publics
7. *entrepreneur:* looking for improvement opportunities, taking the initiative in new projects and developments
8. *disturbance handler:* mediating and resolving disputes and disruptions among work groups

9. *resource allocator:* determining how the division's resources are to be distributed
10. *negotiator:* managing formalized and informal bargaining with both internal and external groups

Mintzberg's classic list stands the test of time, although one could argue that shifts in importance of given subroles have taken place. Also, different nurse executives spend different amounts of time on these subroles. Yet, it is difficult to imagine an effective nurse executive ignoring any one of them entirely.

Katz (1974) offered a different perspective on executive roles, identifying just three:

1. *remedial role:* acting to correct deficiencies and past inefficiencies
2. *maintaining role:* preserving a steady balance.
3. *innovative role:* seeking new projects and new directions

Katz (1974) asserted that the remedial role required conceptual and technical skills; the maintaining role needed primarily human skills; and the innovative role demanded both conceptual and human skills. Katz's roles are reminiscent of Mintzberg's (1973) strategies:

1. *entrepreneurial:* active search for new opportunities; spontaneity in managerial opportunism; proactive, dramatic leaps forward in the face of uncertainty
2. *adaptive:* reactive decisions, remediation, reducing conflict; negotiating with the environment; incremental decision making and problem solving
3. *planning:* anticipatory decision making; reliance on rationality and scientific techniques; goal setting with systematic plans for goal achievement

External circumstances affect one's selection among these classic strategies. Today's health care environment encourages a switch from the planning (e.g., MBO) to greater use of both adaptive and entrepreneurial strategies.

Katz's roles perceive the executive through organizational eyes, specifying the nature of the executive's work—remediation, maintenance, or innovation—as it relates to the organization. Greiner (1972) goes a step farther, creating roles for the organization rather than the executive. In this organic interpretation, organizations grow and evolve, going through the following sequence:

1. *organization:* entrepreneurial and technological orientation; informal and frequent communications; direct interaction with the market
2. *direction:* formal systems introduced; accounting, purchasing, work standards, inventories; communication formalized; functional specialists and managers differentiated
3. *delegation:* characterized by decentralization; direct control by top executive lost; powers distributed
4. *coordination:* decentralized units merged; companywide programs of control established; certain specialized functions centralized

Combining the notion that organizations have specific stages at given times with the idea that executive roles may be defined in relation to the managerial approach, the following role categories can be identified among nurse executives:

1. *innovator:* starts new programs, new methods, new ideas; role characterized by creativity and new expressions
2. *expander:* interested in growth and expansion, increasing the size and scope of the division; moves are highly political
3. *refiner:* neatens up the division, straightening up loose ends, formalizing policies and practices, refining systems, and providing a rationale for decisions and functions
4. *stabilizer:* maintains harmony and equilibrium, balancing the various interests and group demands and providing for smooth continuity of operations
5. *revolutionary:* tears down outmoded structures and practices, instituting methods, policies, and practices radically different from those in existence earlier

Each role has particular strengths associated with it. The innovator is creative and visionary, not tied to the past. He looks to new ideas and new methods, creates new goals, and enjoys dealing with unique problems. The expander is good at building bridges—making the personal and political linkages that will advance the division, building the communication networks that will open doors. The refiner puts the pieces together in logical patterns, applying the fine strokes that develop the intellectual glue to make everything fit together. The stabilizer excels in handling issues and resolving problems that threaten to upset the balance of the well-running machine. The revolutionary excels in nest cleaning, getting rid of unnecessary red tape, outmoded practices, or any other excess baggage.

Organizations may need these diverse talents at different times in their own growth, and the success or failure of the nurse executive may be a reflection of the match or mismatch of his talents to the organization's immediate needs. A successful pattern of executive performance in one situation may be disastrous in another situation. Some nurse executives are sensitive to their strengths. "I only stay until a place is running well; then I start looking for a new job with a challenge." Or "I only apply to institutions with well-developed programs."

One danger is when a nurse executive interprets a position in line with his strengths instead of the organization's needs. For example, if a nurse executive has exceptional interpersonal skills, he is likely to view all organization problems as interpersonal. Or he may imagine that an organization needs a complete overhaul if he is an instinctive revolutionary.

Expanding Nurse Executive Roles

The nurse executive role is undergoing extensive change in this period. The characteristics demanded of a nurse executive are, perhaps, more shared than was once the case. In large and small institutions, a competitive shrewdness is required, an ability to deal with rapid change, an entrepreneurial spirit, and a comfort in dealing with many diverse individuals and groups internal and external to the organization.

Furthermore, there are now at least two common executive positions: that of nurse executive (often labeled as nursing vice president [NVP]) in a given institution (free-standing or within a multi-institution corporation) and that of chief nurse executive officer (CNEO) for a multi-institution corporation.

The CNEO, stationed at corporate headquarters, relates to the NVPs of the individual institutions within the corporation in several ways. Sometimes, the subordinate NVPs work in a matrix, reporting to both the corporate CNEO and the separate institutional administrator. Sometimes, the CNEO has direct line authority for the NVPs. At other times, the corporate CNEO relates to them in a staff cooperative relationship, with no direct authority over them. The latter situation, depending on the structure of the corporation and the job requirements for the CNEO, can be challenging. It is difficult to be accountable in any position in which persuasion is one's only level of authority.

Sometimes, a single CNEO presides over staff in two or more institutions in which she plays the dual role of CNEO and NVP for the respective organizations. Without exceptional assistants at each organization, this role conceptualization is difficult.

TRANSFORMATIONAL NURSING LEADERSHIP

In a day when the environment is subject to sudden and unaccountable changes requiring a swift response, the management literature has accommodated to the reality, moving from old models that dictate what a manager should *do* (e.g., the old POSDCORB) or even the predictable plan-ahead MBO orientation to so-called transformational leadership.

The change is a shift back to an older model, namely, from what the leader does to who the leader is and how he motivates those led. Like the older MBO orientation, the transformational role focuses on the leader, but with the followership being the measure of effectiveness (this is the new aspect).

In transformational leadership, the leader and the followers have the same purpose, and it tends to be lofty. They raise one another to higher levels of motivation and morality. Barker (1991) noted that the scientific method has fallen short in controlling and explaining world events, and consequently, a new view of humanness is emerging. People bring to the workplace a new set of beliefs and values that spring from the new paradigm.

The old paradigm was characterized by logical decision making and rationality. This fit the old descriptions of the manager's role—POSDCORB, the managerial cycle, MBO. Transformational leadership, in contrast, recognizes that there is more to the job than performing a set of functions, no matter how effectively. The new paradigm looks at relationships among the leader and group members. It values mutuality and affiliation, acknowledges complexity and ambiguity, advocates cooperation instead of competition, emphasizes human relations and process instead of task, accepts feelings, values networking instead of hierarchy, and values intuition and empowerment of all employees.

The transformational leader mobilizes others; leaders and followers grow and develop together. As one set of needs and values are satisfied, new ones surface and contribute to personal and professional growth. In transformational leadership, it is easier to see results than process (it is fluid). The focus is on goals, joy in work, enthusiasm about patients and the care they receive, commitment to the organization as a mutual endeavor, and a sense of accomplishment.

There are many strategies natural to the transformational leader, including:

- creating a vision
- building a social architecture that provides meaning for employees (how the vision will be institutionalized)
- sustaining organizational trust
- recognizing the importance of building self-esteem

Transformational leaders are less hide-bound than the older manager models. The model fits what is happening in today's world. Because we are in the midst of a major shift in the environment, we need the fluidity to interpret, create, and grow with change. Transformational leadership is a better match with these characteristics of strategic planning than are the older models. Like strategic management, transformational leadership operates with broad strokes and is capable of shifting gears quickly. Table 34–1 compares older models of leadership (or management) with transformational leadership. Transformational leadership, although applied to the person and not the institution, is reminiscent of Greiner's organismic approach to describing the organization.

processes (planning, organizing, so forth). Similarly, the management cycle (plan, organize, direct, control) focused on process. The counterpart to these processes in nursing care is the so-called nursing process. Like the management cycle, it focuses on processes in a serial sequence. Mintzberg's ten leadership roles focused on content aspects of the role, abstracted from the environment in which they are displayed.

Context did not matter so much when the world changed slowly. But today, context is everything. The change from MBO to strategic management and the change from older manager profiles to transformational management

Table 34–1 Comparison of Old and New Leadership Patterns

Old Structures	New Structures
Nursing practice Goal-driven (comprehensive patient care)	Resource-driven (environmentally sensitive)
Management models Management by objective (MBO)	Strategic management
Manager Rational planner (focus on what one does [e.g., POSDCORB, MBO])	Transformational leader (focus on what one *is* and values, and who one empowers, and what one envisions)

SUMMARY

Management models of any era reflect two elements: (1) how far the field of management has developed, and (2) the era itself. Today, our models are changing because of environmental presses imposed on the health care field by outside influences.

Any comprehensive management model has three components:

1. *content:* what is acted on—the pieces of the model
2. *process:* movement (i.e., what is done to the content pieces)
3. *context:* nature of the environment where the phenomenon (management) happens

Few models are comprehensive; most concentrate on one or two of these elements. POSDCORB was a partial model focused on

typify responses to context. Those changes complement the change from goal-driven to resource-driven care.

It is vital that the nurse executive critically examine his role conception and role performance. He should take an activist's position in regard to the role, making it the sort of role he wants it to be rather than the role as others expect it to be enacted. Every role has elasticity, and this enables the nurse executive to manipulate and alter the role. Role is an excellent concept through which to consider such various elements of management as managerial skills and abilities, functions, organizational status, and strategies.

REFERENCES

Barker, A.M. 1991. An emerging leadership paradigm. *Nursing and Health Care* 12, no.4:204–207.

Blake, R.R., and J.S. Mouton. 1968. *Corporate excellence through grid organization development*. Houston, Texas: Gulf.

Fiedler, F.E. 1964. A contingency model of leadership effectiveness. In *Advances in experimental social psychology*, vol. I, ed. L. Berkowitz, 150–190. New York: Academic Press.

Greiner, L.E. 1972. Evolution and revolution as organizations grow. *Harvard Business Review* 50, no. 4:37–46.

Gulick L.K. 1937. Notes on the theory of organization. In *Papers on the science of administration,* ed. L.K. Gulick and L. Urwick, 1–45. New York: Institute of Public Administration.

Herzberg, F., et al. 1957. *Job attitudes: Review of research and opinion*. Pittsburgh: Psychological Services of Pittsburgh.

Katz, R.L. 1974. Skills of an effective administrator. *Harvard Business Review* 52, no.5: 91–102.

Korman, A.K. 1973. Consideration, initiating structure, and organizational criteria—a review. In *Perspectives on organizational behavior,* ed. P.F. Sorensen, Jr., and G.H. Baum, 134–135. Champaign, Ill.: Stipes.

McGregor, D. 1960. *The human side of enterprise*. New York: McGraw-Hill Publishing Co.

Mintzberg, H. 1973. Strategy-making in three modes. *California Management Review* 16, no.2:44–53.

Mintzberg, H. 1975. The manager's job: Folklore and fact. *Harvard Business Review* 53, no.4:49–61.

Nelson, C.W. 1957. *The leadership inventory*. rev. ed. Chicago: Industrial Relations Center, University of Chicago.

Ouchi, W.G. 1981. *Theory Z*. New York: Avon Books.

Stogdill, R.M. 1974. *Handbook of leadership: A survey of theory and research*. New York: Free Press.

SUGGESTED READINGS

Aurelio, J.M. 1993. An organizational culture that optimizes stress: Acceptable stress in nursing. *Nursing Administration Quarterly* 18, no.1:1–10.

Bader, G.E., & O'Malley, J. 1992. Transformational leadership in action: An interview with a health care executive. *Nursing Administration Quarterly* 17, no.1:38–44.

Beckhard, R., and W. Pritchard. 1992. *Changing the essence: The art of creating and leading fundamental change in organizations*. San Francisco: Jossey-Bass, Inc. Publishers.

Bell, E.A., and B.D. Bart. 1991. Pay for performance: Motivating the chief nurse executive. *Nursing Economics* 9, no.2:92–96.

Block, P. 1993. *Stewardship: Choosing service over self-interest*. San Francisco: Berrett-Koehler Publishers.

Clark, K.H., et al. 1991. Turning the organization upside down: Creating a culture for innovation and creativity. *Nursing Administration Quarterly* 16, no.1:7–14.

D'Argenio, C. 1991. Management training effects on nursing manager leadership behavior. *Nursing Economics* 9, no.4:249–254.

Dunham, J., et al. 1991. Nurse executives: Decision points in their careers. *Nursing Economics* 9, no.3:149–158.

Herron, D.G., and L. Herron. 1991. Entrepreneurial nursing as a conceptual basis for in-hospital nursing practice models. *Nursing Economics* 9, no.5:310–316.

Hollander, S.F., et al. 1992. The intrapreneurial nursing department: Nature and nurture. *Nursing Economics* 10, no.1:5–9, 14.

Johnson, L.M. 1992. Structures, strategies, and synthesis: The nurse executive as social architect. *Nursing Administration Quarterly* 17, no.1:10–16.

Johnson, M., et al. 1991. The Iowa model: A proposed model for nursing administration. *Nursing Economics*, 9, no.4:255–262.

Johnson, P.T. 1989. Normative power of chief executive nurses. *Image* 21, no.3:162–167.

Koerner, J.G., and S.S. Bunkers. 1992. Transformational leadership: The power of symbol. *Nursing Administration Quarterly* 17, no.1:1–9.

Kramer, M., and C. Schmalenberg. 1991. Job satisfaction and retention: Insights for the '90s—Part 2. *Nursing 91* 21, no.4:51–55.

Krugman, M.E. 1990. Nurse executive role socialization and occupational image. *Nursing & Health Care* 11, no.10:526–530.

McCloskey, J.C. 1990. Two requirements for job contentment: Autonomy and social integration. *Image* 22, no.3:140–143.

Murphy, M.M., and V. De Back. 1991. Today's nursing leaders: Creating the vision. *Nursing Administration Quarterly* 16, no.1:71–79.

Nyberg, J. 1991. The nurse as professsnocrat. *Nursing Economics*, 9, no.4:244–247.

Porter-O'Grady, T. 1992. Transformational leadership in an age of chaos. *Nursing Administration Quarterly* 17, no.1:17–24.

Smith, M.C. 1993. The contribution of nursing theory to nursing administration practice. *Image* 25, no.1:63–67.

Smith, T.C. 1993. Management skills for directors of nursing. *Journal of Nursing Administration* 23, no.9:38–49.

Wolfson, B., and S.N. Nerdlenger. 1991. Nurse entrepreneurship: Opportunities in acute care hospitals. *Nursing Economics* 9, no.1:40–43.

Yourn, S.W. 1992. Educational experiences of transformational nurse leaders. *Nursing Administration Quarterly* 17, no.1:25–33.

35

A Look at Relationships

Much of the nurse executive's job concerns relationships with superordinates, organizational peers, subordinates, and individuals and groups outside the employing organization. As a major officer of the organization, she is involved with others in managing the affairs, directions, goals, and activities of the organization as a whole. In other circumstances, she is involved with these persons as an advocate of the nursing division or at least as an interpreter to others of the nursing function within the organization. In other situations her function is to coordinate and facilitate intraorganizational or divisional operations. An additional function is her role as a public figure representing both the organization and the nursing profession in external groups.

RELATIONS WITH ONE'S BOSS

In the newly developing complex forms of health care organizations, it becomes harder to tell who is whose boss. Sometimes, nurse executives report in matrices to two or more bosses. For simplicity, this discussion reviews the relationship that still predominates, in which the nurse executive officer reports directly to the chief executive officer (CEO) of the institution.

In any such relationship, the nurse executive must have a clear understanding of what the

CEO requires of her, but she cannot expect her boss necessarily to have captured these expectations in clear prescriptive documents. Usually, the nurse executive is expected to be partially responsible for creating the job description and selling the role content to the boss. The demands and content in the job may change radically over time, as the relationship of the organization to its environment changes.

The nurse executive must know the changes that are taking place from the CEO's perspective as well as from her own. It is not an era in which the nurse executive can work independently with a focus on the nursing division with minimal attention to the rest of the institution. Because of the need for total institutional response in today's environment, the nurse must be a vital part of the central management team. This position must be both formal and informal.

The nurse executive ensures her institutional participation when she negotiates for employment in addition to building a productive working relationship with the CEO and organizational peers. A productive working relationship requires regularized and continuous communication. If the CEO does not establish such a pattern, the nurse executive should initiate it. Although it is ideal to work with a superordinate who can provide friendship or even mentoring, this is not always possible. The nurse executive needs an open, honest, direct relationship with her boss, but this does not have to involve a personal friendship.

What matters most in the relationship is the forthright and mutual exchange of vital information. The nurse executive must take whatever steps are required to see that she receives the proper corporate input as well as gives it. And she must keep her CEO informed as to the state of the nursing division (whether or not he wants to know).

The nurse executive needs to be clear about what is necessary to get the job done. Sometimes, nurse executives are expected to achieve results without the necessary resources. In these cases, the CEO will need to be educated. The nurse executive never need apologize for identifying the resources she requires to do the job.

Because of the effectiveness of many nurse executives, the chief nurse executive officer role often is expanded to include responsibilities beyond the nursing division. Such a move recognizes the skills of the nurse executive as well as maintaining a lean management team at the top. The frequency of this pattern indicates the wisdom of putting supportive services under the same administrative framework as the service (nursing) that they support.

EXECUTIVE LEVEL TEAMS

Much has been written recently about the need to develop highly synergized teams for the executive group. Yet, it is all too common that executives are involved in competitive relationships and put their own individual needs above those of the organization. Robbins (1990) conceptualized the organization as a conglomerate of many tribes involved in tribal warfare, each with a high degree of self-interest. Unfortunately, this describes all too many organizations.

Organizations surmount this problem if executive roles are well defined and the executive team understands the mission and shares the vision. Then, they can operate as a well-oiled machine both in times of crises and when doing the routine work of the organization. However, reaching this level of operating is a tremendous challenge.

In contrast to groups from other organizations, health care executive teams are comprised of a highly heterogeneous people from a wide variety of backgrounds, displaying a wide variety of behaviors in the executive team. For example, clinicians and nonclinicians bring very different backgrounds to issues such as caring and professional ethics. Executives come from many different backgrounds, and many different collegiate programs, as well as having different motivations for being in health care. People will bring to this group sexual identity/role beliefs, religious and humanitarian beliefs about health care, and beliefs about where health care should be going in the future. The group is likely to be highly competitive because it is comprised of people who have acquired executive status through high achievement motivations and competitive natures.

The nurse executive often comes to this group as the only clinician and the only female. Often, she is older and better educated, with more professional success under her belt. Nurse executives often get to their positions by having worked through the ranks for a long time. Some of these characteristics are drawbacks, some are advantages. One drawback is that there are still some administrators who are not comfortable with a female executive. These situations require a carefully designed strategy to make the relationship work.

One advantage is that the nurse executive is usually the most knowledgeable person on the executive team about group process. She has had more education and experience in developing interpersonal relationships because of her clinical background. She also may know how to facilitate and bring diverse groups together.

Although it is an honorable goal to have teams working well at the executive level, often it is easier to develop teams in other parts of the organization. Katzenbach and Smith (1993), the authors of *Wisdom of Teams,* demonstrated that executive teams come with so many hidden agendas and diverse personalities that it is not surprising that they work less efficiently than teams at lower levels.

Another danger in operating in teams is that people can become too closely affiliated with a team and not have the freedom to disagree or bring up issues as they occur. Janus (1972) described this phenomenon of "group-think"—as a person becomes tightly bound to a team, often it becomes impossible for him (despite having very good information) to express these views in a way that will be accepted if they differ from the prevailing views. Peer pressure in tightly synergized teams often prevents the team from hearing the very things they most need to hear. Although synergized teams are a great idea, they are very difficult to achieve, and there is a danger they may not be able to do the work necessary for the organization.

It is not uncommon for the nurse executive to be perceived as a loner and not a team player. Often, her schedule is burdened with many responsibilities because she has the largest and most complex organizational component. Also, her role is different from those of the other executive team members, and occasionally it is not understood or appreciated. Successful nurse executives are adept at marketing themselves as a team player and at helping the rest of the organization understand and support the complexity of their role.

OTHER RELATIONS WITH PEER MANAGERS

Not all relationships with peers take place within the context of performance teams. Day-to-day operations require many types of informal exchanges. Perhaps the chief thing to be said concerning peer relations is that the nurse executive needs to be clear as to the players, their roles, and their powers. One needs to be sensitive to the hierarchical subtleties of the organization. This does not mean that one fails to deal with lower-level managers in non-nursing divisions; it simply means that one deals from a position of strength. The nurse executive who can be intimidated by the dictates of a department-managing executive (e.g., the purchasing officer) is abdicating the powers of her office.

Nor can the nurse executive rely entirely on an organization chart and titles in figuring out

the powerful players in an institution of any complexity. She must be sensitive to institutional signals of power. Do others always seem to know when a major event is afoot before the nurse executive? Who knows first? Do the nurse executive's support services reflect appropriate status compared with those who are ostensibly her peers on the organization chart? Does she have adequate corporate support in the form of a personal administrative secretary and a budget for corporate-level activities? Is her office on the right floor, and in the right location? If the signals do not match the responsibilities, the nurse executive should set about systematically to improve them.

An important peer relationship is that of the nurse executive and the physician chief of staff. This physician may or may not be an organizational employee and administrator. Sometimes, this is an honorary position rather than a paid organizational one. More often than in the past, however, this position is held by a paid administrator. Whatever the structure, the chief of staff is the peer with whom the nurse executive seeks to work out interprofessional practice issues. It is important that the relationship be one of mutual problem solving rather than of competition.

Because of the added stresses in today's health care environment, the two professions sometimes do take on adversarial qualities. Joint practice committees can greatly ease competitive problems within the organization. They create forums where professionals meet for mutual problem solving. In one-on-one relations with the chief of staff, the nurse executive aims to create a cooperative collegial stance.

Frequently, debates between the two professions occur around the appropriate roles of each in an organizational setting. Resolutions should be clear concerning the authority of physician assistants, nurse practitioners, and various technicians. Other issues concern the management of unwritten orders, practice errors on the part of both physicians and nurses, and general attitudes of each profession toward the other. Some of these items defy resolution by standing procedures or committee. In an environment of mutual respect, such problems can be resolved.

The nurse executive cannot accept a patronizing attitude on the part of the chief of staff. One way of creating the appropriate quality between the two professions is for her to be clear about who makes decisions for nursing. Nursing prerogatives should not be yielded as a way of solving interprofessional problems.

In some instances, the nurse executive reports directly to the chief of staff or to a president who is a physician. In an era when physicians are moving back into ownership positions in health care facilities and back into organizational roles, we may expect many institutions to demonstrate this pattern.

RELATIONS WITH PHYSICIANS

Relations with the medical staff become more and more important as systems of medical practice interrelate with the general system costs. Because medical practice has a direct effect on costs and reimbursement, the nurse executive may have more negotiations—and more potentially problematic relations—with the medical staff than was the case in the past. In larger institutions, these relationships may be with chiefs of specialty practice. In many cases, much education is involved. Some physicians focus their resistance to external controls on the nurse executive, who is trying to cope with these changes as best she can.

Indeed, it speaks well for nursing that so many collegial relationships are firmly and positively established. It also reflects a slowly changing ethos in physician education. The nurse executive must create structures that support the nursing staff in interprofessional tensions. Evolving economic competitions and a shortage of nursing personnel do little to ease such tensions.

The collegial relationship between the nurse executive and the physician must be extended in principle throughout the organization. Positive interactions with physicians are more than mere pleasantries. Research points to the fact that patient care is far superior in facilities that have collegial relationships between nurses and physicians. For example, several studies now show that the mortality is lower in intensive care units

if nurses and physicians have excellent relationships than in units where they do not. So, not only is it a matter of importance to stabilize relations, but it becomes an essential ingredient of the practice. The nurse executive must infuse the organization with a clear message that excellent nurse–physician relationships are expected.

Some nurse executives use grass roots, unit-level nurse–physician collaborative projects to foster the necessary relationships. An example is a project in which nurses proposed that teenage patients could be prepared for very complex scoliosis surgery at home. The particular physician group was reticent but agreed to a test project in which a nurse coordinator dealt with the teenagers by phone. The successful project not only won physician approval but shaved 1 day off the length of stay for all these patients. This sort of reasoned approach to disagreements creates an environment in which everyone can win.

One function in which nurses and physicians must work together successfully is quality management. Nurse–physician cooperation in this arena has been made essential by the Joint Commission on Accreditation of Healthcare Organizations' move to a single set of patient outcome standards rather than separate standards for each profession. The lesson is an important one: we all share the same patient. Creation of case management designs for care delivery has the same effect: bringing medicine, nursing, and other professions together for planning.

RELATIONS WITH NURSE PRACTITIONERS

The nurse executive is likely to have many relationships with nurse practitioners. First, she may employ some, perhaps in several different settings, with diverse assignments. Many institutions (large and small) have found nurse practitioners very cost-effective. Some institutions have even extended them admitting privileges. (Presbyterian in New York City claims to be the first.)

In other instances, the nurse executive may deal with nurse practitioners who are employed in the institution directly by physicians or by a physician-run administrative unit. Administrative rules should determine the rights and privileges of all such nurse practitioners, as well as physician's assistants. And these rules must be communicated to the nursing staff so they will know how to relate to these individuals.

It is advantageous if the nurse executive can keep track of all the nurse practitioners within the institution. It may take a special inquiry to track down those who might escape her notice because they are not on the division payroll. It is usually appreciated if professional courtesies can be extended to these nurses, who may feel isolated in their roles. They often welcome participation with other nurses in continuing education programs and various nursing celebrations and ceremonies.

RELATIONS WITH THE PROFESSIONAL NURSING COMMUNITY

Any nurse executive has an opportunity for professional leadership. Only by making and maintaining professional links to nurses outside the institution, however, can this stature be achieved. It is through professional groups that the nurse executive builds her reputation as well as a network of peers in similar job positions. Such networks are highly supportive to all nurse executives. Most major cities have formal groups of nurse executives. In more isolated locations, the relationships may be less formal.

More extensive communications with peers may be reinforced through writing, speaking, research, and continuing education events. An active professional life is a requirement for the nurse executive if she is to be a good role model for subordinates. Indeed, the nurse executive's achievements in the profession bring credit on the institution and should be an expected part of her role performance.

RELATIONS WITH VARIOUS COMMUNITIES

The nurse executive needs to establish working relationships with many communities—

those in geographic proximity, those that house the institution's clients, and those that relate through various organizational interfaces. The latter include governing boards and benefactors as well as groups (e.g., churches) that may have legal ownership rights in the institution. What is most important is that the nurse executive carefully identify all these relevant communities and systematically set about to make appropriate relationships with each.

The nurse executive who is making any substantial changes in the organization needs to be aware of how each community will view these changes. Public relations for both the institution and her division are critical elements in community relations.

In the geographic community, support may be reciprocal. For example, one nursing division runs a summer program employing teenagers from the economically depressed community, introducing them to career options in the health professions. Paybacks from such efforts have been many. In one instance, the interpersonal relations of a nurse executive with a community activist group smoothed the way for a building campaign that might otherwise have been blocked or impeded. In another instance, community support helped a nurse executive sell her boss on establishing the institution's first nurse-run clinic.

Involvement in nonnursing health groups (citizens' groups, insurance company scholarship committees, occupational health programs) gives the nurse executive a broader conception of the health needs and interests of her community. Similarly, action with political groups increases the nurse executive's vistas. Nor should her linkages be limited to health-oriented activities. Many female nurse executives find enjoyment and benefit from belonging to women's executive groups.

Relations with the institution's trustees address another critical type of community because this group has such power over the operations of the organization. Some nurse executives have achieved appointment to the trustee group. Others work by cultivating good working relationships with board members. Others are active in evaluating candidates for board appointments. Certainly, a nurse executive fares better if there is prestigious nursing representation on the board.

In some cases, the nurse executive must work diligently to gain access to the trustees. Often, a door can be opened when the nursing division has some major achievement to announce. If the nurse executive requests an opportunity to make a presentation to the board, she is likely to get an approval. Whatever method the nurse executive uses, she should strive to get to know those who function at these higher levels of institutional politics.

The nurse executive also should learn how the institution's board functions. Some boards simply ratify the goals of the CEO, although they are becoming less common. Others are deeply involved in the affairs of the institution.

The nurse executive also will want to cultivate potential benefactors, grantors, or others who may contribute in some meaningful way to the development of nursing or of the institution. Although fund raising is seldom a defined job function for a nurse executive, expectations are increasing in relation to this function.

Today's health care environment places larger demands on the nurse executive for the external aspects of role performance. The chief nurse executive of a major institution may spend most of her time in outside contacts and public relations, using an associate for the internal operations of the nursing division. When an institution is large enough to require that a nurse executive focus primarily on external responsibilities, the nursing staff need to understand and appreciate this role.

RELATIONSHIPS WITH SUBORDINATES

As a manager, the nurse executive does much of her work through subordinates. Because this is the case, it is important that she scrutinize the nature of the roles she gives to them, managers and staff alike. To a great extent, the content of these roles is up to the executive. As long as she stays within the constraints of licensure laws and statutes governing employment, she can use her personnel creatively to achieve goals.

She will be concerned not merely with development of the individual roles but how those roles interface with each other. New arrangements are common today, as is the emergence of new roles—the case manager, the nurse practitioner, and the nursing technician, for example.

In addition to adding new roles, nursing has increased the number of specialty roles in an organization. Some functions that used to be incorporated into other roles have been separated out into full-time organizational positions. The roles of nurse researcher, quality management director, risk manager, nursing systems manager, management information specialist, discharge planning officer, and nursing budget manager typify the growing list.

Also, old roles are being modified by new structures. For example, staff nurse roles are empowered by participation in self-governance models and head nurse roles have added a major business dimension to the role responsibilities.

Nursing roles are further intensified and complicated by the high number of linkages with non-nursing staff demanded of today's care models. Ultimately, these increases in the communication/coordination lines will benefit the profession. Because the roles are shifting, incumbents are bound to feel the stress of change. Many studies have shown the growing complexity and stress in the head nurse role, for example. The nurse executive must be cognizant of these stresses and strains and consider them when making any reorganizations.

Professional Authority

One differentiation that has grown increasingly important in dealing with nursing staff is the difference between a nurse's organizational authority and her professional authority. Professional authority rests on the nurse's clinical expertise, not her organization role (staff nurse, head nurse, supervisor). Today's models rely heavily on the concept of professional autonomy, and nurses are expected to practice at the top of their clinical capacities.

At one stage, the argument for making part of the nurse administrator's curriculum clinical was that she could not manage persons who had more clinical knowledge than she did. Today, every administrator works with many staff personnel who have skills she lacks. Indeed, one of the critical skills an administrator requires today is the ability to manage lots of experts, each with unique skills and knowledge.

Because few managers (including the nurse executive) are likely to have sufficient expertise with which to assess all these specialists, these personnel must be held accountable on the basis of patient outcomes and managerial goals. Improved outcomes are expected for patients receiving the specialist's care. Case managers may be held accountable, not only on improved patient outcomes but for the timeliness and cost-effectiveness by which the outcome goals are achieved.

Communication

The most important way in which the nurse executive relates to subordinates is by active building of communication links. The staff must be kept informed and educated as to the new complexities of corporate health care and how they affect the institution. Without that education, they will not feel a part of the endeavor, and they will not understand the strategies that are put in place.

Communication is so important that it must not be left to chance. Systematic lines must be established, including in-house newsletters, memos, reports, E-mail, staff meetings—whatever works. Some information may be sent down the chain of command, but the executive will need to assess the effectiveness of this channel.

At times, the difficulty in communicating with staff revolves around the fact that the issues with which the nurse executive deals are so familiar to her that she forgets staff members do not know about them. A personal journal may help her keep track of information that needs to be shared.

Mostly, staff need to understand why things change. Given the rationale, staff are usually graceful about living with even less than desirable changes. Without explanations, the opposi-

tion builds. The best approach is to assume that staff are reasonable, intelligent people who need and deserve explanations as the organization evolves and changes while coping with today's world.

SUMMARY

For the nurse executive in an institution of almost any size, the demands of the job include working on many upward, lateral, and downward relationships. As the health care environment changes, these linking functions are expanding and assuming greater and greater importance. Indeed, the nurse executive role is rapidly evolving into two roles: an internal operations one and an external relations one. In her dissertation, Wasserman (1985) still found executives acting primarily from both of these two perspectives. Today, it is the rare nurse executive who can simply play a role with a downward focus and be successful.

Today's nurse executive works with groups she did not even know in past years—insurers and local media, for example. All the relationships of a nurse executive need careful planning with attention to communication lines.

REFERENCES

Janus, I. 1972. *Victims of group think.* Boston: Houghton Mifflin Co.

Katzenbach, J., and D. Smith. 1993. *Wisdom of teams.* Boston: Harvard Business Science Press.

Robbins, H. 1990. *Turfwars.* Glenview, Ill.: Scott, Foresman & Co.

Wasserman, C. 1985. *Task demands and attention patterns of chief nurse executive officers.* Unpublished dissertation, Teachers College, Columbia University.

SUGGESTED READINGS

Baker, C.M. 1981. Moving toward interdependence: Strategies for collaboration. *Journal of Nursing Administration* 11, no.4:34–39.

Balassone, P.D. 1981. Territorial issues in an interdisciplinary experience. *Nursing Outlook* 29, no.4:229–232.

Berger, S. 1984. Outside directors bring experience, ideas to Holy Cross health system. *Modern Healthcare* 14, no.12:130, 132.

Bibb, B.N. 1982. Comparing nurse-practitioners and physicians: A simulation study on processes of care. *Evaluation and the Health Professions* 5, no.1:29–42.

Blouin, A.S., and N.J. Brent. 1993. The chief nurse officer as board member: Selected legal and ethical issues. *Journal of Nursing Administration* 23, no.12:14–15, 54.

Bunsey, S., et al. 1991. Nurse managers: Role expectations and job satisfaction. *Applied Nursing Research* 4, no.1: 7–13.

Butler, A. 1984. Exploration of roles in nursing homes: The medical director, nurse executive, and administrator. *Nursing Home* 33, no.1:24–28.

Davis, L.L. 1983. Professional collaboration in health care administration. *Nursing Administration Quarterly* 7, no.4:45–51.

Field, P., and J. Larsen. 1989. Management behavior of one community health nurse supervisor. *Journal of Advanced Nursing* 14, no.3:234–239.

Mills, M.E., and M.S. Tilbury. 1993. Collaboration: The CNE-CFO connection. *Nursing Administration Quarterly* 17, no.4:17–25.

Oncken, W., Jr., and D. Wass. 1990. Management time: Who's got the monkey? *Journal of Nursing Administration* 20, no.12:6–9.

Walker, D.D. 1992. Friends of nursing: A strategy for transforming the community-nursing relationship. *Nursing Administration Quarterly* 17, no.1:34–37.

Zurlinden, J., et al. 1990. Situational leadership: A management system to increase staff satisfaction. *Orthopedic Nursing* 9, no.2:47–52.

36

Legal Considerations and Labor Law

In her role as executive, the nurse calls up many different areas of expertise. However, it is equally important to know when a situation requires more knowledge than she can possibly acquire. When it comes to legal aspects of practice and management, it is often the better part of wisdom to consult the experts. Any institution should make available to the nurse executive legal experts who can advise and direct her on everything from labor law, contract law, and malpractice to occupational safety requirements. Like prisoners who build reputations as "jailhouse lawyers," experienced nurse executives may become versed in many legal aspects, but most will be wise to consult with the pros on legal matters.

This chapter looks briefly at the domains of law that have a major impact on the role of the nurse executive. In the space of a chapter, those domains are merely identified, not detailed. Even though she uses the legal staff, the executive needs to try to stay updated in the most recent case and administrative law. Today, changes are rapid in all arenas of society; the law is not an exception, and technological change is making many old laws obsolete before they can be replaced with new directives.

New value systems also demand change in the legal structure. Take, as a simple example, the living will of a patient requesting no heroic measures in his care. What is the status of this will? Will it protect the practitioner who follows the patient's directive? Will it penalize the practitioner who rejects the request? Today, the sentiment is shifting toward upholding such written preferences, but states vary widely as to the legal status of such a document, and in many circumstances, durable power of attorney is to be preferred to a living will. (These two elements, durable power of attorney and living wills, are considered the main vehicles for advance directives.)

Often, we think of laws simply as constraints. In an era such as this one, we come to appreciate them fully as resources. When one finds any situations in which ambiguity reigns, in which precedent has not yet been set, or in which opinions and values conflict, then one comes to appreciate the function of law as a resource.

Extant laws delimit our decision making. They are directive of managerial actions in many situations. When appropriately applied, they protect us from vulnerability to suit. When they are absent, the job of the nurse executive is much harder.

SOURCES OF LAW DIRECTIVES

The nurse executive and her organization are subject to laws derived from various sources.

These include statutory laws—federal, state, and local—and regulations of administrative agencies—also on various levels. She also may be subject to suits for civil wrong (torts) or criminal wrong. Although they are not absolute, in such cases, decisions of judges may be heavily influenced by prior relevant cases (precedents).

From the perspective of the nurse executive, the best practice of law is the practice of prevention. She attempts to regulate her organization to avoid possible sources of conflict. She attempts to be in conformity with extant statutes and administrative regulations.

Statutory law applies to the health care agency and its managers in a hierarchical fashion, with federal statutes holding precedence. For those areas not covered by federal law, the states may create their own statutes. Similarly, municipalities may enact additional laws that do not conflict with laws made at higher levels. Conformity to federal laws alone requires extensive knowledge of many statutes. For example, a nurse executive may in the course of her job make decisions affected by the Patient Self-Determination Act, the Occupational Safety and Health Act, Social Security amendments, the Consumer Product Safety Act, the Health Maintenance Organization Act, the Child Abuse Prevention Act, the Comprehensive Drug Abuse Prevention and Control Act, the Fair Labor Standards Act, Medicaid and Medicare, and the Federal Rehabilitation Act, to name a few.

Although such acts are passed for the protection of all (or groups of) citizens, they tend to be cumulative in nature. Usually they are made more complex by amendments, and seldom are any removed from the books. The same pattern occurs at state and local levels. Additional laws, such as licensure of professionals, remain the privilege of the states, as dictated in the Constitution.

Administrative Agencies

Any law must be administered, and legal bodies create administrative agencies to manage given pieces of legislation. These agencies de-

rive rules and regulations designed to implement the intent of the given laws. Although such rules and regulations may be challenged, they have the weight of law. On the federal level the nurse executive may be involved with agencies of the National Labor Relations Board, the Federal Trade Commission, or the Health Care Financing Administration, to name a few.

Some national legislature enactments assign administration to the states. Further, when federal law is administered on the state level, applications may be different from state to state. Here, a nurse executive may find herself dealing with different Medicare and Medicaid regulations in every geographic career move she makes. For example, although Medicaid is a federal statute, each state determines its own poverty level and hence who qualifies under the law.

If one surmounts the maze of statutes and administrative rules and regulations that are required, one comes to another group of quasi-legal guidelines. The Joint Commission on Accreditation of Healthcare Organizations (JCAHO) illustrates this type of regulator. The JCAHO accreditation process is voluntary, but approval is required by so many funders and beneficial programs that few organizations can afford the luxury of not "volunteering." Many specialized settings have their own accrediting agency or group, using standards appropriate to the setting and the client population.

Newly developing forms of health care increase the legal complexity. Multi-institution corporations are subject to additional regulations in commercial law. And when a corporation grows through vertical integration, it may find itself needing to learn a whole new set of laws and regulations. For example, if a corporation that previously managed only acute care hospitals adds nursing homes and extended care facilities, it must learn its way around the complex federal regulations for skilled nursing facilities and for intermediate care facilities.

Tort Law

There is still another legal arena that the nurse executive must consider: tort law. Here, she may have to deal with cases of patient injury and staff malpractice. With patients, she must guard against professional negligence and acts of commission on the part of her staff. Because of the legal principle of *respondeat superior,* she and her institution may be held liable for acts of employees who commit malpractice within the performance of their assigned duties.

The potential cases boggle one's mind; nurse employees may be held liable for any nursing procedure that results in injury, including drug errors, following erroneous physician orders, incorrectly interpreting telephone orders, inaccurately counting sponges in surgery, failing to prevent burns and personal injuries, and using defective equipment, to name a few. Further, the *Darling* case ensures that the nurse will be liable if she fails to strive actively to prevent physician malpractice.

Educating Staff

Clearly, nursing staff require education concerning their legal responsibilities. It usually falls to the nurse executive to see that patient situations regulated by law conform to it. These situations include securing informed consents for treatment and explaining to the patient his rights concerning advance directives.

The nurse is also required to report certain cases (e.g., gunshot wounds, communicable diseases, criminal acts resulting in injury). And she must walk the delicate line between the individual's rights to privacy and the community's right to protection. For example, the nurse must know who can and who cannot be informed if a person tests positive to human immunodeficiency virus, a policy like many others that may vary from state to state.

All this takes place in an environment that must guard the patient's right to privacy (while using computer systems that make record access a challenge any good hacker can surmount). These situations are relatively clear at law.

There are still many unresolved problems at law simply because the technology changes faster than the law can keep up. Take human reproduction, for example, and the issues involving abortion, viable fetus age, surrogate motherhood, ownership of frozen sperm and embryos, and transplant of fetal tissues. As soon as norms of behavior are set—let alone court precedents—a more advanced technology comes along, creating yet another set of issues. And this is just in one specialty: obstetrics.

Personnel Administration

Administrative vulnerabilities also occur in personnel management. The nurse executive needs a clear idea of what she can and cannot do to, with, or for employees. With the wrong decisions, she may be liable to charges of assault and battery, false imprisonment, invasion of privacy, defamation, or other forms of infringement on the employee's civil rights.

Further, she must consider issues of sexual harassment at all levels of the organization, sometimes including her own. Cases are now reaching the courts in which nursing vice presidents are suing institutions for being offered different retirement/separation packages than their male counterparts. At the divisional level, the nurse executive must see that staff are educated and sensitive to gender issues, that suit-engendering behaviors do not take place.

Other personnel questions have to do with the individual's right to be protected from illegal search and seizure. Can the nurse executive, for example, have an employee's locker searched if the employee is suspected of theft? What can or must be done for a nurse judged to be drug-impaired? What level of proof is required to fire an incompetent employee? What are the rights of a nurse who advises a patient concerning therapies other than those advocated by the physician?

To these issues, one can add those regulated by contract law. What sorts of contract should be negotiated for maintenance and repairs on major equipment? What contracts with nursing education programs protect all parties? What contracts or agreements should or could be made for interinstitutional exchange of services?

The nurse executive works in an environment fraught with legal jeopardies, bordered by legal constraints and directives. In such an environment, the executive must try to stay on top of the legal issues most likely to affect nursing practice in her institution. And she must have immediate access to good legal advice when she needs it. The environment is simply too complex to hold the nurse executive accountable for being a do-it-yourself lawyer. Not only does she need access to legal counsel, but the counsel should be appropriate to her problem. Seldom does the same attorney have expertise in contract law, labor relations, and tort law, for example. The nurse executive should have access to all the legal services required in her complex environment.

LABOR RELATIONS

Much of the managerial job is that of working with and through others, and this involves labor relations. The nurse executive must understand laws relating to the organizing of workers into unions, the negotiation of a labor contract between employees and management, and the administration of a contract by the nurse executive.

This is only part of the task. She must also consider the intermix of personnel relations and labor relations, with the former based on constitutional law and the latter originating in contract law. Although good personnel relations do not necessarily protect an institution from contract disputes, poor personnel relations leave an institution open to unionization, many grievances, and costly suits.

Errors in Personnel Relations

Three personnel systems affect staff attitudes toward unionization and grievances: the wage and salary administration system, the performance appraisal and disciplinary system, and the supervisory system.

Inequitable salary distribution is a major factor. A worker may be drawing a high salary, but if a coworker with less seniority and less re-

sponsibility draws a higher one, he will be discontent. In a nursing division, inequities may lead to unionization or, when a house is already unionized, in attempts to dictate salary by labor contract. When unions enter into salary distribution, the principle of seniority is inevitably advanced.

Although seniority sounds like a principle a nurse executive could live with, it is not that easy. First, salaries fixed by seniority ties the executive's hands as to merit pay, and that removes one of her performance incentives. Worse, once a principle of seniority takes precedence in job retention—a logical extension of pay by seniority—the successful operation of the institution may be jeopardized.

An example is an acquired immune deficiency syndrome (AIDS) unit where an intelligent, committed head nurse had worked diligently to build a well-working team. Her staff gave excellent care and each member was devoted to working with AIDS patients. Then, the institution experienced downsizing. Because of a labor contract based on seniority, nurses on closed units were allowed to "bump" nurses with less time in the system.

Nurses on this unit were vulnerable—they were among the more recently hired, the unit being only 3 years old. In an era when nursing jobs were scarce, the bumping privileges were exercised. More than half the staff of the unit were replaced with nurses from other specialties as distant as obstetrics and orthopedics.

For the most part, the replacement nurses resented having to work with AIDS patients and could not wait for other opportunities to open up in the system. The spirited working team of the unit was destroyed. Then, bit by bit, the nurses who had bumped them returned to their regular units as vacancies opened up by attrition. This left the unit in flux for more than a year. At about the time the unit stabilized, another downsizing occurred, initiating the process all over again. The difficulties experienced by the AIDS unit were played out on many other units as well—all in the name of seniority.

The goal of equity (as intended by a seniority system) may be easier to apply in the employee disciplinary system. If some employees constantly ignore policies (e.g., those relating to tardiness and absenteeism) without any penalty while others are penalized according to the rules, then morale sinks. Because inequity of treatment is a major factor inciting unionization and grievances, nurse managers simply cannot implement policies discriminately.

An institution needs a good grievance procedure available to the employee who believes he has been unfairly judged or disciplined. The grievance procedure should be clear and simple to follow; it should not have too many steps until final resolution is achieved. If a licensed practical nurse has a dispute at the unit level that is not settled to his (or his union's) satisfaction, it should not be necessary that it be heard at every intervening level—head nurse, supervisor, department director, vice president for nursing, and president. Most grievance procedures sidestep the usual chain of command, shortening this procedure. Often, the final hearing officer is appointed from the personnel department, although this is not invariable. The nurse managers of an institution must not deviate from the established pattern for grievance hearings.

The executive must see that the grievance procedures are applied precisely. Most grievance procedures have time limits for how soon after an incident a grievance must be filed and for how soon after a hearing the hearing officer must respond. The procedure must be applied without exceptions.

Because the hearing officers in grievance cases are managers of the institution, hearings must not be loaded in favor of management. If the grievance is merely a *pro forma* event, with the outcome easily forecast, then the procedure will cause more discontent than would exist without it. Where there is such bad faith, *pro forma* hearings result in a large number of expensive arbitration cases. When there is not a union contract, unfair grievance hearings may result in moves to unionize. Unfortunately, some hearing officers are so threatened by employee action that they are prejudiced in favor of the grieving employee. In this case, the institution makes a travesty of management by undercutting their power. The aim of any grievance hearing should be that of fair resolution.

Managerial Principles for Labor Relations

When labor contracts already exist or when the potential for contractual relations exists, the nurse executive must know what laws are applicable. All private hospitals, both profit and nonprofit, fall under the provisions of the Labor Management Relations Act (LMRA). The act incorporates the National Labor Relations Act (NLRA), the Wagner Act of 1936, the Taft-Hartley Amendment of 1947, and the Health Care Amendment Act of 1974.

If the nurse executive is in a federal institution, then labor relations are covered by Executive Order 11491 as amended and the Federal Personnel Manual. This order functions in the federal public sector much as the LMRA does in the private. However, the provisions of the two documents are not identical, so the nurse executive will need copies of the legislation that affects her institution. If the nurse executive is in an agency in the public sector but under a state or political subdivision rather than in a federal institution, then she must check on the laws of her state to find out the status of collective bargaining. Both the LMRA and the aforementioned executive order make collective bargaining mandatory. When collective bargaining is *not* mandatory, the agency still may elect to enter into bargaining on a voluntary basis.

The nurse executive must know whether she must bargain with an elected union and what enabling rules she must follow. She should have access to an expert labor relations consultant if she is new to the collective bargaining process. She needs consultation long before negotiation begins and should seek consultation at the start of any unionizing activity. Some institutions handle unionizing within the personnel department, but if part of the nursing staff are involved in unionizing, there will be impacts on the nursing division that go beyond the interests and attention of the typical personnel department.

Often, the nurse executive seeks expert help only after a contract has been negotiated that is virtually impossible to execute. One director who had relied on others to negotiate a contract discovered the agreement allowed all vacation time to be taken at the employees' discretion. This seriously affected her budget, incurring unanticipated replacement salaries.

Finally, the nurse executive must realize that labor relations are bilateral; they divide people into two camps—managers and employees. Labor relations work on the principle of balance created by the push and pull of the vested interests of the two sides. Many nurses and even nursing organizations are hesitant to admit to this division between worker and manager. It fights against the sense of unity created among professional colleagues. It can also be difficult to determine who is in management and who is in staff. Indeed, a recent case raises new issues by calling a bedside nurse a manager.

The nurse executive recognizes that her role as manager necessarily gives her a unilateral position at the negotiating table on management's side. If she is ambiguous in an attempt to show her unity with the nursing staff, all sides will suffer from an imbalance in the bilateral relationship. Labor relations are based on the principles of conflict and negotiation, not on principles of synergism and cooperation, and this is difficult for some nurse executives.

PHASES IN LABOR RELATIONS

The process of establishing a labor contract will be reviewed in four steps: the organizing phase, the recognition phase, the contract negotiation phase, and the contract administration phase.

Organizing Phase

The organizing phase takes place when a union builds a base of support among workers. Managerial responses to this activity depend on whether the institution legally must bargain with a duly elected union, whether the management favors unionization (or *this* union), and whether unionization is perceived as inevitable or preventable.

The typical management response to incipient union organizing is to try to defeat the move-

ment. Counteractions may involve correction of wrongs—if any—that led to the union activity and attempts to propagandize against the idea of unionizing. If an organization waits until the threat of unionization to correct blatantly unfair policies, the action may come too late.

When a nurse executive is involved in an anti-union propaganda campaign, she must be careful not to overstep legal boundaries. Under the LMRA, she cannot institute employee surveillance (e.g., identifying employees entering a meeting on unionizing), interrupt employees promoting unionization on their free time and on property where the work of the organization is not being disrupted, nor allow biased disciplinary action against leaders of the unionizing movement. Under the law, she can stop unionizing activities when they impinge on the work of the institution and when they use the work hours of employees.

The organizing phase of unionizing includes solicitation (oral encouragement to form a union) and distribution (written encouragement to form a union). Groups organizing under the LMRA are able to demand an election if they can produce signed cards showing that 30 percent of the employees of the given class are interested in holding an election. Although such an election cannot be held more than once a year, any group with a constituency can constitute a union. Where more than one union is interested in representing a group, the winner of the election will get sole representation rights (providing that unionizing is not voted down).

The Recognition Phase

A union is recognized as the sole representative of an employee group if it wins the majority of votes in an election, no matter how many or how few qualified voters actually vote. Often, employees think that not voting speaks against unionizing. Given the way that votes are counted, failure to vote works in the union's favor and staff should be made aware of this fact.

In the recognition phase, one may ask who is to be recognized? A union group is considered to be formed by a community of common interest. In the health field, it is typical that groups divide between professional and nonprofessional roles.

Ideally each small group would like to have its own union because each group thinks that its issues and needs are unique. However, if each and every group were granted the right to bargain separately, management would be forced to spend unreasonable time and resources in bargaining. The National Labor Relations Board decides who must be in the same union to limit the number of bargaining agents in any one institution. In nursing, it may be difficult to identify where management responsibility starts and employee functions leave off. Is the primary nurse a manager? What about the case manager? Further, employees may fill a managerial function (team leading) one day and a staff position (bedside care) the next.

Under the LMRA, a supervisor/manager is anyone with the authority to make personnel decisions such as assignment, hiring, suspending, promoting, and firing, or even anyone who has the right *to recommend such action.*

In the recognition phase, the institution must recognize as the bargaining agent any legitimate union that wins election under the appropriate procedures and laws. When an agent is recognized, under the LMRA, the institution cannot legally refuse to enter into the next stage: collective bargaining.

The Contract Negotiation Phase

Major issues in negotiation, from the manager's perspective, include managerial rights and employee salaries. Because nurses have been very successful in winning increased salaries in recent years, often "increases" are asked for in benefits.

Workers often try to win concessions in nonsalary issues such as every other weekend off, greater medical benefits, or more paid education days. These are not really divorced from cost; they have major cost implications. Many proposals hope to limit managerial flexibility. If the nurse executive must allow one-half of her staff off every weekend, for example, weekend qual-

ity of care may be jeopardized. Unions also try to limit management's right to reassign staff. If the nurse executive agrees to a contract that does not allow her to move staff according to patient acuity, she will have to hire a larger staff. The nurse executive must look at the real cost when she gives up such managerial prerogatives as flexibility in scheduling and assigning of staff.

Obviously, as nursing moves into an age of specialization, flexibility declines naturally. For example, one cannot assign a regular medical-surgical nurse to a specialized intensive care unit and expect her to assume responsibility for the specialized care that goes on there. One can, however, assign such a nurse to such a unit if she is to work there under the supervision of a nurse who knows that specialty and if the transferred nurse is accountable only for performance of those routine nursing acts with which she is familiar.

The nurse executive or her agent should sit at the bargaining table to ensure that others do not give away nursing managerial prerogatives without recognizing that they are doing so. For example, a non-nurse negotiator may not recognize the potential impact on care of an every-other-weekend-off policy. Certainly, no contract should be signed without the approval of the nurse executive if it deals with nursing personnel. The nurse executive will want to watch developments as contracts are negotiated outside of the nursing division as well. If another group of workers bargains out of a given duty, the assumption may be that the nursing division will pick up the task. Nursing is the hub of the organization's services; it is usually affected by changes made in any other section of the institution.

Dynamics of Collective Bargaining

The nurse executive who sits on a negotiating team for the first time needs to be prepared for the negotiating process itself. She must recognize the process as an adversarial one in which the other side may use unpleasant tactics. Unfortunately, personal attacks are used at times. The nurse executive should be prepared to cope with such tactics, although this is easier to say than to do, and many nurse executives refuse to sit at the negotiating table because these tactics tend to alienate them from their nursing staff. It is a difficult problem, and the director who cannot deal with such tactics with a cool head probably does not belong at the table. Nevertheless, it is important that nursing top management be represented and that the nurse executive follow the happenings in the negotiations in detail.

Negotiations take place with each side giving up some lesser goals to achieve its major goals, negotiating in good faith. Give and take does not mean, however, that management must give in to unreasonable demands. Management must consider labor's demands; it need not cave in to them. And certainly, management should get something for every item it gives to the other side.

A word about unions: Union leaders are elected on the basis of the benefits they obtain for their membership. Although the professional union claims it is bargaining for patients' rights as well as staff members' benefits, it is typical that when those rights and benefits clash, the union opts to support staff benefits, claiming that it is management's job to find a way to achieve high-quality care.

The Contract Itself

The nurse executive must be careful concerning what is included in the contract. For example, if the contract inadvertently mentions certain personnel documents, a director may subsequently find herself unable to change even a job position description without agreement by the union (because those outside documents are legally included in the contract by reference). Conversely, one might fail to include some critical clause, such as a managerial rights statement, a scope clause, or an exclusionary clause.

The contact itself primarily covers such items as salaries, fringe benefits, and working conditions. Some nursing contracts also refer to controls on patient care quality that may be exerted by the employee. There are different levels of employee participation in setting standards for care. Recently, some contracts have included

clauses limiting an employee's assignment. For the executive, this is a double-edged sword, beneficial in demanding a better staffing ratio, disastrous in emergencies when additional staff simply cannot be found.

Clear language is essential in a contract. It prevents disagreements between management and labor concerning the issues included. If the contract's language is ambiguous, it will present as many problems as it solves. The contract must be carefully checked for contradictory clauses, another potential source of future problems.

One important clause in almost every contract is the arbitration clause. In exchange for a guarantee of no strike during the life of the contract, management agrees to arbitration of disputes that are not satisfactorily resolved in the grievance procedure. In an arbitration, an outside party makes the judgment in a dispute, and both parties—labor and management—agree to abide by the arbitrator's decision. Two methods are used in seeking an arbitrator: Either an arbitrator is sought for each separate case, or the two sides agree on a permanent arbitrator to hear all cases within the institution. The second method allows the arbitrator to become more familiar with the institution and thus more likely to be able to resolve disputes to everyone's satisfaction.

The Contract Administration Phase

Once a contract has been negotiated, the administrator is responsible for seeing that its provisions are upheld. The nurse executive will need to know intimately any contract that she administers as well as to educate new managers to the necessity of preserving the contractual agreements. The nurse executive cannot afford a manager who fails to implement the contract carefully, for consequent grievances and arbitrations could be costly.

The nurse executive does not derive her right to make managerial decisions from the contract. Her relations with union representatives only concern those matters legitimately within the contract. Two major responsibilities fall to the nurse executive: to see that the contract provisions are upheld and to provide the appropriate grievance channels when there are disagreements as to whether the contract was enacted. When grievances are not satisfactorily resolved through the usual channels, most contracts provide for arbitration. Only matters contained within the contract are subject to this route. Any items not contained within the contract remains a managerial prerogative. There are at least two major sources of arbitrators: the American Arbitration Association and the Federal Mediation and Conciliation Service. Both will provide lists of possible arbitrators and their qualifications. Ideally, an arbitrator with previous experience in the health field would be selected.

LABOR LAWS AND COLLUSION

In the day-to-day relations with the union during the life of the contract, the nurse executive must remember that certain actions that she might think of as merely cooperative are actually illegal. For example, to support the union by providing telephones, offices, or meeting rooms for union activities is illegal under LMRA. There is a question of legality concerning collecting dues for the union by payroll deduction plans; some questions also are raised concerning the sending of employees to continuing education programs that will put money into union coffers.

Shared governance is another issue. There is controversy concerning employee involvement in these programs and how far they can go legally in terms of organizing a staff. It is difficult when the legalities seem to fight against what seems desirable on other principles, namely, employee involvement programs. Historically, the law has acted to balance the powers of the worker and management.

However, to get around the laws that gave the workers the right to engage in collective bargaining activities, some companies organized sham unions in an attempt to get workers to eschew real labor unions. Congress specifically prohibits employers from establishing a labor organization. Employers are banned from establishing organizations in which workers discuss wages, working conditions, and other employment-related topics. It has been construed by many administrators that employee involvement programs such as shared governance will be seen in this light.

In 1993, the National Labor Relations Board ruled against a company that created an employee involvement program—Electromation, Inc., a small nonunion organization producing electrical components. A similar ruling went against DuPont, as the courts determined that the activities of their employee involvement programs met the definition of a company-run union. There are similar cases under investigation at this time.

From these deliberations, one may infer that there are certain things not within the purview of the employee involvement program (e.g., shared governance). Discussions of raises, bonuses, and cash awards would clearly increase the risk of appearing to be a company-initiated union.

The activities of the employee teams can safely be oriented toward improving the work process and the quality of both the processes and outputs of the units. The trend in successful corporations and hospitals is to eliminate the labor–management split and to have the distinctions between managers and workers blurred. In high-performing teams, creative quality and productivity can be achieved if people with various talents can get together and in synergistic relationships. Because the courts have sounded a cautionary note, the nurse executive must be fully cognizant of the employee involvement activities and make sure they address the mandates of the court.

RISK MANAGEMENT AND THE ROLE OF THE NURSE EXECUTIVE

The nurse executive holds tremendous responsibility for ensuring that the hospital is secured from the risk of a financial loss incurred through suits for patient and employee injuries. Risk management programs are organized to prevent injury and to minimize financial losses if injuries do occur to patients. Risk management programs usually are directly related to the quality and safety programs. The nurse executive can develop an effective and legally secure nurse management program by developing a joint program with the risk management and legal departments.

The first task for the nurse executive is to analyze where the exposures lie in the institution and take action to evaluate the risks. The nurse executive who has had exposure to qualitative and quantitative research methods will have many tools at her disposal to determine the probable and possible vulnerability. With a thorough analysis, programs can be put in place to prevent problems, to reduce the frequency of abuse, and to minimize risk. For example, the nurse executive can determine, through review of data such as incidence reports and monthly reports, if the instance of falls in the hospital is greater than what should be expected. A falls management program can decrease the number of falls and injuries from falls. Other significant risk areas, such as medication errors, have also been found to be sensitive to prevention programs aimed at reducing the risk of error.

Once an error occurs, the potential financial loss can be lessened greatly with aggressive and intensive work with the patient and the family to work through the situation. The nursing staff can be very adept and therapeutic in situations such as this. When a crisis occurs, there is often a mutual withdrawal on the part of the staff and the patient. Instead, if the staff remains in very close contact with the patient and family, working closely to help the people through the crisis, the likelihood of a suit and subsequent financial loss can be minimized.

The most effective risk management program is a prevention program that is incorporated into the practice of each and every nurse. Patient care units can take pride in the reduction of patient and employee injuries that happens with an aggressive risk management program. By having the staff develop a sense of pride in their work and search for means of continuous quality improvement, an aggressive and effective risk management program will be the outcome.

It is most effective if programs are put in place throughout the organization striving for excellence and zero defects. The socialization toward excellence begins in the hiring process. It must be made clear in the interview that the organization has exceptionally high standards of quality and is very active in preventing problems for patients and staff. The candidate must hear that those who work in the facility are expected to be intimately and actively involved in the preventive programs; they must thoughtfully criticize practices, making and implementing suggestions for change that will reduce the risk of injury to patients and families. Orientation programs and frequent outcome-oriented inservice programs reinforce these concepts in this culture.

Despite having very good programs in place, in our litigious society, a nurse executive may not escape the threat of lawsuit. Having to defend oneself in court is a very intimidating and stressful experience for the nurse executive or any member of her staff. When staff are involved, the nurse executive should arrange for them to be coached so that they can do their best, both on their own behalf and on behalf of the hospital. No nurse should ever feel that she walks alone when confronted with an aggressive legal system that challenges her abilities. Needless to say, coaching does not include changing a witness' testimony.

The successful nurse executive should be able to demonstrate a continual decrease in risk management problems. With the proper programs in place and with a culture of aggressively preventing problems, risk management will be incorporated into everyone's thinking.

WORKING WITH THE LEGAL STAFF

Health care facilities have people from many walks of life and many disciplines who have been taught to think in many different ways. The thought patterns of clinicians can be assumed to be fairly similar because of their professional socialization. However, differences exist between the way that attorneys and nurses arrive at their conclusions. In an article by Weiler and Rhodes (1991), two nurse lawyers compare and contrast the differences between legal methodology, the nursing process, and quantitative research. The two professions use very different methodologies to arrive at recommendations for nursing practice. The main difference is that the lawyer does not use the hypothesis testing process and does not fixate on the newest findings. Indeed, in law the best authority to answer a question might be a century old. There is no right or wrong way to solve problems. But it is imperative that the nurse executive be aware that many of the issues become problems because of the differences in the socialization and patterns of thought of different groups.

SUMMARY

Given the demands of a litigious society in a time when circumstances and the law are both changing rapidly, it behooves the nurse executive to develop a mind-set that serves to prevent legal problems from happening. This involves active indoctrination of staff into their legal responsibilities as well.

The nurse executive must acquire as much personal knowledge as possible, then rely on the help of experts in the important domains of legal practice that affect the work of the nursing division.

REFERENCE

Weiler, K., and A.M. Rhodes. 1991. Legal methodology as nursing problem solving. *Image* 23, no.4:242–244.

SUGGESTED READINGS

Acord, L.G. 1982. Protection of nursing practice through collective bargaining. *International Nursing Review* 29, no.5:150–152.

American Nurses Association, Commission on Economic and General Welfare. 1981. *American Nurses Association's economic and general welfare program—Dynamics of the local unit.* Kansas City, Mo.: ANA.

American Nurses Association, Commission on Economic and General Welfare. 1981. *American Nurses Association's economic and general welfare program—A historical perspective.* Kansas City, Mo.: ANA.

American Nurses Association. 1986. *Enforcement of the Nursing Practice Act.* Washington, D.C.: ANA.

American Nurses Association. 1993. *Legislative and regulatory initiatives for the 103rd Congress.* Washington, D.C.: ANA.

American Nurses Association. 1993. *Sexual harassment.* Washington, D.C.: ANA.

Baumgart, A.J. 1983. The conflicting demands of professionalism and unionism. *International Nursing Review* 30, no.5:150–155.

Bolton, Z. 1990. OBRA. *The PADONNA Journal* 3, no.4:6–7.

Buffington, C. 1993. The impaired nursing professional—What nurses need to know. *ASLTCN Journal* 4, no.2:6–7, 19.

Clark, M.D. 1991. Toward safer nursing practice. *Nursing Management* 22, no.3:88–90.

Cohen, S.S. 1990. The politics of Medicaid: 1980–1989. *Nursing Outlook* 38, no.5:229–233.

Cournoyer, C. 1989. *The nurse manager and the law.* Gaithersburg, Md.: Aspen Publishers, Inc.

Crisham, P. 1990. Living wills—Controversy and certainty. *Journal of Professional Nursing* 6, no.6:321.

De Vries, C., and M. Vanderbilt. 1993. *The grassroots lobbying handbook: Empowering nurses through legislative and political action.* Washington, D.C.: American Nurses Association.

Fiesta, J. 1994. *20 legal pitfalls for nurses to avoid.* Albany, N.Y.: Delmar.

Fleming, C.M., and M.C. Scanlon. 1994. The role of the nurse in the Patient Self-Determination Act. *Journal of the New York State Nurses Association* 25, no.2:19–23.

Gale, B.J., and B.M. Steffl. 1992. The long-term care dilemma: What nurses need to know about Medicare. *Nursing and Health Care* 13, no.1:34–41.

Hague, S.B., and L.E. Moody. 1993. A study of the public's knowledge regarding advance directives. *Nursing Economics* 11, no.5:303–307.

Kowalski, S. 1993. Assisted suicide: Where do nurses draw the line? *Nursing and Health Care* 14, no.2:70–76.

Murphy, E. 1991. Celebrating the Bill of Rights in the year of *Rust v. Sullivan. Nursing Outlook* 39, no.5:238–239.

O'Quinn, J.L., and P. Hulme. 1993. After HIV testing: What's next? *Nursing and Health Care* 14, no.2:92–94.

Powers, J. 1993. Accepting and refusing assignments. *Nursing Management* 24, no.9:64–66, 68.

Schwarz, J.K. 1992. Living wills and health care proxies: Nurse practice implications. *Nursing and Health Care* 13, no.2:92–96.

Shalala, D.E. 1993. Nursing and society—The unfinished agenda for the 21st century. *Nursing and Health Care* 14, no.6: 289–291.

Sieracki, C. 1993. Organizational liability prevention: Automated profiles. *Nursing Management* 24, no.7:60–64.

Suppes, J.M. 1993. Self-regulation in the nursing profession: Response to substandard practice. *Nursing Outlook* 41, no.1:20–24.

Tammelleo, A. 1993. Failure to restock crash cart: Delay and death result. *Regan Report on Nursing Law* 34, no.4:1.

Weber, G. 1993. Tips on implementing the Patient Self-Determination Act. *Nursing and Health Care* 14, no.2:86–91.

37

Gauging Success of the Nurse Executive

It is mandatory that the nurse executive be able to identify and judge outcomes for his program of nursing. Accountability for outcomes is becoming the watchword for assessing success for the nurse executive and for the facility itself.

QUANTITATIVE MEASURES

External groups are demanding more quantification of the quality of care. For example, health maintenance organizations have nothing by which to differentiate hospitals except for their hard data on quality of care when the price of care is the same. In some situations, managed care organizations are willing to pay more for quality if it can be demonstrated. The nurse executive can benefit greatly from a regular "report card" that tells where his program stands and what future direction it must take to meet higher quality standards. If the nurse executive regularly and routinely gauges success, the entire organization is likely to adopt this orientation. Continual improvement becomes ingrained in the culture.

Much of the executive's work requires a goals orientation—to develop a vision and a program, to determine standards, and to develop a strategic plan. An outcome-oriented program requires

goals and predetermined levels of achievement at which each goal will be met. One of the most important measures of success that the nurse executive has at his disposal is his ability to structure reports of projects in ways that give this information. The concept of a report card applied to all operations will allow the nurse executive to compile monthly, quarterly, and annual evaluations that gauge success.

Quantitative measures of the quality of care can take many forms. With the advent of continuous quality improvement programs and the influence of statisticians and researchers in this arena, we have all become familiar with a process of measuring, taking action, and remeasuring. Clinical outcome measures can be tracked through the quality management program dictated by regulatory bodies such as the Joint Commission on Accreditation of Healthcare Organizations (JCAHO) and Medicare. Positive outcomes can be measured as can negative outcomes such as numbers of pressure sores, falls, medication errors, and infection rates. Tracking these data can reveal trends. These data give concrete confirmation when the nurse executive's programs are improving the quality of the outcomes.

The efficiency of the clinical programs can also be measured in areas such as length of stay, average cost per case, and other generic broad-based measures. Efficiency can also be measured by looking at institutional processes. For example, measuring the accuracy of sputum cultures, the laboratory turnaround for cultures, and the administration of antibiotics within the prescribed time frames are all measures of efficiency that indicate if the program is improving.

Benchmarking is a process in which the nurse executive looks for best practices and compares his program against them. Once he achieves the level of the best, the challenge is to go beyond. Another way of benchmarking is against one's own past record. For example, medication errors can be benchmarked against medication errors last year with the assumption that they will show a continuous improvement and decrease of incidences over time. Benchmarking also can be done against peers. In this example, the medication errors can be benchmarked against a similar unit either within the hospital or at another comparable facility.

Benchmarking can also be done against competitors. Measures compared between competitors have become a factor in determining where managed care companies will take their business. When the cost is similar, the facility with the best track record is the one that is awarded the contract. Therefore, it is important to know what competitors are achieving and, consequently, what they are marketing to payers as their quality outcomes.

The nurse executive's job is to position his programs so they can compete against others in the community successfully in the era of managed competition. Benchmarking can also be done against regional, national, and international programs. Care managers have become acutely aware in the past few years that, even though we spend a great deal of money in health care, our outcomes in several areas are not as good as those achieved in other countries. It is important for us to have a broad view of success measures elsewhere to determine how we can meet and surpass these best practices.

Once an executive has the information about where he stands by benchmarking with another group and if he determines that his results are not as good as the other group, action must be taken to improve outcomes. First, he must de-

velop a hypothesis to explain the differences. Once this analysis has been done according to continuous quality improvement methods, action plans can be developed and evaluated to determine if the actions planned and implemented in fact change the data and the results improve. This continual process of striving to improve outcomes should eventually narrow the gap between the best practice and that of the nurse executive's staff.

Although benchmarking gives quantitative data supporting enhanced quality of care, measuring success does not stop with these assessments.

QUALITATIVE DATA

In addition to quantitative data, there are qualitative measures that identify excellence in outcomes. Although quantitative measurements of the sophistication of the staff might include the number of nurses with specialty certification or specialty to general registered nurse (RN) ratios, educational levels of RNs, turnover statistics, and other quantitative measures, the executive will also derive a qualitative sense of sophistication by the level of discussions on the units and in meetings, the character of the staff's published papers, and other "soft" data of this sort.

There may also be indirect measures of quality, such as having state-of-the-art equipment for care needs. Implementation of critical paths would also lead one to believe that quality would be higher in this facility than one that does not yet have these programs. Although these factors may not correlate with quality of care directly, they can be taken as strong indicators. Having an infrastructure in place that can recognize problems when they happen and take action also gives evidence of quality.

PERCEPTIONS AS OUTCOMES

Not only does the actual achievement count, but the perceptions of achievement form the greatest part of the truth. The nurse executive may be doing an exceptional job, but if the opinion makers do not perceive this, it is to little avail. If, however, the executive knows what people's perceptions are, he can implement programs to change them. It is important for the nurse executive to know the perceptions of important decision makers and to see that their perceptions of the nursing division are favorable. Truth is in the minds of people who judge the success or failure of the nurse executive.

The nurse executive has many customers whose opinions count. These customers pass judgment on his outcomes. Opinion makers include people such as the staff, physicians, the chief executive officer, other department heads, patients, outsiders such as deans and nurse executives of other nursing programs, and the organization's own trustees. The list is lengthy.

By regularly and routinely sampling the opinion of these customers, the nurse executive will know what the perceptions are and where the work of changing perceptions must be done. Employee opinion surveys, patient satisfaction questionnaires, external peer review processes involving deans and nurse executives from other programs, and other types of surveys are appropriate ways of obtaining information about how the nurse executive and his programs are perceived. At times, this feedback can be painful, but the process provides useful information on which action plans should be developed both to change the realities and the perceptions.

To be successful in the job, the nurse executive must be customer-focused. Perceptions must be highly valued and action plans developed to address issues. In far too many cases, the nurse executive has been doing a good job but has not paid attention to the perceptions being produced. There have been situations in which the nurse executive has been caught totally unaware of negative perceptions. Surveys, informal inquiry, and other ways of testing the water tell the nurse executive how the program is being perceived. If the perception is wrong, the next step is to change it.

COSTS OF ACHIEVING QUALITY CARE

There are extensive costs involved in achieving quality care objectives. Any time an objec-tive is not achieved, the work must be redone. When a patient with a hip replacement falls out of bed and has to go back for surgery, the costs are enormous. In health care, not only are rework costs expensive but institutions are more and more exposed to lawsuits that add to the cost of the rework. In the book *Principals of Quality Costs*, Campanella (1990) categorized the cost of quality in categories, including

- *prevention costs:* dollars spent in education and training, quality improvement, and team meetings aimed at improving the processes to prevent costly problems
- *appraisal costs:* costs incurred by measuring, evaluating, and auditing (examples would be the cost of continually monitoring JCAHO and Medicare compliance and benchmarking against other programs)
- *failure costs/internal:* costs incurred when the processes do not meet standards, such as the cost of medication errors and infections
- *failure costs/external:* costs incurred after delivery of a service such as the readmission of a patient, the successful lawsuit of an employee for a wrongful discharge, patients demanding after discharge that their bill be reduced because of perceived poor quality
- *total quality costs:* summation of the difference between the actual costs of the service and how much the cost could be reduced if the possibility of defects, substandard service, and failure to reach standards could be eliminated

The nurse executive can gauge success by continually examining the cost of quality in these areas and reducing it over time. Financial efficiencies can also be measured by various ratio analyses. For example, numbers of full-time equivalents (FTEs) per occupied bed, cost of FTEs per occupied bed, labor cost by patient day, supply cost by patient day, and many other indicators are financial ratios that can serve as benchmarks. Over time, the ratios should improve if the nurse executive is successful.

SUMMARY

Summarizing the qualitative and quantitative data in a report format will provide information to the nurse executive about trends, and can be used to develop his programs. It is useful to share as much data as possible with customers so that they have both a qualitative and quantitative view of the success of the nurse executive's program. Some data, however, cannot be shared because of issues of confidentiality and fear of legal exposure.

Staff in particular need to understand where they have been and where they need to go to continually improve the processes. It is imperative that the nurse executive have mechanisms in place to help the staff benchmark their practice against other groups. In today's competitive environment, it is essential that the nurse executive have qualitative and quantitative information available to compete in the marketplace.

The predictions are that over the next few years, quality care outcome measures will be one of the most important criteria for anyone who works in health care. As this area of measurement becomes more sophisticated, the nurse executive has great opportunities to improve his organization's practice. It is important to gauge nursing division success for the organization and for the nurse executive's personal success.

REFERENCE

Campanella, J. 1990. *Principals of quality costs.* 2nd ed. Milwaukee: America's Search for Quality Control Press.

38

Nurse Executive of the Future

To say that "times are changing" is an understatement. Health care is in the middle of a paradigm shift and a revolution in our thinking concerning how we should deliver care. The kind of concerns we have about illness and health will be much different in the future than they are now. The information revolution and the globalization of business force us to look beyond our walls to a future filled with international challenges and demanding radically different thinking in terms of how we do business. The role of the nurse executive will not be immune from this. Health care in hospitals has remained virtually unchanged since the present structures and organizations came into place based on the industrial model of the 1920s. No longer will these highly bureaucratized, departmentalized organizations, locked inside their walls, serve us for the future. The nurse executive will be working in a much different situation, and her role will change.

MOVING FROM SINGLE FUNCTION TO MULTIPLE FOCUS

Integration will be the watchword of the future. No longer will the nurse executive be accountable for a single division with a single focus (i.e., merely to provide nursing care). Vertical management will be replaced by horizontal management, in which the nurse executive will need to partner and network, not only with other divisions in the organization but outside the walls of the health care facility. Horizontal management will mean managing as the customer goes through the organization. Using a patient-focused design under capitated arrangements, the customer/patient will be reviewed in a whole new way from outside the walls of the hospital. To manage in the future, people from various disciplines will need to move across organization boundaries. The nurse executive will be challenged to see the big picture and work beyond the walls of the division. The roles of the future will involve moving around, between, and across divisional/departmental lines rather than operating within them.

The organization of the future and its nurse executive must be fluid. In *Fifth Generation Management*, Savage (1990) talked about businesses being organized in concentric circles rather than on hierarchical models. Alliances, partnerships, and relationship management will be the watchword for the nurse executive of the future.

FROM INTERNAL ORIENTATION TO "CUSTOMERIZED/ MARKETIZED" ORIENTATION

In the past, it was sufficient for the nurse executive to run the internal division very well. She did not have to worry about where the patients were coming from or how the division of nursing fit within the competitive forces of the city. Peters (1992), in *Liberation Management,* coined the terms *marketizing* and *customerizing* to indicate that the future for organizations will be determined by their ability to be responsive to the market and to understand the customers' needs.

The markets are changing dramatically in health care. We have moved to a resource-driven model in which the payers are in the driver's seat and are able to shape the way health care will be delivered. Customers, the patients, physicians, payers, and others, have many options. The nurse executive is obligated to understand what the customers want and to shape services around the customers and the market.

CATCHING THE HUSTLE

Successful organizations of the future and the nurse executives who manage in them will be the ones who can best interpret the environment, react fast to external changes, and make internal changes accordingly and quickly. In essence, the organization that is nimble will be best able to meet the challenges of the customers in the market. Nurse executives who cannot move the organization quickly as forces in the environment dictate will not long survive in the fast-paced health care system.

MANAGING BY OUTCOME/ DEMANDING EXCELLENCE

"Results-driven" management will be the job description of the nurse executive, and the measure of success will be driven by the outcomes produced by that nursing staff. The nurse executive who is driven by the pursuit of excellence will be in great demand as health care institutions learn to differentiate levels of quality and to demand excellence. For example, tolerating a static number of medication errors will not be possible in a results-driven environment that differentiates itself from others based on quality.

RETHINKING HEALTH CARE

With advances in genetics and related fields, health care of the future will shift toward preventing and managing chronic diseases rather than the present focus on acute care models. According to Goldsmith (1992), a health care futurist, one will know at birth one's genetic program for health. One will manage that genetic mapping to avoid or better cope with the inevitable. Health care will not be what it is today.

RE-ENGINEERING EVERYTHING

Nurse executives will know intimately and well the principles of process improvement and will learn to continually think through the framework of re-engineering. For example, we now treat gallbladders much differently with laparoscopic surgery but often have not re-engineered the hospital to cope with the change. Every innovation presents an opportunity to rethink. Continually rethinking and asking unthinkable questions about why we are doing certain processes certain ways will be an essential quality for the nurse executive of the future.

Sacred cows such as change-of-shift report and patient care conferences will have to be carefully rethought to determine the most effective way of getting the job done or, in fact, of not doing the job at all. Many of our processes were never designed in the first place but serendipitously happened. The results were complicated processes, inefficiencies, and duplications everywhere. Everything in health care will be reopened for re-engineering in the future.

DEVELOPING ENTREPRENEURIAL ORGANIZATIONS

The nurse executive will not be able to direct everything that is necessary in the future. Self-managed teams who believe that they own their work and their unit and are share-holders in the organization will do the work that the organization needs done. Entrepreneurial units and people who understand what needs to be done will replace workers who need continual direction and challenge.

THE HARDEST THING: TECHNOLOGY FOR THE INFORMATION REVOLUTION

Health care has not made the investment in information technology that other businesses have. Consequently, clinical and business decision support systems are rare, and much of our clinical information is still stored on paper in most hospitals. Tracking the outcomes of specific clinical treatments is laborious in most instances to say the least. Yet, nurse-sensitive outcomes must be tracked by information technology, and the nurse executive of the future needs to be the expert in leading the development of these systems.

The health care system of the future will be an organization in which the people, technology, and processes are integrated, with the nurse executive playing a strategic role in the information revolution in health care.

EDUCATION OF THE NURSE EXECUTIVE OF THE FUTURE

With such a broad-based role in the future, the nurse executive needs breadth in her education. The question will be, "How can the nurse executive obtain the knowledge necessary?" There will be many educational tracks to becoming a nurse executive. As the role of the nurse executive broadens in the future, the education of nurse executives must keep up with the position demands. The nurse executive of the future cannot be just a technocrat in the areas of nursing and business.

A sound clinical background will provide an advantageous foundation from which to build the nurse executive's practice. Grounding in the hard sciences of clinical nursing is important; the soft sciences that support the practice of nursing and health care such as sociology, psychology, and anthropology are mandatory for the nurse executive of the future. She will need to be a renaissance person to handle the challenges of the role.

With solid clinical expertise, she will then need grounding in the business side of the role. The knowledge and ability to use financial management skills, to analyze how finances have an effect on the clinical side as well as the administrative marketing, and other aspects of business management will be crucial to the nurse executive of the future. With the resource-driven model, the ability to manage resources effectively will be more and more crucial.

Beyond the hard sciences of clinical, financial, and business sciences, the nurse executive of the future would be well advised to step out of the traditional boxes and learn from nontraditional studies, to learn to see the world through other models and to question what needs to be done for the future. Experiences and studies that challenge and awaken the creative side of the brain will continually keep the nurse executive open to new ideas.

Opportunities to become immersed in totally different cultures and reading in areas far distant from the practice of management help the nurse executive bring more creativity to the job. Studies in philosophy and models of thinking and knowing open up new vistas.

The discipline of the left brain must also be challenged by continual studies in areas such as a second language, advanced financial management, or advanced work with software programs. The nurse executive's knowledge base is one of the greatest assets she has, but this asset will be continually challenged by the fast changes that will be coming in health care.

There is no one way of obtaining an education to be the perfect nurse executive of the future. But the successful nurse executive will continually challenge herself to get outside the traditional boxes and seek out the experience of mentors in a wide variety of areas.

SUMMARY

The nurse executive of the future needs to learn to love change. It must be embraced and celebrated; it must be seen as an exciting challenge. The world of health care for the future will be faster and much more competitive and will challenge us to rethink our sacred cows and to re-engineer everything that we do. The times they are a-changing, and this will be all right for the nurse executive of the future.

REFERENCES

Goldsmith, J. 1992. The reshaping of healthcare. Part 1. *Healthcare Forum Journal* 35, no.3:19–27.

Peters, T. 1992. *Liberation management.* New York: Alfred A. Knopf, Inc.

Savage, C. 1990. *Fifth generation management: Integrating enterprises through human networking.* Maynard, Mass.: Digital Press.

SUGGESTED READING

Denton, D. 1991. *Horizontal management: Beyond total customer satisfaction.* New York: Lexington.

Index